AF601898

Purple Biotechnology

The Editors

Dr Viralkumar B. Mandaliya is an Assistant Professor – Research at Gujarat National Law University, Gandhinagar. He was awarded with "Bharat Shiksha Ratan" by Global Society for Health and Educational Growth, Delhi, and "Young Scientist" by Venus International Foundation, India. He hold numerous member positions of Scientific and Educational Society and Council. He has pursued several short term courses from WIPO, Geneva; agMOOCs, Ministry of HRD, GOI; EUIPO, Spain. He has numerous publications (national and international), book and book chapters, paper-presentations to his credit.

Dr Anjani Singh Tomar is Associate Professor of Law at GNLU. She is recipient of 5 Gold medals from Devi Ahilya Vishwavidyalaya, (DAVV) Indore, for holding merit positions in LL.B. (Hons) & LL.M. exams. She is also holder of M.Sc. degree in Clinical Bio-Chemistry from Holkar Science College, DAVV, Indore. She passed her NET (Law) exam in 2008 & received Ph.D. degree in 2010. She has an experience of more than 11 years as a faculty in Law. She has written books on variety of subjects including labor law, information technology, taxation laws, intellectual property laws etc. She is editor of leading journal of the country, The GNLU Law Review. She has published the papers in leading journals of the country as well. She has also worked as faculty of law at Indore Institute of Law, Indore, & University of Petroleum & Energy Studies, Dehradun.

Purple Biotechnology

— *Editor* —
Dr Viralkumar B. Mandaliya
Dr Anjani Singh Tomar

2019
Daya Publishing House®
A Division of
Astral International Pvt. Ltd.
New Delhi – 110 002

ISBN: 9789388173940 (Int. Edition)

Published by : **Daya Publishing House®**
A Division of
Astral International Pvt. Ltd.
– ISO 9001:2015 Certified Company –
4736/23, Ansari Road, Darya Ganj
New Delhi-110 002
Ph. 011-43549197, 23278134
E-mail: info@astralint.com
Website: www.astralint.com

Digitally Printed at : Replika Press Pvt. Ltd.

Acknowledgements

Team members would like to acknowledge the Government of Gujarat for graciously accepting the research project "The Key Development in Biotechnology and its Impact on the Society, and Creation of Techno-legal Awareness towards the Recent Trends in Biotechnology" to be conducted by GNLU. We are equally obliged & thankful to Director, Gujarat National Law University, Prof. (Dr.) Bimal N Patel, Professor of Law, who have posed his confidence & trust in our team and have given us this opportunity to bring our research into success. We are also thankful to Dean, Research division, Prof. (Dr.) Ranita Nagar, who has been a source of encouragement to us. We would like to thank all the members of Research Division, with special reference to Mr. Rahul B. Pandya, who has been instrumental in the completion of the research project and this book. We would also like to acknowledge the administrative support given to us by the Registrar's office, GNLU.

The entire project and the book could not take up the shape without the hard efforts put in by our Project Assistant, Ms. Urvi Vacchheta. She, being the active support to us, has really worked very hard to bring our project into reality. We are very thankful to her whole hearted contribution, in every aspect of our project.

We express our sincere thanks to all the contributing authors for their contributions that resulted in this book. We also express our sincere thanks to Astral Publishers especially Mr. Kanav for his support and suggestion to bring it in a form of book.

We would also like to thank all our friends and family members who have directly and indirectly supported us to bring out this book.

We are most thankful to the contributions made by Dr. Bindu Vijay, Asst. Professor of Science & Tech. at GNLU in completion of this book.

Preface

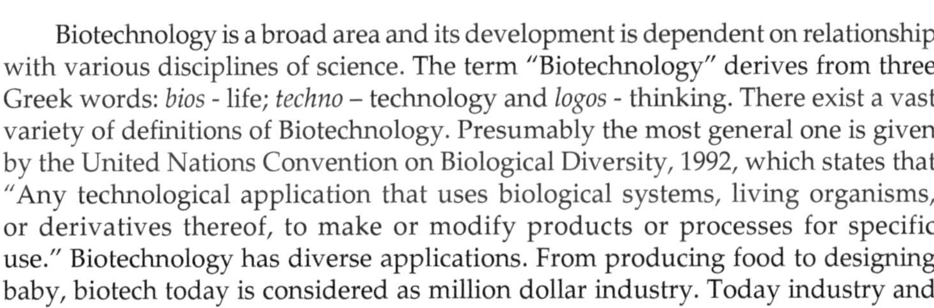

Biotechnology is a broad area and its development is dependent on relationship with various disciplines of science. The term "Biotechnology" derives from three Greek words: *bios* - life; *techno* – technology and *logos* - thinking. There exist a vast variety of definitions of Biotechnology. Presumably the most general one is given by the United Nations Convention on Biological Diversity, 1992, which states that "Any technological application that uses biological systems, living organisms, or derivatives thereof, to make or modify products or processes for specific use." Biotechnology has diverse applications. From producing food to designing baby, biotech today is considered as million dollar industry. Today industry and researchers use biotechnology as a tool in their process to a greater extent in a diverse manner.

This diversity has, in turn, brought about the need for a system to classify biotechnology uses based on common features or final purpose. As a result, nowadays there exist **five** main groups in biotechnological applications, which have been identified by a color system.

Red Biotechnology brings together all those biotechnology uses connected to medicine which includes producing vaccines and antibiotics, developing new drugs, molecular diagnostics techniques, regenerative therapies and the development of genetic engineering to cure diseases through genetic manipulation. It also includes reproductive technologies.

White Biotechnology comprises all the biotechnology uses related to industrial processes - that is why it is also called "industrial biotechnology". It includes the use of microorganisms in chemicals production, the design and production of new materials for daily use (plastics, textiles, etc.) and the development of new sustainable energy resources such as biofuels.

Green Biotechnology is focused on agriculture as working field. It includes creating hybrid varieties, new plant varieties and transgenic plants of agricultural interest using modern biotechnology, producing biofertilizers and biopesticides etc.

Purple Biotechnology deals with different domains of Intellectual Property such as Patents, Trademarks, Copyrights and Geographical Indications. It is connected with inventions and trade in biotechnology, especially in an economically globalised scenario, where technology transfers by way of intellectual property protection is now part of global trade.

Blue Biotechnology is based on the exploitation of aquatic and marine resources to create products and applications of industrial interest. Sea has covered ¾ of the planet where diversity of sea creatures is enormous. The researcher has explored a huge portion of the ocean and a lot of species, yet many mysteries are waiting to be discovered.

The present book on the topic "**Purple Biotechnology**" aimed at finding out the issues and challenges in Intellectual Property of Biotechnological Innovations and how they can be addressed. The contribution were invited from the people involved in the field of Intellectual Property Rights. The articles have covered the substantive matter from India and abroad. We believe that this edited book will be useful not only to scientific community but also to others who are involved in policy making.

Editors

Contents

Chapter 1

IPR Protection in Agriculture

***Sonali Behera*[1] *and Abhisek Dash*[2]**

[1]KIIT School of Biotechnology, Bhubaneswar, Odisha 751024
[2]KIIT School of Law, Bhubaneswar, Odisha 751024
e-mail: 1583001@kls.ac.in

ABSTRACT

A new report on 22 March, 2018 sounds the alarm regarding surging levels of acute hunger. Some 124 million people in 51 countries were affected by acute food insecurity during 2017 –Global Report on Food Crisis. Food/crop hoarding, improper export restrictions across the countries, public stockholding for security purposes, exploitation of the plant varieties for increased yield and the like, lead to food crises over the countries. Ostensibly, Intellectual property doesn't really environ multinational companies, law firms, industrial design rights, trademarks, copyrights, patents just, it has its wings stretching to agriculture as well. Intellectual property is to safeguard the creations of human intellect and to not exploit it in any manner. It necessarily acts as the rewarding body for any new innovations of human intelligence. This will let monitoring of human manhandling of the commercialism of any innovation.

Number of IPRs are relevant to agricultural section, for protecting agricultural goods and services produced in the sector. However, IPRs include patents which prevents the interference of any third parties from commercially exploiting the newly found type. Plant Breeders' Rights (PBR) under Agreement on Trade Related Aspects of Intellectual Property rights, is an internationally recognized system, which allows the breeder to hold intellectual property rights in the propagation of a new variety for commercial use. To be eligible for PBR, the variety should be novel, distinct, uniform and stable. Identification of the grain type and quality type is done by the national offices after examination, then grant the rights over the new variety for certain period of time. This gives a legal capture of the breeder over the new variety for the stipulated time within which no third body can make an unauthorized use of the variety.

India, however not one amongst the participating countries in the International Union for the Protection of New Varieties of Plants. In such case, Protection of Plant Varieties and Farmers' Rights Act, 2001 was enacted in India to safeguard new plant varieties. The objective here is to recognize the efforts of the farmers, the conservers and their contribution to the agro-biodiversity, investing in the seed industry for better varieties of the breed which would result in higher quality of yield and preventing encroachment upon the rights of the farmers. This Act gives the rights to the farmers to sow, resow, grow, cultivate, trade, import, export the variety and complete legal hand over it, prohibiting its unauthorized activities. Onions from Lasalgaon will get the Geographical Indication (GI) tag soon as the horticultural bureau of the state has begun the procedure to allow the uncommon status to the item delivered in the locale. The advancement and improvement of GI is a device for local advancement and to secure the legacy of a specific place. This will enable the makers to advertise their items and win more income. The Classical IPR's relevant to agriculture are patents particularly on biotechnological inventions, Plant Breeders' Rights, Trademarks, Geographical Indications and Trade Secrets.

Keywords: *IPR, Patent, Plant Breeder's Rights, Geographical Indication*

Introduction

India, an agrarian country, is an abode to people who have dire respect for their religion, customs and rituals. We are such ideal keepers of values, that we neither think twice before chopping off the head of a muslim guy who loved a hindu girl, nor burning a hindu girl down cause she entered the church. It is like we have a part of Sikander Butshikan (cruel emperor, hands down) within us. Our history books also did tell us about The Indus Valley Civilization (flourished during 3rd and 2nd millennia BC). Archaeologists have found Indus people kept cattle, pigs, sheep and goats for food. Cows provided milk and meat. Farmers grew fruits such as dates, grapes and melons and field crops such as wheat and peas. Not to forget, even Adam and Eve (First man and Woman) were told to eat trees only. So, plants, crops and agriculture has been there ever since our ancestry was set up. Any manhandling with the religious policies lead to strikes, massacres, honour killings and subsequent words but manhandling of agricultural policies result?

NEW DELHI (May 3, 2017): The centre informed the Supreme Court on Tuesday that despite a multi-pronged approach to improve income and social security of farmers, over 12,000 suicides were reported in the agricultural sector every year since 2013[1].

So, apparently there is no outburst of temporary heroic behaviour of superpatriots of our country by burning tyres, declaring curfew, calling for strikes, like it happens if a historic event is filmed plus minus fictionally in a 400 crore Sanjay Leela Bhansali movie but there is Loss, Deprivation and Detriment of a human life which was dutifully spent composting, planting, watering, weeding, harvesting and delivering, dripping drops of non-corrupted sweat and investing true man power.

---

1 Over 12000 farmers suicide per year Centre to SC, times of India, https://timesofindia.indiatimes.com/india/over-12000-farmer-suicides-per-year-centre-tells-supreme-court/artic leshow/58486441.cms, Dhanajay Mahapatra (2017 May 3).

Agriculture, though fighting a tough battle, is anyway still contributing to the food security and health of a nation. Before Industrial Revolution, agriculture was the primary source of economy. We have always been told and taught about sustainable development, nature friendly and peaceful method of livelihood for which our primary duty should be to keep up the agro-economy of our country at par with food requirement, sound health and poverty inclining mass. Protecting the rights of people engaged in agriculture, spreading awareness of the existence of the agricultural laws would ensure constant supply of food to look upon the nutritional index of the population availability of useful medicines for the health profile of the mass and ensuring employment of the generation. Agriculture being primary source of food which carbohydrates directly supplies protein, fats, oil, vitamins, minerals and growth factors for growth, development, nourishment and utmost value a healthy and robust lifestyle. Medicinal herbs are profitable cash crops.Bramhi, Aswagandha, Amla, Aloe-vera, Jatamanshi, Guggal, Jatropha, Kesar, Parsley, Patchouli, Stevia just to name a few are the medicinal crop of utmost beneficiary qualities. Enzymes alkaloids, laxatives, glycosides are all obtained from agriculture source which even gives us a scope for further development and research in the field of medicine and food additional. Agriculture despite being the greatest source of revenue in most countries, it is still amongst the most neglected sector of the economy, neither the government inverts in research and development for prospective, various new technologies and plant varieties. Despite agriculture having so much importance in many sectors, food production will always stand top most among all the other sectors. Food, the most essential element of the very existence of humans, with globalization, urbanization and the mass conversion of agriculture lands into commercial or residential lands has given rise to farmers loosing their cultivable land which has indirectly resulted in food insecurity, price surge of food products and acute hunger all over the world, increasing the poverty rate. According to Global Reports on food crisis lack of developed technologies, lack of research and protection in the field of agriculture has lead to food insecurity among developed nations. Many factors contribute to food insecurity/crisis people hoard food crops, mutilate with genes for better production. More than a century ago, the textile industry started using protein fibers from animals and vegetables such as casein from milk and zein from corn to make new kinds of fabrics.

Agro-market size during 2017-18 crop year, food grain production is expected to reach a record of 277-49 million tonnes. Agrochemical and pesticides, rice, vegetable, seeds, fruits, tea, pulses, nuts and Kernels, dried fruits, cashews, grain, coconut, poultry food, supplements, wheat, coffee, coir product, cereals, animal fodders, plant and animal oil *etc.* are just to name few which contribute to the agromarket of our country[2].

Not just the common needs, agricultural products and agri-waste also meets the in the not-so-common applications of human welfare. **Ecofemme**- reusable cloth pads made from organic cotton, **Anandi**- 100 per cent compostable pads made from

---

2 Agriculture in India: Information About Indian Agriculture and Its Importance, https://www.ibef.org/industry/agriculture-india.aspx, April 2018.

locally souced agri-waste. **Saathi-** made from entirely biodegradable banana fibre, **Heyday**- made from biodegradable and highly absorbent bamboo and corn fibre.

Section-1

Intellectual Property Rights and Innovation in Agriculture

Innovation is the constant change in whatsoever field taken. So does agricultural field require innovation for growth, survival and success of human existence.

Innovation never really means creativity, it means changing and improving a process, breed, variety or product. This is how Intellectual property right come into the field of agriculture.

Since innovation requires, intellect, investment, research and development, implementation and management, growth period, collection of results, all at par with the current technologies and better than the already established predecessor, single handed rights will protect the originality of an individual's planar to staple ideas and honour the efforts put into it all the while. This way IP protection encourages investment in innovation and helps to safeguard the continuous research; as a result acting as a source of support for any developments taking place in the field of agriculture. It helps IPR owners to make their product open to the market without the fear of exploitation and illegal use. IPR is not only restricted to law firms, multinational companies, industrial design rights, trademark, copyrights, patents, but with the changing scenario, its scope has even stretched to primary sector of ever economy, *i.e.*, the agricultural sector. Agricultural sector deals with a number of laws for the protection of agricultural goods and services provided by this sector.

Biotechnology and information and communications technologies (ICTs) are expected to make revolutionary changes by developing modified agricultural crops of better quality and yield which has high productivity and adaptability with a wider diversity to combat the problems of poverty, food insecurity, malnutrition and diseases.

Patents are generally granted for novel, non-obvious and inventions having industrial applications, which generally give the patent holder legal right to exclude the third party from using or commercially getting benefited from the product, for a limited period of 20 years. Many countries do not allow patenting on living organisms. In agriculture, biotechnology patents may cover for example, plant transformation methods, vectors, genes *etc.* and patenting transgenic plants and animals. Patents are the most crucial form of protection in agricultural biotechnology[3].

Plant breeder's right was originally initiated to protect traditional breeding methods used to develop new plant varieties. Sui generis is a relatively weaker mode of protection as it does not exclude other breeders from using the subject matter for

---

3 IP and innovation in agriculture, https://www.innovationpolicyplatform.org/content/ip-and-innovation-agriculture, 2018.

further development. Geographical indications is a protection of the geographically produced materials which have a distinct quality relating to the geographical area.

Introduction of IPR in India

Ministry of Agriculture, vide Letter No.11-71/88-SD-1 dated September 16,1988, brought out '**New Policy on Seed Development**', with the aim of providing to the farmer the best planting materials available in the world so as to increase productivity and there by increasing farm income and export earnings. Soon the private sector started demanding for rights in agriculture which smoothly got the public sector and the government to discuss about the same (which was earlier objected by the public sector for they believed the private companies would encroach upon their breeding material). Reports and discussions suggested that India should implement rights for the farmers and the breeders in accordance with the (UPOV) International Union for the Protection of New varieties of Plants. Enormous protest against implementing Trade-Related Aspects of Intellectual Property Rights (**TRIPS**) with a valid argument that it only encompasses agricultural innovations of breeders and corporations, but ignores informal innovations of farmers and communities, especially in developing countries. In the background of this debate on plant breeders' right in India, the government formulated a draft of a bill to grant Plant Breeder Rights in 1993/94.

The bill provided for plant breeders' rights through provisions based on UPOV.

However, The farmers right under this draft was defined as:

1. Farmers' privilege as a right not only to save and exchange seeds but also to sell seeds (except branded)
2. Benefit sharing based on compensation and operating through a mechanism where communities/farmers can make claims for such compensation
3. Farmers Rights as ownership: the idea that farmers must be able to register their varieties.

Section-2

Plant Breeder's Right

To begin with, TRIPs' agreement on plant varieties don't allude to or consolidate any previous licensed innovation assentions, including the 1978 and 1991 UPOV Acts. This oversight stands out pointedly from different fields of licensed innovation, for example, licenses, copyrights and trademarks, for which TRIPs explicitly requires WTO Members to conform to the models of security contained in previous IPR understandings, for example, the Berne Convention for the Protection of Literary and Artistic Works and the Paris Convention for the Protection of Industrial Property. Because of this exclusion, WTO Members are neither required to wind up individuals from UPOV nor to institute national laws reliable with either UPOV Act keeping in mind the end goal to agree to their commitments under TRIPs. (Be that as it may, certain "Treks in addition to" settlements do force either of these prerequisites, see para. 2.3.1.6 underneath) Although the drafting history of TRIPs does not clarify this notably extraordinary treatment of plant assortments, it appears to be likely that consistence with UPOV was not required in light of the fact that so few WTO Members were gathering to UPOV and the individuals who were couldn't concur whereupon of its two latest Acts should fill in as the standard for security[4].

Second, article 27.3(b) grants WTO Members to secure plant varieties utilizing one of three unmistakable methodologies: (1) patent law, (2) a viable sui generis framework or (3) a blend of components from the two frameworks. Hence, not at all like most different territories of licensed innovation secured by TRIPs, article 27.3(b) explicitly gives Members noteworthy watchfulness to pick the way in which they will ensure plant assortments and it mulls over that prudence might be practiced contrastingly by various states.

This carefulness and the open door for disparate results it induces has critical outcomes. From one perspective, TRIPs' inability to fuse and expand upon the prior UPOV Acts may have "a deharmonizing impact," with states inside the UPOV framework establishing one sort of plant varieties insurance law and states outside of that framework authorizing an alternate sort of law (which could possibly take after each other). This could make noteworthy complexities and vulnerabilities for plant raisers looking to showcase ensured varieties in various locales. Then again, this endorsed decent variety of lawful methodologies enables WTO Members to adjust the assurance of plant raisers' rights against the other vital and contending societal objectives distinguished in Part I, a considerable lot of which are found in other worldwide understandings. Seen from this point of view, article 27.3(b) gives a truly necessary "safe space" for governments to blend clashing standards and strategies - a space that is inadequate in different zones of the TRIPs Agreement.

TRIP's obliges, with a couple of special cases, that patents be accessible in all fields of innovation for developments that are new, include a creative advance (or identically, are not clear to people of normal ability in that field) and are modernly material (or comparably, are valuable). Once more, with constrained exemptions, TRIPS sets out that patent proprietors must be given the privilege to prohibit others from making, utilizing, offering or offering available to be purchased the licensed development, including items straight forwardly got through protected procedures. It, be that as it may, enables constrained special cases to patent rights, including the give of mandatory licenses under specific conditions.

Excursions likewise unequivocally permits prohibitions of patentable developments that are in opposition to open request or ethical quality, including those that are biased to the wellbeing or life of people, creatures or plants or to the earth when all is said in done. In any case, creations barred on these grounds, should likewise be restricted from business abuse in that locale. Further, such innovations can't be rejected only in light of the fact that their utilization is precluded by local law. As it were, these developments must be resolved to be biased on a case-by-case premise before they can be avoided from patent allow.

4 International IPR agreements regulating plant varieties and plant breeders's rights, http://www.fao.org/docrep/007/y5714e/y5714e03.htm, 2017.

The arrangements of most significance to the AGRICULTURAL division is Article 27.3(b) of TRIPS, which permits the prohibition from protecting of plants and creatures and basically natural procedures for their generation, regardless of whether such innovations are generally qualified for licenses. It does, be that as it may, require the protecting of qualified creations covering 'microorganisms' and 'microbiological' or 'non-organic' procedures and items thereof. These terms are not characterized, leaving extensive degree for understanding. Excursions likewise requires the organization of a 'powerful' sui generis law for the [5]insurance of plant assortments. Not at all like on account of different IPRs, TRIPS does not oblige consistence with the previous universal arrangement on the assurance of plant assortments, UPO, nor does it set down in any further detail the extension or span of such security. Treks, nonetheless, requires this sub-segment, 27.3 (b), to be returned to in 1999 and such a survey is at present in progress in the TRIPS Council of the WTO.

Unmistakably, at the time of the talks on TRIPS, the US and the EU varied on their ways to deal with patenting of biotechnological developments. While the US trusted that 'anything under the sun made by man', aside from individuals, was patentable, the EU was thinking about solid inside protection from patents on living beings. The US had been conceding patenting of living materials since the point of interest choice on the patentability of miniaturized scale living beings in 1980. It conceded its first plant patent in 1986 in Ex parte Hibberd and its first creature patent on the acclaimed Harvard oncomouse in 1988. In any case, since the level headed discussion had not yet been settled in Europe, it was consented to hold a negligible assention while resolving to return to this arrangement inside four years from the section into power of TRIPS *i.e.* by 1999. It was normal that with the death of the European Biotechnology Directive, under dialog at the season of the transactions, there would be extension to push for tolerating the patentability of all qualified biotechnological innovations, including of qualities, plants and creatures. With the quick selection of transgenic plants in numerous nations over the most recent couple of years, the modest number of fruitful multinational farming biotechnology organizations, beginning for the most part in the US, are especially inspired by the overall reception of plant licenses. They contend that Plant Breeders' Rights (PBRs), with raisers' exception and ranchers' benefit, are not adequate to recover their tremendous ventures on R&D to build up these inventive items. Undoubtedly, there is prove that private area interests in the improvement of new plant assortments has, without satisfactory IPR assurance, for the most part occurred in crops amiable to the generation of half breeds and even PBRs are not adequate to guarantee appropriability.

Transgenic or hereditarily changed yields are an exceptionally late marvel all around. Between 1996 to 1998, the worldwide region under such products has expanded fifteen times, from 4.3 million sections of land to 69.5 million sections of land, reflecting incredibly high reception rates by ranchers by models of new

---

5 Jayashre Watal (1999) Intellectual Property Rights and Interest of Developing Countries, Conference of agriculture and new tread agenda, WTO 2000.

advances in the farming division. The fundamental achievement has come in upgrades to herbicide resilience and creepy crawly protection of yields. The five primary transgenic trims in 1998 were, in plunging request of significance, soybean, corn/maize, cotton, canola/rapeseed and potato. Soybean and corn alone record for 82 per cent of the worldwide territory under transgenic crops. 74 per cent of the worldwide territory is in the US, with 15 per cent in Argentina, 10 per cent in Canada and the rest of Australia, Mexico, Spain, France and South Africa[6].

The potential for the advantages of horticultural biotechnology for creating nations go past the adaption to neighborhood states of the present age of transgenic crops created in different markets to take care of issues of bug assaults or weeds. This innovation can possibly tackle a portion of the issues of ailing health, ailment and low agrarian efficiency that are specific to creating and minimum created nations. For instance, it was as of late reported that hereditarily adjusted rice may help decrease press insufficiency frailty or vitamin A deficiency. Also dry spell safe plants or those that endure large amounts of soil danger could assist enhance yields and prompt more prominent nourishment security. Unmistakably this potential must be completely tapped and this innovation additionally created for the advantage of mankind. While solid IPR insurance, joined with other fitting arrangements, may help grow such a potential, there are fears that the subsequent items may not be accessible or might be dreadfully costly for most purchasers in these nations. These feelings of trepidation are exarcebated by the current pattern on mergers and acquisitions in the seed and life sciences segments. The ten biggest worldwide seed firms control 30 per cent of the seed deals on the planet. Progressively, the new seeds being produced are controlled through IPRs that have a place with these best companies. Then again, so far farming examination and seed dispersion in creating nations has been overwhelmingly in the hands of the general population part. Nonetheless, open division look into is experiencing an intense deficiency of assets in a large number of these nations. Progressively, private firms, generally remote firms or joint endeavors, are venturing up their examination endeavors in these nations. These organizations are hesitant to present new assortments that can be appropriated effectively by other opponent seed organizations without solid IPR assurance. By and by, in nations like India, which are yet to embrace even PBRs, these organizations bind their examination to mixtures. Indeed, even here, seed of single cross crossovers of maize are not being promoted as a result of the still high cost of seed generation and the absence of IPR security.

Changes in IPR administrations, especially as identified with the agricultural division are especially pertinent to the way global agrarian research is sorted out through the focuses of the Consultative Group on International Agricultural Research (CGIAR) and the National Agricultural Research Organizations (NAROs)[7]. Creating nations have been reliant on the CGIAR framework for the free trade of

6 Jayashre Watal (1999) Intellectual Property Rights and Interest of Developing Countries, Conference of agriculture and new tread agenda,WTO 2000.

7 International IPR agreements regulating plant varieties and plant breeders's rights, http://www.fao.org/docrep/007/y5714e/y5714e03.htm, 2017.

germ plasm and logical learning. About 15 per cent of the examination spending plan of the CGIAR focuses is dedicated to hereditary designing and these focuses have turned out to be enter players in farming biotechnology. However few licenses have yet been connected for by these focuses and by and large restrictive advances might be utilized without formal assent. This is for the most part a direct result of a noteworthy absence of recognition with IPRs. There is currently expanding assention that these focuses should take out guarded licenses keeping in mind the end goal to stake out their cases and guarantee access to it.

Section-3

Patents in Agriculture

Patents gives the exclusive right for a stipulated period of time through legal systems to have a control over one's invention and prevent the exact duplication of the invention by a third party.

According to the Indian Patent Act 1970 and subsequent Patent (Amendment) Act, 1999 and 2002, patents could be applied mainly for agricultural tools and machinery or the processes for the development of agricultural chemicals. However, agricultural and horticultural methods (Process patent) and products of agriculture which delivered rise in economical value of the country, helped in the nutritional index of the mass, containing medicinal values, potential of combating diseases did not encrypt the patent. This went on until the Patent Amendment Act, 2005 was passed, which gave the rights to patent over the products of agricultural inventions (Product Patent). Later as a signatory of TRIPS, *sui generis* system pf protection of plant varieties was adopted which enables an owner to design the own way of protection of a plant variety and product. Thus, patents will now been granted for seeds, plants, micro-organisms, cells and even GMOs and animals. Agricultural patents constitutes ~2 per cent of the total patents of Indian patents.

Sl.No.	*Patents*	*Use*
1.	Product patent	Asserts rights over a product.
2.	Process Patent	Patent on a process or method.
3.	Use Patent	In order to use a particular product for a specified use.

$$\text{Activity Index (India)} = 100 \times \frac{\text{Indian patents in a particular block/ total patents in that block}}{\text{Total Indian Patents/total patents}}$$

Activity Index gives us the information regarding India's performance with respect to the world's performance in the field of alkaloids for different years.

Patents can be levied upon genes, genes of a plant which is novel

International Patent Classification as a tool has been used to obtain a specific level of precision in relation to activities related to agriculture. The bibliographic references contain information on patent number, publication date, IPC number, inventor's name, applicant's name, inventor's country, title, *etc.*

Some of the patenting activities in IPC classes are-

IPC Class A01B

The patents (11) were granted to Indian applicants for developing agricultural and gardening tools set, seed-cum-fertilizer drill, human-propelled tiller, ploughing-cum-sowing implement, mattock cultivator, rotary tilling device, shaft-driven timing system for internal combustion engines, improved plough with a mounted adaptor, adaptor for plough and improved process for manufacturing tractor discs.

IPC Class A01C (Planting, sowing and fertilizing)

Out of 15 patents Indian applicants received 10 for developing portal digital soil salinity tester, air screen cleaner machine, preparing *in situ* compost, machine for cleaning and grading of seeds, preparation of synergistic fertilizer composition from agricultural compost and agricultural waste, groundnut planter, animal-driven agricultural apparatus, manufacturing a slow-release urea fertilizer by nitrification inhibition, sowing device and composition for increasing herbage and essential oil yield in Palmarosa.

IPC Class A01D (Harvesting and Mowing)

Indian applicants received patents for self-driven crop-orienting two-wheeler and three-wheeler harvester; machine for harvesting sugarcane; trimmer; sugarcane-harvesting knife, harvester for harvesting crops; lawnmower and machine for separating out cotton from cotton pods[8].

IPC Class A01F (Processing of Harvested Produce, Devices for Storing Agricultural or Horticultural Produce)

Four patents were granted to India for multi-crop thresher, novel container for storing plant products, storage pot and improved process for the preparation of a *pseudobactin* useful for storing agricultural/horticultural produce.

IPC Class A01J (Manufacture of Dairy Products)

4 patents were granted to India for continuous production of cheese free from aspartic protease, manufacturing paneer; while foreign applicants for the production of immobilized milk-clotting protease, method of preparing milk, producing shredded cheese, no fat cheese analogue and container for fast cooling used for preservation of milk.

IPC Class A01H (New Plants or Processes for Obtaining them, Plant Reproduction by Tissue Culture Techniques)

8 patents were granted to India for nutrient medium composition for enhancing shoot sprouting from bamboo species and excised embryo-axis of cotton,

---

8 The Indian Seed Act and Patent Act: Sowing the Seeds of Dictatorship AUTHOR: Vandana Shiva Publication: Znet DATE: 14 February 2005 URL: http://www.zmag.org/content/showarticle.cfm?SectionID=56 and It emID=7249.

transformation of plant/tissue, rhizobial preparation for enhancing nodulation activity and grain yield in legumes, cold extruded composition, and synergistic composition as growth medium for fungi and bacteria.

According the recent trend in agricultural patenting, major patents were done in the field of herbicides, pest-repellents or attractants. The Patents (Amendment) Act, 1999 offers Exclusive Marketing Rights (EMR) in agricultural chemicals, which helped foreign multinationals to exclusively market their agricultural chemicals in India for a period of 5 years, subject to the right granted in the country and marketing approval on/after 1 January 1995.

Patenting DNA Genes

Patenting DNA genes was however objectionable by a many for it meant considering life (DNA - Hereditary material from one generation to another) as a commodity and a 'gene machine' which could be exploited for profit. Nevertheless, genes are being patented which are novel and the plants possessing it, the seeds and their progenies.

According to Section 3(j) of the Indian Patent Act, the following is not an invention:

"Any process for the medical, surgical, creative, prophylactic or other treatment of human beings or any process for a similar treatment of animals or plants or render them free of disease or to increase their economic value or that of their products."

The second amendment of the above act deleted the term 'plant'. Thus, genetically engineered plants have got the allowance to be patented. India law of Article 27.3 (b) of TRIPS Agreement. Article 27.3 (b) of TRIPS states:

"Parties may exclude from patentability plants and animals other than micro-organisms, and essentially biological processes for the production of plants or animals other than non-biological and microbiological processes. However, parties shall provide for the protection of plant varieties either by patents or by an effective sui generis system or by any combination thereof. This provision shall be reviewed four years after the entry into force of the Agreement establishing the WTO."[9]

This is considered as a loophole for our country in the name of scientific boon as Monsanto being a drafting hand in TRIPS agreement, has made a way to India's patent laws.

Seed Act, 2004: Seed act, 2004 aims at preventing the farmers from saving/hoarding seeds from the private seed industries, dealing in seed exchanging and seed reproduction. The motive behind this act was to foster the rise of high quality seeds at the community level. The act regulates by imposing fine of upto 25000/- on the farmers who have unregistered seeds with them and rights to the Seed Police to break into the huts and fields of the farmers for checking of their unregistered possession. Thus, this act in every way worked for the betterment of the private

9 International IPR agreements regulating plant varieties and plant breeders's rights, http://www.fao.org/docrep/007/y5714e/y5714e03.htm, 2017.

seed industries without doing any good to the farmers, resulting in the suicide of the farmers as they drowned in debt and loss of seeds.

Farmers' rights in the Indian PPVFR Act, 2001:

1. Denied right to sell a branded seed of a variety under this act. They are free to save, sow, re-sow, use the seeds and the products of the seeds, including seeds of protected varieties.
2. The legal Indian bodies which provide growth hormones for the making the crop disease resistant and giving better yield should be benefited in the gain of the farmer, thus benefit-sharing should be practised.
3. The farmer is eligible of obtaining compensation if the seed received from the seed industry fails as was stated to give results.
4. Farmers have the right to access registered seed of varieties at a fair price.
5. Farmers who have contributed positively to crop improvement strategies are rewarded from the national gene fund.
6. If a farmer's variety is to be used by the third party, authorization from the farmer is mandatory.
7. A farmer is well protected from accidental infringement if proven that he is unaware of the existing rights.

Along with the private sectors, farmers are being promoted to conserve and make use of the rights made for them and effectively contribute to the balance in private sectors and farmer's rights.

Section-4

Geographical Indication

Geographical indications are valuable rights, which if not adequately protected, can be misused by dishonest commercial operators to the detriment of both the consumers and the legitimate users.

The TRIPs endorses least gauges of insurance of GIs and extra security for wines and spirits. Articles 22 to 24 of Part II Section III of the TRIPS recommend least guidelines of assurance to the geological signs that WTO individuals must give. India, in consistence with its commitment under TRIPS, has taken authoritative measures by authorizing the Geographical Indications of Goods (Registration and Protection) Act, 1999, which happened on September 15, 2003 and the Geographical Indications of Goods (Registration and Protection) Rules, 2002[10].

According to the (Indian) Geographical Indications of Goods (Registration and Protection) Act, 1999 "Land Indication", in connection to merchandise, implies a sign which distinguishes such products as horticultural merchandise, common merchandise or made merchandise as beginning, or made in the domain of a nation,

10 Pradyot R. Jena (2015), Does Geographical Indication (GI) increase producer welfare, https://www.researchgate.net/publication/228453155_Does_Geographical_Indication_GI_increase_producer_welfare_A_case_study_of_Basmati_rice_in_Northern_India.

or a district or region in that region, where a given quality, notoriety or other normal for such merchandise is basically owing to its topographical starting point and on the off chance that where such merchandise are fabricated products one of the exercises of either the generation or of handling or readiness of the merchandise concerned happens in such region, area or territory, all things considered.

GIs have been utilized as a part of India for a wide assortment of items, for example, Basmati Rice, Darjeeling Tea, Kangra Tea, Feni, Alphonso Mango, Alleppey Green Cardamom, Coorg Cardamom, Kanchipuram Silk Saree, Kohlapuri Chappal, and so forth.

By enrolling a geological sign in India, the rights holder can forestall unapproved utilization of the enlisted land sign by others by starting encroachment activity by method for a common suit or criminal objection. Enrollment of the GIs in India isn't obligatory as an unregistered GI can likewise be authorized by starting an activity of going off against the infringer. It is, in any case, fitting to enlist the GI as the testament of enrollment is at first sight confirmation of its legitimacy and no additional evidence of the same is required.

Onions from Lasalgaon will get the Geographical Indication (GI) tag soon as the horticultural bureau of the state has begun the procedure to allow the uncommon status to the item delivered in the locale. The advancement and improvement of GI is a device for local advancement and to secure the legacy of a specific place. This will enable the makers to advertise their items and win more income.

Does GI good increase the level of welfare of the producers ? This question is at the heart of the GI debate regarding whether or not to promote GI at the global level since one of the major arguments in favour of GI is – producers of such goods are mostly smallholder agricultural farmers whose livelihood can be improved by providing the GI protection.

Conclusion

Development cooperation advocates an equitable balance between the legitimate interests of both sides: those of commercial IPR holders on the one hand and those of traditional users and right holders on the other. It advises governments on the use of existing flexibilities of the TRIPS Agreement in the fields of biological diversity, agrobiodiversity, the handling of IPR on plant varieties

REFERENCES

1. Adelman, Martin J. Randall R. Rader, John R. Thomas and Harold C. Wegner (1998): *Cases and Materials on Patent Law*, American Case Book Series, West Group, St. Paul, Minnesota.
2. Barton, John H., William Lesser and Jayashree Watal (1999): *Intellectual Property Rights in the Developing World: Implications for Agriculture*, presented at a workshop on Biotechnology held by the World Bank in June 3-4, at Washington DC.

3. Beier, Friedrich-Karl and Schricker, Gerhard (1996): *'From GATT to TRIPs – The Agreement on Trade-Related Aspects of Intellectual Property Rights'*, IIC Studies, Vol.18, Max Planck Institute for Foreign and International Patent, Copyright and Competition Law, Munich, Germany.

4. Correa, Carlos M (1999): 'Access to Plant Genetic Resources and Intellectual Property Rights', Commission on Genetic Resources for Food and Agriculture, Background Study Paper No. 8, FAO, April, available at http://www.fao.org.

5. Herdt, Robert W. (1999): 'Enclosing the Global Plant Genetic Commons', lecture at the China Center for Economic Research, May 24, available on file with author.

6. James, Clive (1998): 'Global Review of Commercialized Transgenic Crops: 1998', International Service for the Acquisition of Agri-biotech Applications (ISAA), Ithaca, NY.

7. Knaak, Roland (1996): 'The Protection of Geographical Indications According to the TRIPs Agreement', in Beier and Schricker, Eds. (1996), pp. 117-140.

8. Lele, Uma, William Lesser and Gesa Horstkotte-Wessler, Eds (1999): *'Intellectual Property Rights in Agriculture: the World Bank's Role in Assisting Borrower and Member Countries'*, The World Bank, Washington DC, Draft.

9. Lesser, William, Gesa Horstkotte-Wesseler, Uma Lele and Derek Byerlee (1999): 'Intellectual Property Rights, Agriculture, and the World Bank' in Lele *et al.*, Eds (1999), pp. 1-29.

10. Levin, R.C., A.K. Klevorick, R.R. Nelson and S.G. Winter (1987): 'Appropriating the Returns from Industrial Research and Development', *Brookings Papers on Economic Activity*, 3, pp.783-820.

11. Long, Susanna (1996): 'Salient Features of the Patents Act 1994 of Singapore', *International Review of Industrial Property and Copyright Law*, Vol. 27, No. 1, pp. 26-40.

12. Maskus, Keith (1999), *Intellectual Property Rights in the Global Economy*, Institute for International Economics, Washington D.C., forthcoming.

Chapter 2

Section 3(j) of the Patent Act, 1970: Judicial Interpretation and the Impact Thereof

Akanksha Anil

Advocate, Jharkhand High Court, Ranchi, Jharkhand-834033
e-mail: akanksha.anil16_llm@apu.edu.in

ABSTRACT

The chapter seeks to ask whether the interpretation of Section 3(j) of the Patents Act,1970 by the courts have affected the patent trend in India, either in a positive or negative manner. The Patents (Amendment) Act 2002 introduced Section 3(j) which prohibits patenting of "plants and animals in whole or any part thereof other than microorganisms but including seeds, varieties and species and essentially biological processes for production and propagation of plants and animals." fails to define the term "essential biological processes". However in the recent years there have been judicial precedents making some progress in the direction of defining this particular terminology. In the year 2002, the Calcutta High court gave a landmark decision when it held that microorganisms which are not naturally occurring and involve human intervention are subject to patents. If the decision leads to strong patent regime,it would lead to lesser number of patent grants but a higher level of innovation and a weaker patent regime would lead to higher number of patent grants while a lower level of innovation.It is however not clear as to what extent these interpretations have made the patent protection in this respect better or worse. With this concept in mind I intend to study how to determine the impact of these court judgments and what has been the impact on the patent trend in the field of biotechnology in specific.

Introduction

India's biotechnology industry is touching new heights. India is among the top 12 biotech destinations in the worlds and ranks third in the Asia pacific region. India has the second largest number of US Food and Drug Administration(USF

DA) -approved plants, after the USA and is the largest producer of recombinant Hepatitis B vaccine. The Department of Biotechnology and many other autonomous bodies representing the biotechnology sector are working together in order to project India as a global hub for biotech research and business excellence.(Biotechnology industry in India. India brand equity foundation).

A Patent which is an official document granted by the government conveying to the recipient, called the patentee,special exclusive rights named in the document and in the patent statutes serves important role in the promotion of research and development[1]. In the year 2014, the number of patent applications filed in India has witnessed a rise of 23.97 per cent from 2007-08 to 201213, assessment shows that only a meagre 22 per cent of them have been filed by Indian applicants in 2012-13.While 3,663 patents were filed in 2012-13, a majority or 78 per cent were international applications." Citing a report from the WIPO, the deputy controller of patents and designs and head of Mumbai Office stated "According to the World Intellectual Property (WIPO-2012) report,while China's contribution to the rise in patent applications globally has increased from 3.5 per cent between 1995-2009 to 2.7 per cent between 2009-2011.The report shows that while China topped the global list by filing 503,582 patent applications,India was ranked seventh with 2,291 applications".[2][5]

The road to grant of patents isn't an easy one in the Indian Jurisdiction. The Indian Patent Act,via Section 3(j) deals with patenting of microorganisms. Section 3 can be said to be a negative section rather than a positive section. It states a list of things which cannot be patented. Clause (j) of the same section states prohibits patenting of "plants and animals in whole or any part thereof other than microorganisms but including seeds, varieties and species and essentially biological processes for production and propagation of plants and animals."[3] This section fails to give a clear description of what can be included in this umbrella term of 'essential biological processes' and what should be excluded. It is then that our judiciary comes to the rescue and tries to give a clearer picture of what the legislature implied despite its ambiguous language. Despite the hard work undertaken by the judiciary in removing these ambiguities from such provisions, it remains unclear as to whether these judicial decisions impact the patent trend in any way or not.

The chapter therefore aims at exploring the role of judiciary when it comes to patent trends in India and coming to a conclusion of its impact, if any. In determining the effect I shall be looking at the number of patent applications filed and by the number of patents granted by the Indian patent office. The paper has been divided into four sections. The first section gives an overview of the issue in hand,*i.e.*, the ambiguous language of section 3(j) of the Patent Act. This includes the law that existed before the enactment of the relevant section and the ambiguities

---

1 Balasubramaniam,S and Radhakrishnan R (2010). Intellectual Property Rights:Text and Cases. Bookvistas, Delhi.

2 The Indian Express, Mumbai, http://indianexpress.com/article/business/economy/india-sees-sharp-drop-in-patent-applications, accessed on 21st December, 2017.

3 Section 3 of the Indian Patent Act, 1970.

the above mentioned section possesses. The second section deals with the judicial decisions that have aimed at removing the ambiguities discussed in the previous section. The third section deals with patent trend in the field of biotechnology over a period of years. The fourth and final section,*i.e.*, the section on conclusion deals with answering the question as to whether these judicial decisions really have any impact on the patent trend or not. This section will also look into the role played by judicial decisions in other jurisdictions.

Law and the Ambiguity

The history of law on patents in India dates back to the year 1856 when we had the Act VI of 1856 on the protection of inventions based on the British Patent Law of 1852.Under this law certain exclusive privileges were granted to inventor of new inventors of new manufacturers for a period of 14 years. In 1859, the Act was modified as act XV Patent monopolies called exclusive privileges (making,selling and using inventions in India and authorising others to do so for 14 year from the date of filing specification).The year 1872 witnessed the introduction of the Patterns and Designs Protection Act. The Protection of Inventions Act was brought into force in 1883, consolidated as the Inventions and Designs Act in 1888,reintroduced as the Indian Patents and Designs Act in 1911, amended in 1999 and 2005.[4] Patent in India is granted only when it fulfils three requirements, i,e, ***novelty,industrial application and non obviousness.***

Novelty

The European Union adopted the European Patent Convention in 1973 which states that microbiological processes and products are patentable. It implies that the novelty of biotechnological inventions is accepted in the European Union. The convention does not include plants, animals, and essentially biological processes for the production of plants and animals from patenting. This provision was later interpreted to include plant, animals. The US Supreme Court Court and the patent offices have also confirmed to the view that biotechnological inventions are new.[5]Unlike the terms,non obviousness and industrial application the term novelty is not defined under the Indian Patent Act, 1970. However, the 2005 amedment demonstrates the idea of novelty by defining the term "new invention".Section 2(I) defines as follows "new invention means any invention or technology which ha snot been anticipated by publication in any document or used in the country or elsewhere in the world before the date of filing of patent application with complete specification,*i.e.*, the subject matter has not fallen in public domain or that it does not form part of the state of the art". Therefore,novelty can be negated by (a) prior publication or (b) by prior use.[6]

---

4. History of Indian Patent System, http://www.ipindia.nic.in/history-of-indian-patent-system.htm, accessed on 8th May, 2018.
5. Dr. Sreenivasulu, N.S., Dr. Raju, C.R (2008), Biotechnlogy and Patent Law: Patenting Living Beings, Manupatra.
6. Aggarwal Rashmi, Kaur, Rajinder (2017), Patent Law and Intellectual Property in the Medical Field, IGI Global, United States of America.

Industrial Application

Section 2(1)(ac) of the Patents Act 1970 states that "Capable of industrial application", in relation to an invention means that the invention is capable of being made or used in an industry."This criteria is aimed at enhancing industrial and economic progress in terms of the application of new technology or practical sphere of development. The law does not protect information per se,regardless of how novel and no obvious it may be.[7]

Non Obviousness

The TRIPS agreement states that 'patents shall be available for any invention,whether products or processes,in all fields of technology provided that they are new,involve an inventive step and are capable of industrial application. The expression inventive step is equivalent to the idea of non obviousness. Obviousness is a technical question which requires consideration of different technical aspects. An invention,in order to fulfil the requirement of inventive step must be a step further from the existing knowledge in the public domain. It also requires to examine the claimed invention to be viewed from the angle of a person skilled in the relevant field of invention. Obviousness is not judged from the point of view of the person seeking the patent but from the point of view of a person having ordinary skill in the art. The US court in the Graham case held that non obviousness involves a leap forward by the invention over and above the existing knowledge in the prior art. In order to decide the non obviousness of an invention, the court came up with a test.This test imposes three requirements to be fulfilled. They are:

1. The courts must survey the scope and content of the prior art.
2. It must examine the differences between the prior art and the claimed invention
3. There shall be a determination as to the level of ordinary skill in the art.[8]

Biotechnology may be defined as the "synergistic union of the biological science and technologically based industrial arts. In other words, biotechnology is utilization of biological processes, through the exploitation of biological systems,in the development or manufacture of a product or in the technological solution to a real-world problem."[9]

It is relevant to discuss development of India's patent law on biotechnology by looking into the International scenario that played a pivotal role in this development. The United States of America is credited with granting patents on single-cell organisms on several occasions dating back to 1873, when Louis Pasteur obtained

---

7. Kuanpoth Jakkrit (2010), Patent Rights in Pharmaceuticals in Developing Countries: Major Challenges in Developing countries, Tilleke and Gibbins International Ltd., Bangkok.
8. Dr. Sreenivasulu, N.S., Dr. Raju.C.R (2008), Biotechnlogy and Patent Law: Patenting Living Beings, Manupatra.
9. Kumar Abhinav (2008), Towards Patentability of Essentially Biologically Processes, Journal of Intellectual Property Rights, 13: 129-138.

a patent (US Patent No. 141,072) on a purified yeast cell. the *Diamond v. Chakraborty* case stands tall till date being the first judicial pronouncement recognising patents over living things. The relevant law in hand was 35 U.S.C. 101 titled as "Inventions patentable". The section stated "Whoever invents or discovers any new and useful process, machine, manufacture, or composition of matter, or any new and useful improvement thereof, may obtain a patent therefore, subject to the conditions and requirements of this title".The respondent in the above mentioned case filed an application for patent on an invention that involved human made, genetically engineered bacterium capable of breaking down crude oil, a property which is possessed by no naturally occurring bacteria. The application was rejected by the patent examiner and also by the Patent office board of Appeals stat0ing that the relevant U.S. laws on patent does not provide patent protection to living things. However, the Court of Customs and Patent Appeals took an altogether new approach by declaring that "anything under the sun that is made by man" is patent eligible so long as it meets the statutory requirements of 35 USC sections 101, 102, 103, 112, *etc.* Feisee, BIO's Director for Federal Government Relations and Intellectual Property, highlights that with the help of the Supreme Court decision of Diamond v. Chakrabarty and the Bayh-Dole Act, the biotech industry sky-rocketed.Thanks to the forethought of the judiciary, the biotechnology industry, particularly in the United States, was poised for cataclysmic changes after Chakrabarty. [10] Following the microorganism favourable decision in Chakraborty case, the U.S patent office even granted patent for cancer drug. The only condition that the court looked at was that there was human intervention and issues like morality and public order were never considered.

The international treaty on intellectual Property Rights (the TRIPS) also contributed to the development of laws on microorganisms in India.The TRIPS seeks to ensure that the enforcement of intellectual property rights and its enforcement plays a key role in the promotion of technological innovation and the transfer and dissemination of technology. "As a whole, Article 27 of the TRIPS Agreement defines which inventions governments are obliged to make eligible for patenting, and what they can exclude from patenting. Inventions that can be patented include both products and processes, and should generally cover all fields of technology. Broadly speaking, part (b) of paragraph 3 (*i.e.* Article 27.3(b)) allows governments to exclude some kinds of inventions from patenting, *i.e.* plants, animals and "essentially" biological processes (but micro-organisms, and nonbiological and microbiological processes have to be eligible for patents). However, plant varieties have to be eligible for protection either through patent protection or a system created specifically for the purpose ("sui generis"), or a combination of the two. India, being a signatory country to the TRIPS made amendments to its Patent Law in the year 2002 to be in compliance with the above mentioned treaty."[11]A committee on the Government

---

10. Ragavan Srividya (2008), Patent Judicial Wisdom, Natl. Law School of India Review, (2)165.

11. Rujitha T.R, Conceptual Issues in Biotech Patenting,Manupatra, http://www.manupatrafast.com/articles/PopOpenArticle.aspx?ID=0c234c7a-ad1d-75a-881e. 6c73d14c5fa2 and txtsearch=Subject: per cent 20Intellectual per cent 20Property per cent 20Rights, accessed on 3rd May, 2018.

of India's Technical Expert Committee, headed by Dr. Maleshkar was appointed to submit a report concerning two questions,one being whether microorganisms should be grated patent or not. The committee came to the conclusion that TRIPS mandates protection for microorganisms.[12] The 2005 amendment made several changes to the Patent Act, the most relevant being the addition of a new clause(j) to section 3 which excluded inventions on plants and animals other than microorganisms. Section 3(j) when combined with section 3(i) makes it possible to patent biotechnology based tools and processes but at the same time excluding the possibility of protecting any process that is essentially biological for achieving the very same objective.

The enactment of a new clause could not solve all the patenting issues related with microorganism as the language of section 3(j) is highly ambiguous. Section 3(j) provides that plants and animals in whole or any part thereof including seeds,varieties,species, and essentially biological processes for production and propagation of plants and animals are not patentable subject matter. It however allows patents for microorganisms and microbiological processes. The problem,however, arises due to the fact that the legislature used the broad umbrella terms such as 'essentially biological processes', 'microorganisms', 'microbiological processes' without giving a clear list of what is to be included and what is to be excluded under these broad terms. Patents are granted for 'invention' and not 'discoveries'. it is difficult to determine what comes under 'discovery' and what comes under 'invention'.In the West, this problem is resolved by judicial pronouncements and patent office practices on the facts and circumstances of each case rather than through clear cut criteria laid down in the statutory provisions. The doctrine of 'man-madness' would appear to have come in vogue in the judicial decisions of the US to distinguish a 'product of nature' from a 'product of act of man'

[13]The product of nature doctrine dates back to 1889. In *Ex Parte Latimer*, a claim was rejected by the Commissioner of Patents on a new article of manufacture consisting of the cellular tissues of the Southern Pine eliminated in full length from the siliceous, resinous, and pulpy parts of the pine needles and sub divided into long, plant filaments adapted to be spun and woven. In the initial rejection of the claim, the examiner emphasized the identity of the claimed substance and its natural counterpart [14]. Unfortunately, the TRIPS is also silent when it comes to defining these terms. In the absence of any clear definition in the TRIPS Agreement,one needs to adopt the dictionary meaning of the term. All biotechnology inventions involving microorganisms including virus and bacteria are patentable in India. But the animal and plant genes are excluded in India from scope of patent protecting. India is also a signatory to the Budapest treaty. This treaty was brought into force to satisfy the requirement of "sufficiency disclosure".According to this requirement the patent seeker has to file a detailed information on the invention sought to be protected.

---

12 Report of the Technical expert Group on Patent Law Issues, December 2006.

13 Vasudeva P.K, Patentig Biotech Products: Complex Issues, Economic and Political Weekely, Vol 35, No. 2.

14 Prajapati B.J., G.M. Haridas, Senan Suja (2011), Patenting of Microorganisms in India: A commentary, Current Science, 2(100): 159-162.

The Budapest treaty states that where ever this "sufficiency requirement" seeks the deposition of microorganisms, the same should be deposited at the International Depository Authority. India is now obliged to submit the microorganisms sample at the International depository.[15]

In the year 2008, the Draft Patent Manual of India, taking a stand on the difference between discovery and invention stated that a discovery adds to the amount of human knowledge by disclosing something already existent, whereas an invention adds to the human knowledge by creating a new product or processes involving a technical advance as compared to the existing knowledge. For example, a scientific theory is a statement about the natural world. These scientific theories are not considered patentable, no matter how radical revolutionary an insight they may provide, because they do not result in a product or process. On the other hand if the theories lead to a practical application in the process of manufacture of article or substance, they may be patentable. [16].In the year 1999, the Department of Biotechnology established a biotechnology patent facilitation cell (BPFC) to create awareness and understanding about Intellectual Property Rights among the scientists and researchers[17]. In the guidelines issued by the patent office in the year 2014,one of the guidelines was that isolated pure culture is to be patentable since it is not available in nature as such and the term "genetically" modified is restrictive for patenting of microorganisms. The exceptions to the provisions of section 3(j) is genetically modified microorganisms and hence, the same should be applicable in respect of animals as well[18].However the report by the Patent committee and the Patent guidelines cannot have the force of a statute and therefore even though they do bring some clarity to the much ambiguous language, they cannot be considered sufficient to remove that ambiguity.

Therefore in the above mentioned scenario, it can be concluded that though the international regime played an important in the development of law favourable for biotechnological inventions,it remains a fact that the language of the relevant provision is quite ambiguous which cannot be done away with without taking recourse to the interpretation given by judiciary.

Judicial Intepretations

This section of the chapter deals with the judicial decisions made in respect of removing the ambiguity that is employed in drafting of section 3(j) of the Indian Patent Act. The adjudication hierarchy in patent related matters differs from that of other adjudication matters. Patent related matters can be of two types- Patent Administrative cases and Patent Infringement cases. The former deals with the

---

15 Raghuvanshi Salvi Kumar (2017), Patent Regime of India related to Microorganisms: A Critical Analysis, the World Journal on Juristic Polity.

16 Prajapati B.J., G.M. Haridas, Senan Suja (2011). Patenting of Microorganisms in India: A commentary, Current Science, 2(100): 159-162.

17 Raghuvanshi Salvi Kumar (2017), Patent Regime of India related to Microorganisms: A Critical Analysis, the World Journal on Juristic Polity.

18 Department of Biotechnology, Ministry of Science and Technology, http://www.dbtindia.nic.in/patents/

disputes with regard to grant of patent, patent invalidation and upholding, and compulsory licensing of patents and defendant is the Indian Patent office. The latter set of cases are those wherein a third party is involved and the patent holder pursues a case against the patent infringer,for damages or injunction order form the court. In both sets of disputes the hierarchy of the adjudicating bodies falls in this order:

1. Controller of Patents
2. Intellectual Property Appellate Board
3. District Courts and High Courts and
4. Supreme Court.

The IPO examines patent applications and grants them if they confirm to Indian patent laws; maintains records of renewal a specialized forum that was established in the year 2002. It has its headquarter at Chennai and sittings at Chennai,Mumbai, delhi, Kolkata and Ahmedabad. It becomes pertinent to note that the role played by patent offices while giving orders in pre/post grant oppositions are also judicial in nature and working of patents, resolving disputes related to grant of patents.

The IPAB functions by hearing patent related disputes. As per section 77 of the Patent Act, the controller is empowered to function as a Civil Court and his powers under this section extends to issue of summons, administration of oath, requiring the discovery and production of any document,issuing commissions for the examination of witnesses or documents, an even awarding costs. There can be no dispute over the fact that this proceeding is "intrinsic judicial functions"[19]

The district courts function as the first judicial machinery they first hear cases concerning patent infringement in the form of suits. The Indian High Courts hear and decide appeals arising out of the decisions of the district courts. The Supreme Court, decides appeals against the decisions of the district and high courts.[20]

The history of such judicial decisions dates back to the year 2002 (Diminaco AG v. Controller General of Patents)[21] when an issue concerning patenting of microorganisms arose before the Calcutta High Court. This case dealt with the issue of patent of a process for preparation of infectious bursitius vaccine which was to be employed for protecting poultry against infectious bursitis. The patent application was rejected on the basis of section 2 the vaccine used living entity, it did not involve any manufacture and therefore it was not qualified to be invention and hence no patent protection. The decision of the controller was challenged in the High court on the ground that although the process contains live virus, "process for preparation "of any product is a patentable commodity and the Indian law does not bar in patenting of the manufacture of which involves live virus. It was

---

19 Srividhya Ragavan, Patent Judicial Wisdom, 20 Natl. Law School of India Review 2 165 (2008).

20 Patent Enforcement through courts in India,https://blog.ipleaders.in/patent-enforcement/, accessed on 24th March, 2018.

21 Is it unconstitutional for the Patent Office to be the Adjudicatory Authority deciding Oppositions and CL proceedings, https://spicyip.com/2009/03/is-it-unconstitutional-for-patent.html, accessed on 10th May, 2018.

also claimed that the patent protection was claimed only for the "process" and the "end product"as such. The only reason on which the controller's order was based is that the process does not constitute invention without the meaning of section 2(i)(i) of P.A.The order also stated that the process has to result either in an article or a substance. And referring to the dictionary concluded that the said the said invention does not result in any material thing. An inanimate object can be donated as a thing or item but not a living thing. The stand of the respondents was that the process for which the patent is claimed may involve living organism, but the end product produced by the process has to come within the meaning of manufacture and it cannot contain any living organism. The Honourable Calcutta High Court observed that one of the most common test to determine whether in a particular test the process of manufacture involved in the invention ought to be patented or not,is the vendibility test. The said vendibility test is satisfied if the invention results in the production of some vendible item or it improvises or restores former conditions or a vendible item or its effect is the preservation and prevention from deterioration of some vendible product. In other words, a vendible product means something,which can be passed on from one man to another upon the transaction of purchase and sale. The court held that the controller erred himself in law by holding that merely because the end product contains a live virus, the process involved in bringing out the end product is not an invention. The dictionary meaning of the word manufacture does not exclude the process of preparing a vendible commodity which contains a living substance and in a case like this where there is no statutory meaning of manufacture, the dictionary must be accepted.[22] The judiciary while giving judgement on a particular matter is influenced by several factors. Just before the May 2002 Dimminaco AG decision, the South African AIDS crisis showcased the importance of the Indian generic drug industry and its biotechnology potential to the world. So, the same logic that would have applied to the American judiciary to promote biotechnology applied to India as well[23].The Diminaco case[24] is considered to be the break through case in the field of biotechnology since it opened doors for biotech industries to patent inventions involving live microorganisms on the condition that it involved human intervention.

The next landmark case that sought to do away with the ambiguities involved in the terms used in section 3(j) of the Patent Act is the Monsanto case (decided on 13th July,2013) wherein the IPAB gave a clearer view as to what "essentially biological processes" means. The Indian Patent Office had refused the grant of a patent to Monsanto for an invention described as "a method of producing a transgenic plant with increased heat tolerance,salt tolerance, or drought tolerance" based on the following key grounds: 1. that the subject matter of claims was considered to lack inventive step in view of prior art documents cited in the office action 2. that the

---

22 Judicial System for Protection of Intellectual Property in India, http://legasis.in/Legist/April2014/html/judicial_system.html

23 Robinson, douglas, and Nina Medlck (2005), diamond v. Chakrabarty: A Retrospective on 25 Years of Biotech Patents, Intellectual Property and Technology: 12-15.

24 (2002) I.P.L.R. 255(Cal).

claims in the application were not considered to qualify as an invention. The reason offered for rejection was that the structure and function of a cold shock protein was disclosed in the cited prior art, and was, therefore, obvious to a person skilled in the art to make a transgenic plant The claimed invention was considered unpatentable as it was regarded as a mere application of an already known cold shock protein in producing cold stress tolerant plants as well as plans tolerant to heat,salt and drought conditions. It was held that the claims in the Monsanto patent application fell under the proscription of Section 3(j) of the Patent Act. The primary reason offered for rejection under this ground was that th claims related to "essentially biological processes" of regeneration and selection,which in turn included growing of plays in specific conditions.'Challenging the controller's decision, Monsanto filed an appeal before the. The IPAB upheld the decision delivered by the Indian Patent Office. The IPAB was in consensus with the first three grounds listed by the Controller but disagreed with the fourth ground. It significantly, overruled the patent office's findings on Section 3(j). The IPAB affirmed that the claimed method of the case being considered included an act of human intervention on a plant cell and produced in that plant cell some changes, which took it outside the proscription of Section 3(j).

The Delhi High Court in May,2017 decided the case of Monsanto v. Indian Seed Companies. At the centre of Delhi high Court judgement was claim 25 of the Indian patent no. 214436 which read as follows: Claim 25: A nucleic acid sequence comprising a promoter operantly linked to a first polynucleotide sequence encoding a plastid transit peptide, which is linked in frame to a second polynucleotide sequence encoding a Cry2Ab Bacillus thuringiensis δ-endotoxin protein, wherein expression of said nucleic acid sequence by a plant cell produces a fusion protein comprising an amino-terminal plastid transit peptide covalently linked to said δ-endotoxin protein, and wherein said fusion protein functions to localize said δ-endotoxin protein to a subcellular organelle or compartment. The defendants argued that a conjoint reading of section 3(j) of the Patents Act, the National seed policy,2003, the scheme of the plant varieties act and the views of the Ministry of Agriculture in the Government of India addressed to the secretary, department of Industrial Development in Ministry of Industry,New Delhi,makes it clear that there can be no patent on any gene, the moment it becomes art of a plant or a seed. IT was, therefore, argued that the only claim the plaintiffs can make is in respect of "benefit sharing" (in terms of section 26 of the Plant Varieties Act) from such seed companies fro developing new Bt. Cotton Varieties expressing Bt. Trait since the biological processes undertaken by the defendants do not create any nucleic acid sequences nor do they,practice any method by which nucleic acid sequence may be inserted into a plant cell.

The plaintiffs argued that the claim nos. 25-27 being products of bio technology processes, the same are patentable in India. After making detailed references to the legislative history wherein amendments were made to the Patents Act,2002,running parallel to the enactment of the Plant Varieties Act,2001.they argued that section 3(j) of the Patents Act only excludes naturally occurring circumstances and further that non naturally occurring (man made) nucleotide sequence (biotechnolgical invention) does not fall within the scope of Plant Varieties Act. The Court referred to the legislative history behind amendment of the Patents Act,2005 which repealed section 5 from the statute book and the conclusion that is to be drawn from such legislative changes being that the embargo on grant of patents to "products" of "biological or microbiological processes thereby stood removed. Giving the judgement in favour of the plaintiff, the court agreed with the plaintiffs that section 3(j) of the Patent Act, cannot be interpreted without taking into account the effect of changes to section 2(1)(j) and repeal of section 5 so as to deprive the patentee of due reward of human skill and ingenuity resulting in human intervention and innovations over and above what occurs in nature. The suit patent involved laboratory processes and are not naturally occurring substances which only are to be excluded from the purview of what is an invention by virtue of the provision contained in section 3(j).[25]

Determining the Patent Trend

The stages in grant of a patent are as follows:

1. Filing of application
2. Filing of request for examination
3. Publications
4. Examination
5. Pre grant Opposition
6. Grant of Patenting
7. Post grant opposition

There are many methodological problems faced in collecting data to determine the patent trend in a country. There is increasing difference in the number of applications published recently by developing countries such as India in different databases. A large numerical gap is evident in India,especially since 1998.The number of applications filed by Indian nationals in India since 2000 (through PCT or Paris route) is far greater in the case of the Dialog DWPI database than on Espacenet. This would infer that a considerable number of Indian patent applications abroad were not based on priority country therefore,seem to be imperfect country for India.[26]

Within a patent document,several sections can be analysed in order to connect patent to the relevant technology;the International Patent Classification system (IPC) and the national patent classification system;the title of the invention;the abstract describing the invention and the list of claims. One or several classification codes are attributed during the patent examination process.[27]

---

25 Monsanto v. Indian seed companies, http://lobis.nic.in/ddir/dhc/RKG/judgement/28-032017/RKG28032017IA24062016.pdf

26 Yamane Hiroko (2018). Interpreting TRIPS:Globalisation of Intellectual Property Rights and Access to Medicines. Hart Publishing.

27 OECD Information Technology Outlook, http://www.oecd.org/sti/ieconomy/41895578.pdf, accessed on 27th April, 2018.

I have used the International Patent Classification code for biotechnological inventions to determine the patent trend. The IPC serves as a tool to classify patents and utility models according to different areas of technology to which they pertain. It was established by the Strasbourg Agreement in 1971 an dis continuously revised by the IPC Committee of Experts.[28] International classification numbers used for biotech patents, and section 3(j) in particular are C12N, c12Q, c125. I have used data on published patent applications and patent granted in respect of these international classification numbers.

C12N-Microorganisms or Enzymes

Year	*Applications Published*	*Patents Granted*
2002	0	0
2003	8457	1081
2004	8239	711
2005	7980	860
2006	7588	711
2007	6995	519
2008	6239	314
2009	5438	157
2010	752	0
2011	1015	14
2012	3874	0
2013	2759	0
2014	2061	0
2015	1307	0
2016	688	0
2017	80	0

C12Q

Measuring or testing processes involving enzymes or micro-organisms; Compositions or test papers thereof; Processes of preparing such compositions; Condition responsive control in microbiological or enzymological processes.

Year	*Applications Published*	*Patents Granted*
2002	2764	318
2003	2706	293
2004	2388	265
2005	54441	232
2006	2457	187

28 WIPO International classifications, http://www.wipo.int/classifications/en/, accessed on 2nd May, 2018.

Year	Applications Published	Patents Granted
2007	2116	150
2008	1882	80
2009	1644	39
2010	1458	20
2011	1219	5
2012	993	195
2013	811	0
2014	617	0
2015	393	0
2016	211	0
2017	19	0

C12S-Processes using Enzymes or Micro-organisms to liberate,separate or purify a Pre existing compound or composition(biological treatment of water,waste water,or sewage,of sludge;processes using enzymes or micro-organisms to separate optical isomers from racemic mixture; Processes using Enzymes or Micro-organisms to treat textiles or to clean surfaces of materials.

Year	Applications Published	Patents Granted
2002	13	2
2003	12	1
2004	16	1
2005	10	0
2006	9	3
2007	9	0
2008	9	0
2009	9	0
2010	5	0
2011	5	0
2012	3	0
2013	2	0
2014	2	0
2015	0	0
2016	0	0
2017	0	0

Total Number of Applications Published and Patent Granted

Year	*Applications Published*	*Patent Granted*
2002	2777	320
2003	11175	012
2004	10643	977
2005	62431	1092
2006	10054	895
2007	9120	669
2008	8130	394
2009	7091	196
2010	6215	20
2011	5239	19
2012	870	195
2013	3572	0
2014	2680	0
2015	1700	0
2016	899	0
2017	119	0

Interpretation of Data in Relation to the Judicial Decisions

The year 2002 witnessed the judiciary taking stand over the interpretation of section 3(j) in the widest possible way. The Calcutta High court included any process that involves human intervention under the ambit of the word"manufacture" even if that process results in the production of a living entity. This opened a broad window for patentees to get patent over their invention. The number of patent applications filed in this year was 2777 while only 380 grants were made. From the year 2003-2013 (until another landmark decision was delivered),From 2002 -2012, the year 2005 witnessed the highest number of patent applications published as well as the number of grants made. From the year 2006-2012, there is a clear pattern in the number of applications with the number falling year by year. However, there is no clear pattern when it comes to number of patents granted while the year 2010 witnessed just 20 patent grants with 6215 applications published,year 2012 witnessed 195 grants. It clearly shows the number of applications published and grants are not proportionate to each other.

The year 2013 witnessed yet another interpretation of section 3(j) in favour of the patentees. Even though the IPAB gave its decision against the grant of patent, its observation on section 3(j) is of great importance. While the number of applications published from 2013-2017 is definitely lesser than their preceding years but what is shocking is the number of grants is nowhere close to being proportionate. There has been not even a single grant made in respect of applications filed pertaining to section 3(j) since 2013.

The chapter does not conclude that the applications that have not been granted patents have been rejected by the patent office because it may happen that the examination is delayed but what can be concluded is that the patent trend is not affected by the judiciary's approach taken in respect of interpretation of a particular section. Even though the judiciary has time and again taken stance in favour of the wider interpretation of the terms,it can not be said how much impact it ha made in determining the patent trend.

In the recent past there has been a significant drop in the number of patents granted by the Indian Patent Office,not because of a reduction of the Indian inventive activities, but because of a shortage of examiners as well as more stringent guidelines for patent application. The percentage decline in the patent grants from 2008-2009 to 2012-2013 was reported to be 72.96.The Deputy Controller of Patents and Design and head of Mumbai Office,Mr. Rakesh Kumar talking about other possible factors that could determine the patent trend says that there are two reasons for this drop in the number of patent grants. They are:

1. Shortage of examiners as examiners were promoted to controller rank
2. From the year 2009 onwards,quality system was introduced in the patent patent office procedures and various guidelines regarding quality examination.[29][34]

The Indian patent office doesn't always stick to the judicial pronouncements and time and again has transgressed its boundaries by way of issuing guidelines even though these draft guidelines do not have the force of law. There are numerous examples and the definitive language used in the guidelines. This goes against the conventional practice of using manuals and guidelines to only collate judicial interpretation of patent law,in order to update the examiners and controllers on the latest judicial precedents along with patent office practices in past cases. The guidelines also dealt with the patenting of micro organisms under section 3(c) and 3(j) of the Patent Act. Section 3(c) is a standard provision of patent law around the world and prohibits the patenting of scientific principles and discovery of nay living or non living susbstance occurring in nature. The guidelines on its page 12 prohibited the patenting of micro organisms which are directly isolated from nature while on page 16 it states that a co joined reading of section 3(c) and section 3(j) implied that only genetically modified micro organisms are patentable under subject matter. While there has been no judicial pronouncement that mandates these two provisions to be read together, the patent office came up with its rule.

In USA, on the similar lines as India, an invention to be patented should be a process,machine, a manufacture or composition of matter or any improvement thereof. There are three judiciallycreated exclusions to patentable subject matter in USA- laws of nature,physical phenomena and abstract ideas. Patents relating to biotechnology are considered to be eligible subjects as compositions of matter or manufactures. However, what cannot be patented under the broad umbrella of biotech inventions are those that come under the ambit of laws of nature exclusion.

---

29 Policy brief: Co-patenting in India,Flortan Gruber, Centre for Social Innovation, Flirona Pirot, Institute of Software Technology and Interactive Systems.

Unlike the Patent office functioning in India, the U.S. Patent and trademark office (USPTO) while evaluating the products from nature has been forced to tighten its self in light of recent Supreme Court decisions.

After Chakraborty's decision, a large number of patents have been issued on living organisms and other biotech inventions including a patent on a genetically modified mouse. In another case,J.M. AG supply INC., the US Supreme Court held newly developed plant breeds to be patentable subject matter under section 1010 though they had separate protection under the Plant protection and plant varieties protection Acts. The USPTO and the courts have extended patent protection to isolated DNA,RNA AND PROTEINS UNDER SECTION 101 STATING THAT GENE and protein sequences are new compositions of matter resulting from human intervention as opposed to naturally occurring products,which are not patentable. USPTO considers gene and protein sequences as large chemical compounds patentable as compositions of matter. Today,under the United States Patent law every biotech invention is patentable subject matter as long as it can be proved that it has been made by man.[30]

Conclusion

The chapter aimed to look into the impact of judicial decisions on the patent trend in India. I began writing this paper with the hypothesis that judicial interpretations do impact the patent trend and in a positive manner if the interpretation leads to a liberal patent regime. With the data available on the official site of the Indian Patent Office,it can be concluded that the number of patent grants in any year is not affected, either in a positive or negative way. However,it remains unclear from the data available as to whether these applications have been rejected for patent grant or haven't been examined yet.

There can be many factors that have come into fore that determine the grant of patent,such as availability of examiner,rejection of grant on any other ground, *etc.* Compliance of judicial decisions in examination of patent applications and thereafter grant is just one of those factors.

It was also found that while through the judicial interpretations, the courts have tried to widen the window for patent, the Patent office have often come up with guidelines which goes against these interpretations and makes the examination process more stricter, leading to an anti patent environment.

30 Kankanala C. Kalyan, complication in Patenting Biotech Inventions: A peek at US Law, Barain League IP SERVICES.

Chapter 3

Impact of Intellectual Property Rights Protection on Plant Varieties

Amaj Raj Srivastava

Advocate, High Court Lucknow Bench, Lucknow, Uttar Pradesh-226010
e-mail: raj.amansrivastava@gmail.com

ABSTRACT

Over the past several years economic process for development under the exuberance of liberalization, privatization and globalization has been adopted by the global community such as developed and developing countries but at the same time its pose the significant challenges for human development in developing country like India. Among the entire sector the Intellectual property right sector becomes a controversy because of the existing policies and laws are not able to respond the problems associated with the framers of the nation. The Indian government was obligated to extend private property rights to plant varieties under the World Trade Organization's Trade Related Intellectual Property Rights (TRIPS) Agreement. The implications of India's TRIPS-induced Protection of Plant Varieties and Farmers Rights Act for only small producers. The Indian Act gives formal recognition to farmers' rights and work with the principle of benefit sharing. In order to make the balance between intellectual rights protection and economic development by adopting the effective intellectual enforcement But into the present trends in exchange of Germplasm, number of varieties released, breeder and quality plants produced, and number of public private partnerships, indicate the growth of Indian plants industry its cannot be easily upgrade in comparasion with international mechanism. The government of the India extension of private property rights to plant varieties will lead to higher seed prices and could lead to further erosion of genetic diversity in the country, negatively impacting farmers. It is necessary to re-examine existing IPR law and policy related to plant variety for achieving the sustainable development goals and ensuring the rights of the farmer's with the proper focus and effective mechanism on agriculture sector of the country.

Keywords: *Trips, Indian, Plants Variety Protection, Farmer's Rights, UPOV.*

Introduction to IPR

Intellectual property epitomizes the idea that its subject is the matter of mind and intellect. And IPR is a legal fiction whereby the State has created negotiable property rights in intangible assets that is very much similar to the rights vested in the real property.

Originating in Europe and developing over a period of approximately seven hundred years in Europe, U.S., Japan, Australia and Canada, the IPR system is ingenious. A creative individual finds creative ways to adapt to an evolving need felt in the society thereby creating intangible intellectual assets. In most cases, the creator derives a commercial gain by exploiting his intellectual assets that include inventions, artistic work, literary work, logos, trade names, trade secrets, designs, *etc.* These intellectual assets have great significance in commerce and provide distinct competitive advantage over business rivals.

The State grants IPR to the individuals and gives them and their assignees an exclusive right to exercise their invention or creation over a pre-determined period. In return the State demands that the details of the invention or creation be disseminated to the general public for public use after the term of exclusivity has expired, the only exception being trade secrets.

Since the State has primary responsibility of the welfare of her people, almost all IPR systems including the patent system have a series of check and balances which strive for providing a balance between the exclusive rights of the rights holder and the legitimate demands of the society.

Historical Perspective

Granting patent to the inventors, and an exclusive right to their creations for a limited time, has been available since 1790. Until the late 1920s, only the three factors were considered to weigh against patenting plants and plant varieties:

1. Firstly, the sentiment that plant varieties were products of nature and thus not patentable under the general patent statute;
2. Secondly, the view that a new plant variety could not be properly described to comply with the description requirements of the general patent statutes; and
3. Thirdly, the legislature's conclusion that plant breeding was not sufficiently reproducible to allow for stable, uniform, and consistent material suitable for patent protection.

Comparisons between Various Forms of Plant IP Protection

As described earlier, Federal proprietary protection of plants encompasses three forms: plant patents, PVPCs, and utility patents. Trade secrets, governed by State law, represent a fourth mechanism of protection. Although each method of protection differs in some respect, not all methods are mutually exclusive. This section compares the different forms of protection available to plant inventors.

(i) Plant Patents v. Plant Variety Protection Certificates

PPA provides rights, through plant patents, to plant breeders and horticulturists who discover or develop new and distinct plant varieties and propagate them by asexual reproduction. In contrast,

PVPC holders under PVPA are granted protection for discovering or developing new, uniform, stable, and distinctive plant varieties that are propagated by sexual reproduction. Protection under PPA and PVPA complement each other in providing protection for new varieties of plants-asexually reproduced by plant patents and sexually reproduced by PVPCs.

(ii) Plant Patents v. Utility Patents

Utility patents provide protection for plants, including asexually reproduced plants such as those included within PPA, as well as plant parts (*e.g.*, flowers, fruits, and nuts) and hybrids, which are excluded from PPA. Also seeds and plants with defined physical traits can be protected through utility patents. Utility patents for plants, when the requirements can be satisfied, offer broader coverage than would be available for the same plant under PPA.

(iii) Plant Variety Protection Certificates v. Utility Patents

As is the case with plant patents, utility patents offer broader protection for the same plant than would be offered through PVPCs

Section-1

Trade Related Intellectual Property Rights (TRIPS)

The most important component of GATT as far as knowledge and innovation based industrial segments are concerned is the TRIPs Agreement. It was already recognized during the trade negotiations that countries of the world not only differ widely in their economic and developmental status but also in their capability to develop or even utilize modern technology. That was the reason for providing transitional periods (Article 65) in the TRIPS Agreement whereby developing countries had up to a ten year period (2005) and the least developed countries 21years till 2016 for implementation[1].

Some of the articles of TRIPS which are relevant for making legislations of IPR in agriculture are:

1. **Article** 1-members free to determine the appropriate method of implementing the provisions of the TRIPS Agreement within their own legal system and practice;
2. **Article** 7-protection and enforcement of IPR should contribute to the promotion of technological innovation and transfer and dissemination of information;

---

1 Nair M.D. GATT, TRIPS, WTO and CBD: Relevance to Agriculture. NISCAIR Journal of IPR (2011), pages 176-182.

3. **Article 8**-appropriate measures, consistent with the provisions of this Agreement, to prevent IPR practices which unreasonably restrain trade or adversely affect transfer of technology;
4. **Article 27.2** -option to exclude from patentability inventions, the prevention within their territory of the commercial exploitation of which is necessary to protect public order or morality, including to protect human, animal or plant life or health;
5. **Article 27.3** -members may exclude from patentability plants and animals other than microorganisms, however new plant varieties are to be protected via patents or through an appropriate sui generis system of protection or a combination of the two.

Patenting in Agriculture Segment

Patenting of innovations in the agriculture segment has been practiced all through the history of the patent system. In India, the Indian Patents Act, 1970 did not provide for protection of agricultural products; however processes used could be patented even if for a very short period, of a maximum of seven years from the date of filing of the patent application or five years from the date of sealing, whichever was shorter. According to TRIPS Agreement which came into force in India from 2005, inventions in all areas of technology including agriculture are to be protected as long as they satisfy the basic requirements for patenting. Patents are now being filed for agro products, food processing, agrochemicals including fertilizers, and biocides. Such efforts will continue and could have an impact on research in agriculture and food technology areas.

The Indian Patents Act, 2005 stipulates mandatory disclosure of source of the traditional knowledge or bio-resource used in the invention. Presumably this requirement is connected with possible future demands of obtaining prior informed consent for their commercial use and agreement on benefit sharing. While there have been objections from US on this, several other developing countries have followed the Indian model in their national legislations.

Sui generis System of Protection for Plant Varieties

Most of the new innovations in agriculture are related to generation of new varieties of plants and seeds. According to TRIPS, these can be protected under the patent system which in general requires that they meet the standards of novelty, inventiveness (non-obviousness) and utility as in the case of all inventions. Alternatively, they can be protected under a special form of protection (*sui generis*) appropriately legislated.

India has opted for the latter and brought in legislation in 2001 under the Protection of Plant Varieties and Farmers Rights (PPV and FR) Act, 2001. The Act is meant to protect the germplasm of any new plant variety if the novelty, distinctiveness, uniformity and stability (NDUS) criteria are satisfied. An important feature of the Indian Act is that it allows farmers to save, sow and sell seeds even if of a protected (by third party) variety.

Protection of Biotechnology Inventions One of the most controversial issues in recent times has been the evolution and emergence of genetically modified organisms (GMOs), in the agriculture and food segments. TRIPS make it mandatory to provide protection of microorganisms, one of the essential components of biotechnology based inventions. Such processes have the potential to improve productivity of food products apart from the ability to produce more specific and better quality foods. The best known example of a patented technology and product is Monsanto's golden rice which produces beta carotene helpful in the alleviation of blindness. Apart from the health benefits that such foods provide, the technology has the potential to improve the productivity in the agricultural sector.

As of now, a major problem is the high costs of such value added products and possible future hazards of use of GMOs to human and animal health and environment. There are also concerns about the labeling requirements addressed under the Cartagena biosafety protocol. There is a direct correlation between the Cartagena protocol and international trade in living modified organisms intended for development of agriculture.

Geographical Indications Act

In principle, the TRIPS Agreement mandates a minimum standard for protection of Geographical Indications (GIs) under Article 22.2 to be used in cases where there was prima facie evidence of malpractice including misleading the customer to the geographical origin of the product. However, the Agreement specifically mentions under Article 23, that GIs related to wines and spirits have to be protected, whether or not they mislead the customer.

The inadequacy of the law, its interpretation and implementation became very obvious to India when the case of Basmati patents came up against Ricetec of US[2] who claimed that Basmati had already become in a broader sense, a generic product and therefore was not entitled to any special protection. Subsequently, a large number of agricultural and food products have been registered under the Indian Geographical Indications Act, 1999. To what extent these are useful for protecting new agricultural products remains to be seen. In any case they have no legitimate protection outside India, since there has been no general agreement on setting up of international registries of GIs or acceptance of national registries by other members. The situation in the case of wines and spirits is totally different. There is consensus for establishing a register of wines and spirits falling under GIs which the WTO members will consult and take action for registration and protection of trademarks and GIs in accordance with their domestic laws and procedures. The issue of extending this to other products by appropriate amendment to Article 23 has been under the consideration of TRIPS Council and WTO, but nothing tangible has emerged so far.

---

2 India-US Basmati Rice Dispute, case no. 493.

Protection of Traditional Knowledge in Agriculture

Most of the agricultural practices, particularly in developing countries stem from indigenous and traditional knowledge systems, seldom documented. They are extremely valuable for the sustenance of those practices and ensuring food security for large populations. The IP protection systems currently in vogue and stipulated under the TRIPS agreement are unsuitable for protecting such traditional knowledge and practices. Realizing the importance of such knowledge and the need to protect them to afford economic advantage to those in possession of such knowledge assets, several international agencies including World Intellectual Property Organization (WIPO), WHO, Food and Agricultural Organization (FAO); various national governments and national and international non-governmental organizations have been working on developing a fair and equitable system to protect traditional knowledge, indigenous medicinal plants, food crops *etc.*, which will be acceptable to all members of WTO and the global community. India's pioneering efforts to develop a unique Traditional Knowledge Digital Library (TKDL) has been accepted as a model for prior art search by many patent offices around the world. The use of such an authentic database will hopefully eliminate patenting activities in the area of TK, traditional medicines *etc.* The need for recognition of sovereign rights of member countries over their bio-resources resulted in signing of the Convention on Biodiversity (CBD) at the Earth Summit in Rio de Janeiro in 1992 by several countries which are now part of the WTO with few notable exceptions like the USA. The CBD has three basic tenets namely, establishment of the sovereign rights to bio-resources by the countries of origin, modalities for exploitation exclusively by the owners and equitable benefit sharing in cases where third parties exploit these resources.

Trade Secrets TRIPS provides for protection of trade secrets or undisclosed information under Article 39. Trade secrets are protected for unlimited time. However, to qualify for protection, it is to be ensured that information to be protected is actually a secret, has indeed commercial value and every effort has been made to maintain its secrecy. Theoretically, if a farmer wants to keep the undisclosed technology or process used by him in his operations secret, it can be protected under this provision, but in actual practice it is hard to implement these provisions since most, if not all, activities in the agricultural sector are in the public domain with a multitude of stake holders, practitioners and participants.

The United Nations Convention on Biological Diversity

The very first legal framework to provide for balancing the need for conservation and sustainable utilization of plant genetic resources as well as a procedure for ABS was initiated by the FAO in 2001 under the International Treaty on Plant Genetic Resources for Food and Agriculture (ITPGRFA). Prior to this, a UN inter-governmental forum to deal with matters related to the conservation and utilization of genetic resources for food and agriculture under the Commission on Genetic Resources for Food and Agriculture (CGRFA) was set up, which also monitored the implementation of International Undertaking on Plant Genetic Resources (IUPGR), 1983. The IUPGR was the first non-legally binding agreement to deal with international matters related to plant genetic resources. In 1997, CGRFA established working groups on plant genetic resources covering technical and policy issues that facilitated the inter-governmental negotiations for the revision of IUPGR in harmony with the provisions of the Convention on Biological Diversity (CBD).

These two issues were:

(i) The realization of farmers' rights envisaged under the IUPGR, and

(ii) *ex situ* collections held in the international gene banks.

Major Principles and Core Provisions

Basically, the Convention sets out the legal instrument concerning the management of biodiversity at an international level. In this context, it generally restricts the rights of member states and other relevant actors over all biological resources, including plant materials. The Convention reaffirms the sovereign right of states to exploit their own resources pursuant to their own environmental policies, a reflection of the principle of the permanent sovereignty of states over natural resources. The sovereign right of states over their biological resources is limited by the recognition that these resources are a common concern of all humankind.

Furthermore, the Convention provides a set of rules regulating member states' policies concerning access, development, and the transfer of technology related to biological resources. Overall, the CBD provides an international regulatory framework within which rights over plant varieties must also fit. Thus, the Convention is of great importance to the creation of an IPR regime for plant variety protection.

The CBD's policy framework is central in this regard since it constitutes the main instrument concerned with biodiversity management and the protection of knowledge developed by farmers. It acknowledges the potential impact of IPRs on biodiversity management and even provides specific guidance to member states, stating that they should ensure that such IP rights support the objectives of the CBD rather than running contrary to them. Based on the CBD framework, several provisions focus on the protection of agricultural knowledge rights, and the access and equitable sharing of the benefits arising from the exploitation of biological resources.

The most prominent provision that requires the recognition and protection of knowledge relevant to biodiversity protection is CBD Article 8(j)[3], which provides that:

Subject to its national legislation, respect, preserve and maintain knowledge, innovations and practices of indigenous and local communities embodying traditional lifestyles relevant for the conservation and sustainable use of biological diversity and promote their wider application with the approval and involvement of the holders of such knowledge, innovations and practices and encourage the equitable sharing of the benefits arising from the utilization of such knowledge, innovations and practices.

---

3 Article 8(j) of CBD; http://www.biodiv.org

It is recommended that this recognition is implemented via national legislation to protect traditional knowledge relevant to plant genetic resources for the purpose of conserving biodiversity. At least four possible legal contexts have been identified within which traditional knowledge rights can be protected and promoted, as follows:

(i) Biodiversity law
(ii) Traditional knowledge law
(iii) Human rights law
(iv) Plant variety protection law

Plant variety protection law appears to be the most practical of all the various options for national legislation. In fact, in Article 27.3(b) of the TRIPS Agreement, the TRIPS Council also suggests that plant variety protection should be made to promote the protection of innovation and the rights of farmers and local communities in the developing world through the implementation of a more comprehensive legal system for plant variety protection, thereby incorporating some of the access principles of the CBD.

The policy goals of granting IPRs in agriculture through a PVP regime should be made to promote sustainable development. It is important to bring the socio-economic consideration of sustainable development into the plant variety protection system and strike the correct balance between the two objectives of plant protection under the TRIPS and the promotion of sustainable development.

The international regulatory framework for rules related to the protection of plant varieties has been discussed in this chapter. A number of significant points of several instruments have been revealed, including the WTO/TRIPS Agreement, the UPOV Convention, the CBD and ITPGRFA, with a short story of their historical development. The TRIPS Agreement is the most important agreement that has influenced the structure of national IP laws in most countries in the world. It specifically sets out the minimum standard of protection for many forms of IPR for the first time ever. The Agreement requires all WTO members to comply with these forms of IPRs, including plant variety protection, as designated in its Article 27.3(b). The wording of TRIPS Article 27.3(b) grants WTO members the flexibility to protect plant varieties via patents or an effective sui generis system, or a combination of both regimes.

The analysis in this chapter has shown that a legal system of adequate plant variety protection lies in providing breeders with rights, while at the same time, protecting the rights of farmers and local communities. In this sense, two principal components of plant variety protection operate parallel to each other, the first of which includes systematic elements of plant variety protection, either based on the TRIPS patent provisions or the UPOV's plant breeders' rights model. The second system is to provide a *sui generis* form of plant variety protection to supplement the first system. In this respect, a plant variety protection system should contain a number of elements, the first of which relates to rules on new plant variety protection, and it will have a slightly different substance, depending on whether a country models its rules on the UPOV or the TRIPS patent system. Secondly, the minimum term of protection offered to new plant variety protection must not be less than 20 years. This minimum requirement has become the international standard and norm of the term of protection that several countries apply to their national legislation. Finally, plant variety protection should contain some mechanism to cater for the specific needs of local people. This includes legal mechanisms for the protection of the right to traditional knowledge, farmers' rights, and access to plant genetic resources, and benefit-sharing regimes. This "self-serving" *sui generis* approach to the legal protection of plant varieties will enable developing nations to tailor their plant protection regime to suit their unique needs and priorities. Such a legal framework for plant variety protection could form the basis of a plant IP protection regime that would tend to comply with the TRIPS obligations.

Section-2

Intellectual Property Rights on Plant Varieties in India

Innovation has been a way of life for the ordinary Indians. Innovation reflects the ingenuity of the Indian mind to adapt to hardships using resources available in unrelated areas by applying it creatively to solve perceived problems. The learned Indian of ancient India contributed to global knowledge bank and gave treatises on astronomy, surgical systems, a vast store house of medicinal systems and agricultural practices. Most of these sophisticated knowledge systems were created and nurtured by wealthy patrons and wise rulers of ancient India. Now, when India is regaining intellectual sophistication and is emerging as a super power, it is imperative that the ingenuity also translates of the modern India mind regains the recognition accorded to the ancient Indian mind. Fortunately, this recognition of the intellectual ingenuity also translates into economic and social gains through the mechanism of intellectual property rights (IPR).

The concept of IPR in plant varieties gained momentum in India with increased investment of private sector in agriculture and flourishing private seed industry. In 1993, The Convention on Biological Diversity (CBD), gave sovereign rights to the nations over their Plant Genetic Resource (PGR), it raised concerns about breeders' rights, farmers' rights, rights of communities engaged in conservation of biological resources.

India being a signatory to WTO and TRIPS Agreement 1995 has opted *sui-generis* system for protection of plant varieties in compliance with Article 27 Para 3of TRIPS Agreement. The outcome of *sui-generis* system was the enactment of The Protection of Plant Varieties and Farmers' Rights Act, 2001. The major objectives of the Act are to provide an effective system for the protection of plant varieties, the rights of farmers and plant breeders; to encourage the development of new varieties and to recognize and protect the rights of farmers in respect of their contribution made at any time in conserving, improving and making available plant genetic resources for the development of new plant varieties. A variety is eligible for registration under the Act if it fulfills the criteria of distinctiveness, uniformity and stability.

Enactment of Sui-Generis PVP Legislation

Sui-generis is a Latin term meaning unique or special[4]. It offers a unique type of IPR, which is different from the classical IPR like patents. All sui-generis models for PVP that are tailored to the specific needs and circumstances of the countries are legally recognized systems. Plant varieties constitute the principal means of production and growth in agricultural productivity. It is also recognized that the specific needs and circumstances of agriculture in each country vary. This is especially significantly different in developed and developing countries. Therefore it is obvious that PVP in each country needs a specific sui-generis system.

First draft of the legislation on PVP was prepared in Indian Council of Agricultural Research (ICAR) in 1993. The draft was revised several times based on wide dialogue involving Ministry of Agriculture and different stakeholders. A PVP Bill was, however, first tabled in the Lower House of Parliament (Lok Sabha) on 14th December 1999. Lok Sabha assigned the Bill to a Joint Committee of the two Houses of Parliament (JPC) to recommend its suitability for enactment as a new, Sui-Generis PVP Law. The JPC organized a series of country wide meetings at the central level and in different states from December 1999 to mid-2000, heard the public viewpoint and observed more than a hundred petitions that either opposed the Bill or sought some improvements in the same. Recommendations of JPC along with a revised draft were tabled in Lok Sabha in August 2000.

Some of the significant points suggested by JPC could be inferred to include:

(i) Safeguard for the extant varieties in Indian agriculture that would assure-

  (a) sustainability of production in the transition period till the new proprietary varieties gradually overtake the exclusive seed market, and

  (b) continuity of the well-tested, well-adapted inheritance factors of these materials in the future breeding programs of public and private sectors.

(ii) Curbing the possible entry of genetic use restriction technology (GURT) or the terminator technology through PVP route in India.

(iii) Strong protection of conventional rights of Indian farmers in Indian agriculture, and extension of the same to the use of protected varieties.

(iv) Safeguarding Indian farmers from innocent infringements and unforeseen complicacies of the PVP law.

(v) Ensuring compensation for underperformance of protected plant varieties to safeguard the farmers' interests and also as a measure to discourage premature entry of seed and planting material of such protected varieties in the market without proper evaluation for their cultivation and use under Indian conditions.

---

4 Sui generis, http://www.law.cornell.edu

Consolidation of the Bill by incorporating suggestions made by JPC added an elaborate chapter on farmers' rights.

At that stage, Indian farmers were proposed to be recognized, under the new PVP law, as:

(i) Conservers of crop diversity and genetic resources

(ii) Breeders of extant farmers' varieties as well as new varieties

(iii) Cultivators and producers enjoying the conventional right to sow, re-sow, barter or sell the farm-saved seed.

In the enactment process, the PVP and FR Bill was passed by Lok Sabha on 9th August, 2001 and the Upper House of Parliament (Rajya Sabha) on 28th August 2001. The next version of the Bill incorporating further amendment suggestions made by the Members of Parliament got the Presidential nod on 30th October, 2001. Thus assented by the President of India, it became the new Sui-generis PVP law entitled, The Protection of Plant Varieties and Farmers' Rights Act, 2001.

The Protection of Plant Varieties and Farmers' Rights Act, 2001

The existing Indian Patent Act, 1970 excluded agriculture and horticultural methods of production from patentability In order to be in compliance with TRIPS Agreement, the GOI has adopted sui-generis system for protection of plant varieties. This was developed with the intention of integrating the rights of breeders, farmers and village communities, and taking care of the concerns for equitable sharing of benefits. The national government after much deliberation with all enacted this unique legislation. "This is the first time anywhere in the world the rights of farmers and breeders are given concurrent recognition": M.S.Swaminathan, 2001[5]. A number of provisions and concepts contained in the TRIPS, UPOV, the IU and CBD constitute key elements in this legislation. As touchstones of the Indian Act, these elements connect global agreements and national law making process. Thus sui-generis option to construct legislature from TRIPS helped to establish PBR based on UPOV model, concept of farmers' rights from IU and benefit sharing from CBD. The Act does not import the concepts per se but translates these through drafting and assembling, and configures it to be a unique legislation. The Act ensures that the farmers shall be able to raise their own seeds and retain them even to distribute in exchange, among the village community as per se the existing tradition. The researchers shall be able to produce new varieties from the protected varieties. The Act also includes the setting up of a Plant Varieties and Farmers' Rights Protection Authority, National Community Gene Fund, Compulsory Licensing and Protection of Public Interest Appellate Board among others. It offers flexibility with regard to protected species, level and period of protection, when compared to other similar legislations existing or being formulated in different countries. The Act covers all categories of plants, except micro-organisms. The geners and species of the varieties

5 Swaminathan, M.S. 2001 September 15, 2001 "Down to Earth", Pages 48-50.

for protection shall be notified through a gazette, after the appropriate rules and by-laws are framed for the enforcement of the Act.

The process of drafting the PPVFR took more than 10 years. Starting in late 1980s, the first draft was produced by 1993 by Ministry of Agriculture, nodal Ministry throughout the development of the Bill. Three drafts followed in 1997, 1999 and 2000, although the last two were introduced in the Parliament. Based on the UPOV model, the penultimate draft was introduced in Lok Sabha on 12th December, 1999, and later referred to 30-member JPC of both the Houses under the Chairmanship of Shri Sahib Singh Verma, for redrafting the Bill.Both the Houses of the Parliament have passed the PPVFR Bill in August 2001after a long and arduous struggle for the recognition of the rights of the farmers.

Objectives of PPVFR Act

The Act provides for the establishment of an effective system for the protection of plant varieties, the rights of farmers and plant breeders. It encourages the development of new plant varieties. The Act is entitled to achieve following objectives:

(i) To stimulate investment for research and development, both in the public and private sector, for the development of new plant varieties for accelerated agricultural development in the country;

(ii) To facilitate the growth of the seed industry in the country which will ensure the availability of high quality seeds and planting material to the farmers;

(iii) To recognize and protect the rights of the farmers in respect of their contribution made at any time in conserving, improving and making available plant genetic resources for the development of new plant varieties.

Salient Features of Indian Sui-Generis PVP Act

(i) The Act provides an optimum balance between:

- (a) Breeders' rights and farmers' rights
- t(b) IPR and right on genetic resources used to develop a variety, where applicable.

(ii) It provides protection to:

- (a) New varieties
- (b) Extant varieties, including farmers' varieties and the varieties of common knowledge
- (c) Essentially derived varieties

(iii) The Act's procedure to examine varieties for registration is based on novelty, DSU testing and distinct nomenclature

(iv) It provides for benefit sharing from a commercialized protected variety.

(v) It provides for compulsory license when the breeder causes non-supply or short supply of planting material of the variety.

Plant Varieties

Variety

Variety means a plant grouping within a single botanical taxon of the lowest rank which is distinctive, stable and can be defined by the characteristic resulting from a given genotype of that plant grouping. It also includes propagating material of such variety, extant variety, transgenic variety, farmers' variety and essentially derived variety. It does not include micro-organism. Micro-organism is a subject matter of protection under the Patents Act, 1970.

According to section 2(za) of Plant Varieties Act, 2001[6], variety means a plant grouping except micro-organism within a single botanical taxon of the lowest rank, which can be:

(i) Defined by the expression of the characteristics resulting from a given genotype of that plant grouping;

(ii) Distinguished from any other plant grouping by expression of at least one of the said characteristics;

(iii) Considered as a unit with regard to its suitability for being propagated which remains unchanged after such propagation and includes propagating material of such variety, extant variety, transgenic variety, farmers' variety and essentially derived variety.

Propagating material means any plant or its component or part thereof including an intended seed or seed which is capable of, or suitable for regeneration into a plant.[7]

Extant Variety

Extant variety means a variety available in India which is:

(i) Notified under section 5 of the Seeds Act, 1966; or

(ii) Farmers; variety; or

(iii) A variety about there is common knowledge; or

(iv) Any other variety which is in public domain.[8]

Farmers' Variety

Farmers' variety means a variety which:

(i) Has been traditionally cultivated and evolved by the farmers' in their fields; or

(ii) Is a wild relative or land race of a variety about which the farmers possess the common knowledge[9].

---

6 Ahuja,K.V. Law relating to Intellectual Property rights,2015. Page 614.

7 Section 2(r), Plant Varieties Act, 2001.

8 Section 2(j), Plant Varieties Act, 2001.

9 Section 2(l), Plant Varieties Act, 2001.

The term 'farmer' is defined under section 2(k) of the Act to mean any person-

(i) Who cultivates crops by cultivating the land himself; or

(ii) Who cultivates crops by directly supervising the cultivation of land through any other person; or

(iii) Who conserves or preserves, severally or jointly, with any person wild species or traditional varieties or adds value to such wild species or traditional varieties through selection and identification of their useful properties.

Essentially Derived Variety

According to section 2(i) of the Plant Varieties Act, 2001an essentially derived variety in respect of an initial variety is said to be essentially derived from such initial variety when it:

(i) Is predominantly derived from such initial variety, or from a variety that itself is predominantly derived from such initial variety, while retaining the expression of the essential characteristics that result from the genotype or combination of genotypes of such initial variety;

(ii) Is clearly distinguishable from such initial variety; and

(iii) Conforms to such initial variety in the expression of the essential characteristics that result from the genotype or combination of genotypes of such initial variety.

Functions of Authority

It is the duty of the Authority to promote the development of new varieties of plants and to protect the rights of farmers and breeders by such measures as it think fit. The Authority may provide for:

(i) The registration of new extant plant varieties subject to the prescribed terms and conditions;

(ii) Developing characterization and documentation of registered varieties;

(iii) Documentation, indexing and cataloguing of farmers' varieties;

(iv) Compulsory cataloguing facilities for all varieties of plants;

(v) Ensuring that seeds of the registered varieties are available to the farmers and providing for compulsory licensing of such varieties if the breeder of such varieties or any other person entitled to produce such variety does not arrange for production and sale of the seed in the prescribed manner;

(vi) Collecting statistics with regard to plant varieties, including the contribution of any person at any time in the evolution or development of any plant variety, in India or in any other country for compilation and publication; and

(vii) Ensuring the maintenance of the Register.

Criteria for Registration

As per the Act a new variety is eligible for registration if it conforms to the criteria of novelty, distinctiveness, uniformity and stability. However the criteria of novelty is dropped for the registration of extant variety.

(i) **Novelty:** A new variety is deemed to be novel if at the date of filling of the application for registration for protection; the propagating or harvested material of such variety has not been sold or otherwise disposed of by or with the consent of its breeder or his successor for the purposes of exploitation of such variety in India, earlier than one year; or outside India. In case of trees or vines earlier than six years, or in any other case, earlier than four years, before the date of filling such application.

(ii) **Distinctiveness:** A new variety is deemed to be distinct if it is clearly distinguishable by at least one essential characteristic from any other variety whose existence is a matter of common knowledge in any country at the time of filing of the application.

(iii) **Uniformity:** A new variety is deemed to be uniform if subject to the variation that may be expected from the particular features of its propagation it is sufficiently uniform in its essential characteristics.

(iv) **Stability:** A new variety is deemed to be stable if it's essential characteristics remain unchanged after repeated propagation or, in the case of a particular cycle of propagation, at the end of such cycle. Essential characteristics mean such heritable traits of a plant variety which are determined by the expression of one or more genes of other heritable determinants that contribute to the principal features, performance or value of the plant variety.

Non-Registrable Variety

A new variety is not registrable if the denomination given to such variety is not capable of identifying such variety; or consist solely of figures; or is liable to mislead or to cause confusion concerning the characteristics, value, identity of such variety, or the identity of breeder of such variety; or is not different from every denomination which designates a variety of the same botanical species or of a closely related registered species; or is likely to deceive the public; or is likely to hurt the religious sentiments.

Period of Protection

The certificate of registration for a variety including the essentially derived variety shall be valid for a period of nine years i9n the case of trees and vines and six years in the case of other crops. The total period of validity in case of trees and vines shall not exceed eighteen years from the date of registration. And in the case of other crops or extant varieties, it shall not exceed fifteen years from the date of registration.

Rights of Breeders

This Act confers an exclusive right upon the breeder of a registered variety or his successor, his agent or licensee to produce, sell, market, distribute, import or export the variety.

In case of an extant variety, unless a breeder or his successor establishes his right, the Central Government; and in cases where such extant variety is notified for a State, the State Government is deemed to be the owner of such right.

A breeder may authorize any person to produce, sell, market or otherwise deal with the registered variety subject to such limitations and conditions as may be specified in the regulations. Such authorization is to be made in such form as may be specified by the regulations made by the Authority.

Rights of Researchers

The Act confers upon the researchers the right to use any registered variety for conducting experiment or research; and also to use a variety as an initial source of variety for the purpose of creating other varieties.

However, the authorization of the breeder of a registered variety is required where the repeated use of such variety as a parental line is necessary for commercial production of such other newly developed variety.

Farmers' Rights

The farmers' rights of the Act define the privilege of farmers and their right to protect the varieties developed or conserved by them. Farmers can save, use, sow, resow, exchange, share and sell farm produce of a protected variety except sale under a commercial marketing arrangement. Further, the farmers have also been provided protection from innocent infringement when, at the time of infringement the farmer is not aware of the existence of breeder rights. A farmer who is engaged in the conservation of genetic resources of landraces and wild relatives of economic plants and their improvement through selection and preservation, shall be entitled in the prescribed manner for recognition and reward from the Gene Fund, provided the material so selected and preserved has been used as donor of genes in varieties registrable under the Act. The expected performance of a variety is to be disclosed to the farmers at the time of sale of seed or propagating material.

Compulsory License

Any person interested may make an application to the Authority at any time after the expiry of three years from the date of issue of certificate of registration of a variety alleging that the reasonable requirements of the public for seeds or other propagating material of the variety have not been satisfied or that the seed or other propagating material of the variety is not available to the public at a reasonable price, and pray for the grant of the compulsory license to undertake production, distribution and sale of the seed or other propagating material of that variety.

Benefit Sharing

This Act also provides for sharing of benefits accruing to a breeder from a variety developed from indigenously derived pant genetic resources. The Authority may invite claims of benefit sharing of a variety registered under the Act, and shall determine the quantum of such award after ascertaining the extent and nature of the benefit claim, after providing an opportunity to be heard, to both the plant breeder and the claimer. Benefit sharing upholds the principles of equity, rewarding the farmer-conservers in recognition of their profound role in preserving the agro-biodiversity and associated traditional knowledge as well as the PBR right holders. Benefit sharing from the profits accrued from the commercial use of biodiversity is a new concept with little or no functional models across the world.

Comparison between International Conventions and National Legislations

It was in the beginning of the twentieth century that the need for the proper enactment of legislations for the protection of plant varieties was felt. The first International Convention (UPOV Convention) on protection of plant varieties was held in Paris in the year 1961. This Convention for the very first time talked about the plant breeders' rights. The UPOV Convention has undergone revisions in 1978 and 1981. The UPOV Act of 1978 provides the plant breeders the right to sale of new varieties, and it also granted two exemptions. One exemption was for the breeders to use the protected varieties for breeding purpose, it was known as breeders' exemption. And the other exemption was for farmers to use the seeds of protected varieties for cultivation, it was known as farmers' exemption.

The UPOV Act of 1991 took away the breeders' exemption by making way for the payment of royalty to the breeders if the new variety bred by some other breeders bears some resemblance with it.

In the year 1994 the Uruguay round of General Agreements on Trade and Tariffs (GATT) led to the establishment of World Trade Organization (WTO). The most important component of GATT related to IPR is Trade Related Intellectual Property Rights Agreement (TRIPs).

Comparison between UPOV Act and TRIPS Agreement

The UPOV Act and Patent Act under TRIPs can be properly compared on the basis of following provisions, namely:

(i) **Protection coverage:** The UPOV Act provides protection for all plant genera and species. Whereas, the Patent laws under TRIPs provide protection for inventions.

(ii) **Requirements for granting protection-** The UPOV Act requires the following characteristics:

(a) Novelty

(b) Distinctiveness

(c) Uniformity

Whereas, the Patent laws requires-

(a) Novelty

(b) Non-obviousness

(c) Industrial applicability

(iii) Term of protection: The UPOV Acts provides protection for the minimum period of 20 years, but for trees and vines it is for 25 years. Whereas, the Patent law provides protection for a period of minimum 20 years for all the inventions.

(iv) Scope of protection: The UPOV Act provides protection against all commercial transactions, offering for sale and marketing of propagating materials. Whereas, the Patent law provides protection against making, using, selling patented products. It also provides protection against use of patented process.

(v) Breeders' exemption: The UPOV Act contains provisions for providing breeders' exemption. Whereas, there is no such provision of providing breeders' exemption in Patent laws.

(vi) Farmers' privilege: The UPOV Act provides farmers privilege of using protected varieties for cultivation. Whereas, the Patent law does not provide provisions for any such privileges.

(vii) Double protection: The UPOV Act prohibits granting of double protection to registered varieties. Whereas, the Patent law provides that a plant variety can be protected under this Act as well as under sui-generis system.

From the above stated points it can be clearly stated that there are few points of difference between the provisions of UPOV Act and TRIPs Agreement. And for providing better protection to plant breeders and new plant varieties, a nation has to enact a legislation which shall be the combination of both.

Comparison between UPOV and PPVFR Act

Though India has enacted the PPVFR Act by adopting certain provisions of UPOV Act, but still there may be some points of difference as discussed below-

(i) Scope of protection: The UPOV Act provides protection to varieties of all plant genera and species.Whereas, the PPVFR Act protects all crop varieties except those varieties whose commercial exploitation would be a danger for public health and public order.

(ii) Duration of protection: The UPOV Act provides protection for minimum 20 years, but in case of trees and vines for 25 years. Whereas, PPVFR Act provides protection for a period of minimum 6 years and maximum 15 years for all crops, and for a period of minimum 9 years and maximum 18 years for trees and vines.

(iii) Requirements for granting registration: The UPOV Act states for registration or protection granted under this Act a variety has to possess the following characteristics, namely:

(a) Distinctiveness

(b) Uniformity

(c) Stability

Whereas, for registration under the PPVFR Act a variety has to possess the following characteristics, namely:

(a) Novelty

(b) Distinctiveness

(c) Uniformity

(d) Stability

(iv) **Rights granted:** The UPOV Act prevents others from commercializing the propagating materials, and under certain conditions using harvested material.

Whereas, the PPVFR Act grant breeders the right to commercially exploit their registered varieties by selling them. But this Act exempts the exploitation of such varieties whose exploitation may cause danger to public health and public order.

(v) **Seed saving:** The UPOV Act allows seed saving only for listed crops. Whereas, the PPVFR Act allows breeders to deposit seeds of all registered varieties to be deposited in National the Gene Bank.

(vi) **Farmers' rights:** The UPOV Act does not provide any provision related to farmers' rights. Whereas, the PPVFR Act contains a separate chapter regarding provisions of farmers' rights.

Comparison between TRIPS and PPVFR Act

The Indian Act of Protection of Plant Varieties and Farmers' Rights is enacted by adopting the provisions of TRIPS Agreement, but still there are a few points of differences as discussed below:

(i) **Scope of protection:** The Patent law under the TRIPS protects all inventions related to agricultural processes. Whereas, the PPVFR Act protects the discovery and development of the plant varieties.

(ii) **Requirements for registration:** The Patent law require the inventions to possess the following characteristics for getting registered under the Act, namely:

(a) Novelty

(b) Non-obviousness

(c) Industrial applicability

Whereas, for a crop variety to be registered under the PPVFR Act must possess the following characteristics, namely:

(a) Novelty

(b) Distinctiveness

(c) Uniformity

(d) Stability

(iii) Duration of protection: The Patent law provides protection for a period of minimum 20 years. Whereas, PPVFR Act provides protection for a period of minimum 6 years and maximum 15 years for all crops, and for a period of minimum 9 years and maximum 18 years for trees and vines.

(iv) Scope of protection: The Patent law provides protection against making, using, selling patented products. It also provides protection against use of patented process. Whereas, the PPVFR Act provides the breeders an exclusive right to sell or commercially exploit the registered variety, but it restricts the commercial exploitation of certain varieties whose exploitation would be a danger for public health and public order.

(v) Double protection: The TRIPS Agreement provides provisions for double protection as it provides that a plant variety can be protected under the Patent law as well as under sui-generis system. Whereas, the PPVFR Act does not provide any provision for the double protection.

(vi) Farmers' right: The TRIPS Agreement does not contain any provision related to farmers' rights. Whereas, the PPVFR Act contains a separate chapter stating provisions related to farmers' rights.

From the analysis of the above mentioned points of difference it can be stated that there are certain similarities as well as certain differences between the Indian PPVFR Act, UPOV Act and TRIPS Agreement.Though India had adopted the provisions of both UPOV Act and TRIPS Agreement, but it does not follow their provisions strictly, as India had made certain modifications in their provisions for meeting the needs of the nation. The main points of diversions or differences between PPVFR Act and UPOV, TRIPS Agreement are- the provisions related to duration of protection, scope of protection and double protection.

Conclusions and Suggestions

Law is a powerful instrument. But, it can work only in a conducive social environment. This favorable climate can be created only if the right holders and the duty holders are equally responsible. While the right holders are supposed to know their rights, and to act in the right time, the duty holders are supposed to respect the right of others, which created obligation for them. If the right holders are in such a disadvantaged social or economic position, the State is under an obligation to help them in realizing their rights. This principle is equally applicable to the farmers and the plant breeders. It is a great responsibility of the state not only to see that the solid rights are created for the farmers and the plant breeders, but also to see that they enjoy these rights. Though India, has made an attempt to create the farmers' rights, but its position is disappointing, in making these rights available to the farmers.

It is a peculiarity of FR that, it was created as a reaction to the PBR. It was the necessity of the plant breeders themselves that some kind of recognition is given to the farmers so that they can get raw materials for plant breeding. The FR is also an outcome of balancing the rights of the plant breeders and the farmers. When an IPR was given to the plant breeders for their efforts in creating new varieties, and thus adding to the food production, the farmers, who also do the same were to be given some rights. But, a journey through the International laws makes it very clear that no balancing has been done. Because as against the property right of the plant breeders, no right; neither property right nor any other right is given to the farmers. What is given is to facilitate access for the plant breeders. It means that the farmers are made to stand just as mere spectators to see their PGR and TK being accessed by the plant breeders. As a reward for this they are offered something, but not rights. And when the plant breeders develop a new variety based on the same, the PGR of such a variety becomes the exclusive property of the plant breeder.

Thus, the crux of FR in the context of PBR centers round the theme called the farmers' access to the PGR of the plant breeders and the plant breeders' access to the PGR and TK of the farmers. In these two themes, one vital role that is expected from the law is its contribution in deciding the farmers' rights over their PGR and TK.

In chapter two of this dissertation the International treaties and conventions related to IPR, namely- TRIPS, UPOV, CBD and ITPGRFA were discussed. UPOV dealt with the farmers' access to the PGR of the plant breeders. Rather, the farmers' rights to use, save, exchange, reuse and sell the seeds of the protected variety. In that Chapter it was found that UPOV 1978 did not create any restriction on this right of the farmers, as the scope and extent of the PBR was limited to the commercial use of the propagating material. However, UPOV 1991 expanded the scope and extent of the PBR almost to the level of the patent right. As result, even the production, reproduction, and stocking for these purposes, of the propagating as well as harvested material were covered by the PBR.

This prevented the farmers from using, saving, exchanging, re-using and selling the farm saved seeds- the freedom which they were enjoying. This right had always been recognized as a part of their efforts in preserving and conserving the PGRFA and making them available for the world for further development. But, UPOV did not seem to have recognized this right. As a favor the UPOV has only given an optional exception to the State parties to exempt the farmers from using their farm saved seed for further propagation in their own holdings. Thus, even this optional exception did not give the farmers the right to exchange and sell their seeds. Thus, this model sui generis law for the protection of PBR does not respect the FR much. Another international law which deals with the farmers' right to use save exchange and sell seed is the ITPGRFA. In this Treaty Farmers' Rights is recognized formally for the first time in principle. However, its implementation is left to the State parties. State parties are thus to recognize the farmers' right to use, save, exchange and sell the seeds.

As far as the farmers' right over their PGR and TK is concerned, in CBD two recognitions were developed, namely the PIC and benefit sharing. As per CBD, thus the PIC of the indigenous people or the local community who hold the biological resources and the TK are to be obtained. When it comes to the PGRFA, the indigenous or local communities are the farmers. Thus, the PIC of the farmers is to be obtained when access is given to their PGR or TK.

Thus, it can be said that the International conventions provided rights for the protection of plant varieties developed by the breeders along with granting them an exclusive right over the protected varieties. But the International failed to provide equal protection to the farmers cultivating the plants and providing the raw material to the breeders.

However, when we examine the Indian legislations called PPVFRA (India's sui-generis law as per the TRIPS mandate) picture is not very promising. This Act has several positives as well as negatives. Firstly, the Act gives the farmers, the right to use, save, exchange and sell the seeds of even the protected variety. Thus, this can be India's legislation to respect the ITPGRFA mandate. That means India has not blindly followed the model sui generis law called the UPOV. Also, India has gone a step further to give some additional rights to the farmers' right to use, save and re-use the seeds. This right is given in the context of the GURT. India has prohibited the registration of plant varieties which are made using GURT. Also, if the seeds of a registered variety do not give the claimed results, the farmers are entitled to compensation from the breeder. Though there are certain drawbacks to this guarantee, this is a right guaranteed only by the Indian legislation, among any other plant variety protection legislations in the world.

Other very innovative rights which the Indian Act try to recognize are, the IPR given to the farmers over their PGR, and TK, as well as their newly developed varieties. As far as the latter is concerned, the farmer is given the right just as a modern plant breeder, which means he is also given the PBR. Regarding the former, actually the Act was trying to give IPR to farmers over their traditionally bred varieties, and TK.

The benefit sharing under the PPVFRA is bilateral in nature, and it is between the plant breeder and the donor of the genetic material (farmers). The State is not under any obligation to find out the PGRFA and their conservers or preservers under the Act. Unless it is the obligation of the State, benefit sharing will remain only in letters as far as the farmers are concerned, as they are not themselves aware of what they are preserving, and that they are subject matters of protection.

Apart from benefit sharing, PPVFRA also stipulates for a compensation to be given to the farmers who conserved and preserved a particular genetic material which was used for developing a new variety. Actually there is every possibility of benefit sharing and compensation being asked from the plant breeder based on the same genetic material, for the same set of persons. This will invite unnecessary litigations, and this is also another area which requires solution.

Now, as the problem areas are identified, the next part of this Chapter proceeds to suggestions.

The first is to include FR in TRIPS. These rights are the rights over the PGR of the plant breeders, and the farmers' other rights over their PGR and TK. These are to be recognized in a sui generis law for the protection of FR. This means that it is better to separate the Farmers' Rights part and the allied rights from the PPVFRA, and to make them part of the sui generis law. But, before India goes for such a sui generis law, it is essential that there should be a provision for that in the TRIPS itself, as in the case of PBR. Also, there should be an International Convention for the Protection of Farmers' Rights as the model sui generis International law, just like the UPOV. Otherwise, an isolated law like that in India will have only a short life span. Also, FR will not have international development or support.

Second suggestion is that the provisions related to benefit sharing and compensation in the PPVFR Act should be made strict. It should be made obligatory for the states to find and keep a record; who has deposited in the gene fund and what has been protected in the gene fund.

Thirdly, the Indian legislation should amend the Act and increase the duration of protection granted under the Act to be in accordance with the minimum duration set by the TRIPS

And last but not the least; the Indian Act should be amended to make clear provisions regarding Agreement. Protection of micro-organisms and gene patenting.

References

Books

Ahuja V. K., Law relating to Intellectual Property Rights (Lexis Nexis Publication) 2nd edition, (2015).

Black Laws Dictionary.

Narayan P., Intellectual Property Law (Eastern Law House) 3rd edition, (2012).

Articles

Batler M, Cancer Research: Translantic War over BARCA1 Patent Science (2001), pages 292-5523

Claudia C, Plant Patenting Benefit Sharing and the law applicable to the Food and Agricultural Organization, Standard Material Transfer Agreement (2008), Journal of World Intellectual Property, pages1-28

Declaration on TRIPS Agreement and Public Health, Ministerial Conference, Fourth session, Doha 9-14 (2001), WTO

Jorden R. and Button P, Effective system of a Plant Variety Protection in responding to challenges of a changing world: UPOV perspective. NISCAIR Journal of IPR (2011), pages 74-83

Kumar A. and Adrija M, Gene patenting vis-à-vis Notion of Patentability. NISCAIR Journal of IPR (2015), pages 349-362

Lakshmikumaram M, Patenting of Genetic Inventions. Journal of IPR (2007), pages 36-45

Nair M.D, GATT, WTO and CBD: Relevance to Agriculture. NISCAIR Journal of IPR (2011), pages 176-182

Rich G, Escaping the Tyranny of World-Is Evolution in Legal Thinking Impossible? Journal of the Patent Office Society (1978), page 271

Robert J, US gene discovery leads to patent war, British Medical Journal (1996), pages 312-7043

Saini S, Ayme S and Matthijis G, Patenting and Licensing in genetic testing Ethical, Legal and Social issues, European Journal of Human Genetics (2008), pages 510-550

Swaminathan M.S, 2001 September 15, 2001 "Down to Earth", pages 48-50

Web Links

www.biodiv.org

www.cbd.int

www.lawcornell.edu

www.upov.int

www.wikipedia.com

www.wipo.int

Chapter 4

National IPR Policy, 2016: A Substantial Development?

Amrit Subhadarsi

Assistant Professor, School of Law, KIIT Deemed to be University, Bhubaneswar 751024
e-mail: asubhadarsi@gmail.com

ABSTRACT

India stands at a critical juncture regarding intellectual property regulation. Not only have the different domains of intellectual property such as patents, trademarks and copyrights rose to prominence, but the neo-liberal economic policies and their constant interaction with the ideologies imbibed in Make in India, smart cities, artificial intelligence and **high technology industries** necessitate a review of India's IP laws in the context of the above. At the heart of the matter lies the following debate.

The aforesaid ideas and their coming into fruition at a rapid pace make room for analyzing intellectual property through the prism of India's **innovation economy**. The key element being technology, a robust regime for intellectual property protection arises, especially in an economically globalised scenario, where technology transfer by way of intellectual property protection is now part of global trade. Upendra Baxi's idea of 'trade related market friendly paradigm' and the Schumpetarian notions of **dynamic competition**, which is reflective of high technology industries such as pharmaceuticals and telecommunication, compel one to argue for a liberalized regime.

On the other hand, India's socialistic ideals enshrined in the constitution necessitate a pluralist approach, which must take into account all the relevant stakeholders such as innovators, government, licensees and most importantly, public interest. For instance, essential drugs must be made available at cheaper rates, but many US firms are up in arms against India's compulsory licensing regime. The conundrum arises when competing interests clash, namely the constant tussle between socialistic ideals and the advent of neo-liberalistic tendencies.

It is in the above context that India's National IPR Policy, 2016 must be analysed as it raises questions over **sustainable development** on all fronts. The present chapter intends to analyse the policy from the standpoint of the prevalent theories on intellectual property.

The second part tends to deal with elaborating on the text of the present policy. The third part challenges the existing notions such as greater IP leads to greater innovation, the debate between safeguarding innovator's interests in pharmaceutical sector and the public interest, among others. The concluding part suggests reasonable suggestions to address the aforesaid dilemmas.

Keywords: *High technology industries, Innovation economy, Dynamic competition, Sustainable development, Trade related market friendly paradigm.*

Relocating the Intellectual Property Law Discourse in the Innovation Economy: An Introduction

Sustaining the Intellectual Property (IP) Agenda: Evaluating the Trends in Terms of Economic Globalization

The origins of Intellectual Property (IP) show an inherent desire to reward inventors with conferment of intellectual property law protection for limited time. Akin to the concept of the '**human territory imperative' under property law jurisprudence**, intellectual property protection confers one with limited monopoly to exploit the creation made possible by the creator. Much like property law, where the rule against perpetuity is at play to preserve the sanctity and the commercial value of the property, under IP law as well, protection expires after a limited time, thereby making room for the invention or the creation to be made available in public domain.

Despite the above similarities, key differences exist between physical property and intellectual property with regards to their nature and characteristics. **For instance, a piece of land must only be classified as immovable property, however, an artistic work seeking intellectual property protection can qualify both as copyright and a trademark under the law of the land. This indicates the inherent subjectivity in a work,** creation or an invention in order to be classified as intellectual property. Further, in cases of grant of IP protection for new creations and innovations, it must be remembered that IP differs from property rights under conventional property law in the sense that the same idea can be used by many to replicate creations that trace their origin to the idea, without reducing the value of the idea.

These inherent subjectivities are on the one hand, hailed significant for the growth and development of a robust IP law regime, whereas on the other hand, when they interact with the emerging facets of economic globalization in India, such as the advent of IP and competition law jurisprudence in pharmaceuticals and telecommunication, block chain technology, artificial intelligence, adoption of smart cities in the urban infrastructure and technological prowess through the Make in India campaign, they produce interesting implications for sustaining the policies framed from the standpoint of the neoliberal agendas.

So far as neoliberal agendas are concerned, they have played a key role in making IP laws transcend the territorial limitations and become a truly

global phenomenon. On the global front, trade liberalization led to creation of newer markets for most firms dealing with industries like the ones mentioned aforesaid, which in turn meant more generation and commercialization of IP due to the sustained innovation and the constant pursuit of newer markets for many industries. This ensured the emergence of a new economic order where the capitalistic tendencies led to the production of more goods which could be traded across borders.[1]

The movement of intellectual property through different modes was from northern countries to the southern ones. The proliferation of technology transfer clauses in investment agreements is testimony to that because in most cases, technology transfer to the South occurs via FDI.[2] On the domestic front, the liberalization regime 1991 onwards promoted an investment friendly regime and also the emergence of technology transfer thereafter propelled new channels of IP commercialization. **The noted legal scholar, Upendra Baxi, has rightly observed that, the process of globalization can rightly be termed as 'trade related market friendly paradigm'.**[3]

The series of case laws reflecting hands off approach of the judiciary favoring leeway to the executive in economic policy matters has opened the floodgates for a liberalized IP regime. Precedents such as *Delhi Science Forum v Union of India*[4] and *N.D Jayal v Union of India*[5], among others are testimony to the above. Hence, the **judiciary through its decisions has reconstituted and reshaped constitutional and regulatory frameworks governing economic liberalization.**[6]

Enhanced levels of competition among the incumbent cutting across all sectors in the economy has led to the terms 'dynamic competition' and 'disruptive innovation' as the buzzwords. **The former is a kind of competition among market players which strives for constant innovation, which in turn determines the market power possessed by a market player. The latter is a business strategy wherein innovation disrupts an existing market and creates a new one**. Hence, it can be safely presumed that disruptive innovation can be a logical consequence of dynamic competition. With the integration of world economies, there has been emergence of IP ownership patterns cutting across industries, for instance, automobiles, telecommunication, software, pharmaceuticals, among others.

---

1 Subhadarsi A (2017). Trade Facilitation Agreement: Implications for India. Bharati Law Review VI(2): 122-138.

2 Branstetter L, Saggi K (2011). Intellectual Property Rights, Foreign Direct Investment And Industrial Development. The Economic Journal, 121(555): 1161-1191.

3 Baxi U (2003). Globalisation and the future of human rights. Nalsar Law Review 1(1): 6-16.

4 (1996) 2 SCC 405.

5 2003 (7) Scale 54.

6 Mate, M. (2016). Globalization, Rights and Judicial Review in the Supreme Court of India. Washington International Law Journal 25(3): 643-671.

Such high technology industries have also witnessed IP ownership among corporate. It is here that dynamic competition, also termed as Schumpetarian competition, (named after J A Schumpeter) comes into play. **This is so, because in a given industry where there are many incumbent engaged in delivering similar products or services which are backed by innovation, there remains a higher probability of clash between IP and competition law.** Thus, economic globalization and the manifestation in the form of high technology industries have ensured a consistent and a prominent interaction of intellectual property with competition law. Although, seemingly contradictory, there is a growing body of literature through court judgments and scholarly writings which have elaborated **areas for harmony between antitrust law and IP laws. But, the harmony is not perfect as questions remain with respect to the degree of intellectual property protection needed to foster innovation and competition.**[7] This is a true of a number of industries where innovation is the driving force, such as telecommunications.

This industry can be termed as a classic illustration of dynamic competition. The telecommunications industry is witness to **huge expenditure on Research and Development (R&D), sunk costs and enterprise level capabilities**. Enormous amount of time and effort is given towards developing chipsets used in smart phones which then become compatible with a given wireless communication standard, for instance, fourth generation (4G) standard. **When patents are claimed over such standard compliant chipsets, they are called Standard Essential Patents (SEPs).**

These patents are granted recognition as SEPs after they agree to license them on Fair, Reasonable and Non Discriminatory (FRAND) terms. **The conferment of SEP status is beneficial as it endows the patent holder with supreme dominance in the relevant market**. This is best illustrated through *Broadcom Corporation v Qualcomm Incorporated*, wherein the US court of appeals for the third circuit held that when a patented technology is incorporated into a standard, adoption of the standard eliminates alternatives to the patented technology.[8]

In other words, the dominance achieved can cause ripples in competition law if chipset manufacturing companies engage in unfair licensing practices to exploit the downstream licensees, or the handset makers who will incorporate a 4G compliant chipset into their handsets. Such behavior is not merely theoretical and academic, but has encompassed many jurisdictions. Cases such as *Micromax Informatics Ltd v Telefonaktiebolaget LM Ericsson (Publ)*[9] and *Huawei Technologies Co. Ltd v ZTE Corp., ZTE Deutschland GmbH*[10] are two of the prominent precedents emanating from India and the European Union (EU) in this regard. However, interaction with competition law is not the only recent trend with regards to intellectual property law.

---

7 Teece, D.J. (2011). Favouring Dynamic over Static Competition: Implications for Antitrust Analysis and Policy. In: Maine GA and others (eds) Competition Policy and Patent Law Under Uncertainty Regulating Innovation, 1st edn. Cambridge University Press, New York, pp 203-227.

8 501 F.3d 297 (3d Cir. 2007).

9 Case No. 50/2013 (CCI).

10 Case C-170/13 (2015).

With the advent of automation in key industries such as manufacturing, machines and technology is no longer at the mercy of human beings, but has far exceeded its capabilities. **Artificial Intelligence (AI), or the ability of machines to imbibe human capabilities in problem solving, has made its foray into a number of industries, including legal services.** Artificial intelligence is the process of simulating human intelligence through machine processes.[11] There is increasing evidence of law offices using AI for drafting arguments, finding precedents and so on. With such growth of AI, the field of IP laws could not have been bereft of its interaction with it.

For instance, **many commentators have documented how the mingling of AI and creativity can generate interesting implications for global copyright law jurisprudence.** Traditional copyright law has always regarded originality as the key determinant for a work qualifying for copyright protection. This originality has always been attributed to creative works by human beings. However, **the advent of AI has diminished to a considerable extent the utility of creative works by human beings alone, and we see a rise in generation of such works by non human actors.**

Unlike the earlier scenario, where machines were programmed to undertake certain tasks, now they can not only undertake those tasks but outperform human capabilities in replicating more onerous tasks. **For instance, by ingesting works of authorship as training data, computer programs can teach themselves to write natural prose, compose music and generate movies.[12] Though, an interesting development, the question arises as to whether increasing advances in machine intelligence ever lead to a situation in which an AI program can be entitled to its own copyright.**[13] The legal position over this issue is still in a sea of uncertainty in many jurisdictions.

The law of intellectual property is also increasingly interacting with one technology, which may very well turn out to be one of the most promising and fundamental technologies of the 21st century. This technology is called the 'blockchain'. In India, at present, this technology has been more associated with the term, 'bitcoin', a virtual currency which has baffled Indian financial regulators such as the Reserve bank of India (RBI). Though the virtual currency circulation is expected to fizzle out by 2021, the underlying technology, blockchain, is here to stay. The application of this technology has touched the domain of IP law in some areas.

But, before delving into that, a brief introduction about the technology is imperative. Block chain is a recent technological innovation in the form of a peer to peer network based on an open and decentralized system. **This system facilitates completion of transactions and creation of secure and authentic records. This**

---

11 Semmler S, and Rose Z (2017). Artificial Intelligence: Applications Today and Implications Tomorrow. Duke Law and Technology Review, 16(1): 85-99.

12 Sobel B (2017). Artificial Intelligence's Fair Use Crisis. Columbia Journal of Law and The Arts, 41(1): 45-97.

13 Wagner J (2017). Rise of the Artificial Intelligence Author. The Advocate, 25(4): 527-534.

technology is being used by copyright holders to ensure that music licensing contracts are made enforceable through provisions in 'smart contracts'. In other words, the licensing contracts self execute and guarantee timely royalty payments and act as shield against breach of the contract. This is so because, a smart contract is a contract captured in code, which automatically performs the obligations the parties have committed to in the agreement.[14]

Block chain technology has also its implications in other ways. For instance, some commentators have proposed that this technology can come handy, when attempting to solve the 'orphan works problem'. **Orphan works are covered under copyright law, but there is no rightful owner to make claims on such works. As a result, their dissemination becomes difficult. However, usage of blockchain can help generate immutable registers wherein block chain is used to register attempts to find the authors of orphan works.**[15] Block chain technology can also be useful in India's smart cities mission and Make in India campaign and thus contribute to a paradigm shift in approaches towards intellectual property.

Besides the aforesaid, new trends in intellectual property infringement are visible in the cyberspace, which any IPR policy must aim to address. Lastly, a key development can become crucial in shaping the future discourse on intellectual property, namely the Trans-Pacific Partnership (TPP) Agreement, which came into force in 2016. This is a Free Trade Agreement (FTA) among US and eleven other countries bordering the Pacific Ocean, which has its **key objective to ensure economic growth through innovation, trade and employment generation.**

Though noble in its agenda, questions have been raised about the complicated and controversial nature of the advances made in setting international standards for IP through trade agreements.[16] From the above review of major developments on the regulatory and technological fronts, it can be gauged that **even though the fundamentals of intellectual property continue to remain the same, the increasing interactions with innovative business models and emerging technologies have the potential to alter the landscape of intellectual property regulation**. Interesting consequences are bound to result when IP consistently interacts with two key technologies: AI and blockchain.

On the other hand, constant interaction of IP with competition law is not only an emerging trend, but also a prerequisite for a vibrant innovation economy. Even though there are bound to be certain inconsistencies, **India's National IPR Policy, 2016 seeks to minimize such differences because of the goal of balancing socialistic ideals prescribed under the Constitution and the neo liberal agenda in an era of economic globalization.**

---

14 Hsiao J (2017). "Smart Contract on the Blockchain-Paradigm Shift for Contract Law?. Us-China Law Review, 14: 685-694.

15 Goldenfein J, and Hunter D (2017). Blockchains, Orphan Works, and the Public Domain. Columbia Journal of Law and the Arts, 41(1): 1-43.

16 Rogowsky R (2016). Intellectual Property in the Trans-Pacific Partnership. The Brown Journal of World Affairs, 22(2): 123-136.

An economy which aims to achieve the innovation economy status through its flagship programmes such as Make in India, must learn to embrace the aforesaid trends and issues in a holistic manner for benefit of all stakeholders. The subsequent paragraphs will not only outline and elaborate on key provisions of the policy, but will also test the policy both from the standpoint of IP justification theories and the illustrations as mentioned in the above discussion. Though, it is beyond the scope of this chapter to highlight all key developments in the field of IP from an economic globalization perspective, the author believes the above suffice as necessary parameters to test the viability of India's National IPR Policy, 2016.

National IPR Policy, 2016: Analysis and Evaluating the Implementation Issues

Features of the Policy

The Policy lays down the roadmap for effective implementation of IP laws in the country. It is the first comprehensive policy aimed at streamlining the country's existing IP laws. The purpose of the extant policy is not only creation and encouragement of an innovation ecosystem, but also generating awareness about the importance of IP as a reward mechanism for the creator's work. The vision statement makes a pertinent reference to transforming India into a knowledge based economy where knowledge is shared, owned and transformed. The **policy lays down seven key objectives, namely, IPR awareness, stimulating generation of IPRs, the regulatory framework, regulating the management of IP, monetizing the IP, IP enforcement and adjudication, and human capital development.**

As regards the first objective, the policy stipulates that a nationwide program for IP promotion must be laid down in collaboration with all relevant stakeholders such as public and private sectors, industry, academia, Research and Development (R&D) sectors. **It emphasizes that IP awareness must be particularly at the rural level.** The policy further stresses that national policies like Startup India, Digital India, Make in India must be linked with the policy and further, specific programs customized for startups, universities, R&D institutes, inventors and entrepreneurs. The policy prescribes **preparation of course curriculum keeping in mind school students** and distance learning programmes. Further, the policy envisages engaging celebrities as 'ambassadors', creating road shows for generating IP awareness.

The second objective, stresses on **carrying out of IP audits and base line surveys** in collaboration with stakeholders across all industries. Also, there is emphasis on industry-academia interface to generate innovative ideas, **stimulating large corporations with expansive R&D, to create, protect and utilize IPR in India**, encouraging public funded R&D institutes **to contribute towards affordable medicines.** The second objective puts particular emphasis on improvement of R&D through tax benefits, loan guarantee schemes, **usage of Corporate Social Responsibility (CSR) funds for innovation.** The policy emphasizes incentives for IPR for green technologies and **encourages IP generation for cyber technologies** coupled with emphasis on Traditional Knowledge.

The third goal is the regulatory framework on IP laws. Compliance with the socialistic ideals mentioned in the constitution is observed when the policy explicitly states that India will continue to honour the TRIPS Agreement and the Doha Declaration on TRIPS Agreement and public health. To deal appropriately with the legislative framework, there are provisions detailing review of existing IP laws, **effective negotiation of international treaties which lay emphasis on IP, usage of international fora to develop binding international instruments,** especially for TK, Genetic Resources (GR) and Traditional Cultural Expressions (TCE). The policy envisages transfer of clean energy from developed to developing countries to comply with India's UNFCCC obligations. **The policy acknowledges the need for updating the IP laws in consonance with other related statutes such as competition law, FRAND, trade secrets, so on and so forth.**

The fourth objective stresses on effective IPR administration and lays down the machinery to enforce the same. Important stakeholders such as Intellectual Property Offices (IPOs), have now been tasked with the mandate to improve disposal of IPR applications, and usage of ICT to modernize their functions. IPOs have also been encouraged to increase interaction levels with various R&D institutes. To augment creation and generation of IP, the Cell for IPR Promotion and Management (CIPAM), under the Department of Industrial Protection and Promotion (DIPP) has been proposed to be constituted.

The administration of the Copyright Act, 1957 and the Semiconductor Integrated Circuits Layout-Design Act, 2000 has been transferred to the DIPP and consequently the control over the respective authorities for granting registration of the IPs, have been given to the DIPP. The office of the Controller General of Patents, Designs and Trademarks (CGPDTM) has now to be **using best practices for filing and maintenance of records**, taking steps for digitization of the offices in order to facilitate digital filing of documents, conducting periodic audits and implementing quality standards at all stages. The Registrar of Copyrights (RoC) must take steps to digitize records, introduce online search facility, among others. Further, the Protection of Plant Varieties and Farmers' Rights Authority must support increased registration of new varieties and facilitate commercialization of IP for the farmers. Lastly, the National Biodiversity Authority (NBA) must work in harmony with government, IPOs and others to formulate guidelines with respect to biological resources and associated TK.

The fifth aim is to commercialize the IP. This target is to be achieved through encouraging public funded research laboratories, academia, and other institutes to commercialize their research outcomes, **creation of a common database in order to connect buyers, users and funding institutions,** funding options for an IPR exchange, promote licensing, technology transfer, **patent pooling and cross licensing** for effective commercialization, examining availability of SEPs on FRAND terms, **incentivizing reduction of dependence on Active Pharmaceutical Ingredients (APIs) imports and encouraging manufacturing APIs in India,** and utilizing the Technology Acquisition and Development Fund (TADF) under the National Manufacturing Policy for licensing or procuring patented technologies and performance based evaluation for continued funding.

The sixth objective, enforcement and adjudication of IPR, aims to adjudicate disputes through special commercial courts, frequent IP workshops for judges, **undertaking measures to counter attempts of treating generic drugs as spurious**, and assist small technology firms for protection of IP through ICT measures, enhance logistics by improving manpower and technical knowledge, setting up IP cells to tackle IP related offences, and lastly, taking the assistance of Competition Commission of India (CCI) whenever necessary. The final objective is to expand human resources by making IP an important part of all technical institutions' curricula such as legal, technical, medical, and management institutions, **strengthening of IP chairs in higher educational institutions**, among other measures. Through compliance with all the aforesaid objectives, **IP is perceived to be a part of national development strategy.**

Implementation Issues

IP-Innovation Conundrum

A thorough perusal of the policy lays bare an inherently flawed assumption; namely, intellectual property is the genesis for greater innovation and for greater national development. While it is true that IP protection is conferred on a technological innovation or a creative work and therefore seems directly proportional, scholarly literature suggests otherwise. The present IPR policy seems to suggest that IP is an end in itself, whereas, inferences drawn from commentators' arguments suggest that IP is a means to an end. The **pragmatic school of thought justifies that IPR encourages creative and technological advance by providing increased incentives to invent in, invest in and further develop new ideas and without such the invention inducement would be weakened.**[17]

India's IPR Policy, 2016 seems in alignment with this school. But, it is also true that there lies a flawed assumption. It is true that economic incentive can be derived from exploiting the intellectual property protection by either practicing it, simply by licensing it, or by making further improvements on it.[18] However, **there is evidence to show that as and when an industry matures, IP related issues proliferate and dilute the proposition that more IP means more innovation. This is especially true of sectors such as telecommunications.**

For instance, many firms such as Samsung, Apple, Ericsson, among others engage in heavy negotiations for licensing their SEPs to downstream licensees such as Micromax, among others. But, as **most of the former dominate discussions during standard setting for wireless communication and have acquired patents after their commitments to license on FRAND terms, it is trite that when patent standards are low, firms are able to assemble large patent portfolios, which they use to make aggressive licensing demands.**[19] This frequently triggers competition

---

17 Moore DA (1997). A Lockean Theory of Intellectual Property. Hamline Law Review, 21: 65-108.

18 Sichelman T (2010). Commercializing Patents. Stanford Law Review, 62(2): 341-411.

19 Hunt RM (2006). When Do More Patents Reduce R&D?. The American Economic Review, 96(2): 87-91.

law concerns. There have been commentators who have observed that in case of high technology industries, backed by R&D, once a firm acquires dominance; it is more about expanding the patent or the IP portfolio than enforcing an IP on its merit. This creates a situation where higher IP protection does not guarantee more innovation. **When an industry matures, innovation is no longer encouraged; instead it is blocked by the ever increasing appeal to patent protection on the part of insiders.**[20]

Other commentators also voice similar concerns. It has been documented that patents add less value to small firms than large firms because small firms face greater litigation risks.[21] Similarly, other evidence points to the fact that **there is blocking effect of patents held by large firms. This problem afflicts the medical instruments, biotechnology, electronics and computer sectors.**[22] For instance, **cross-licensing agreements can create entry barriers** for new players to enter the market. By virtue of such agreements, **two patent holders agree to license each other their patents upon mutually agreed upon terms and eliminate participation** resulting in market distortions.

This is true of not only industries such as telecommunications, but also glass making, as is evident in *Hartford Empire Co v United States*[23], wherein the US Supreme Court observed that such arrangements violated the Sherman Act. **Licensing agreements stipulate that the licensee is supposed to pay royalties despite exhaustion of the term of the patent**, which can effectively affect competition in the downsteam market. Such agreements have been found to be **more common in the pharmaceutical industry.**[24]

In many industries, the phenomena of exclusive licensing, grant-back clauses, and agreements for royalty payment beyond the patent's term of expiry have been the subject of competition law assessment by different competition law regulators because **in such circumstances drawing the fine line becomes increasingly technical in nature.**[25] This implicitly means unfair usage of patents can only meet aggressive licensing demands, or other methods to extract value from their patents, especially in high technology industries. Hence, more IP does not necessarily mean more innovation. After the relevant industry reaches its saturation point, IP and innovation move in opposite directions. Also, at the same time, a dominant position compels the incumbent to sustain its R&D, whereas the competitors strive to catch up with the dominant market player.

---

20 Ouellette LL (2015). Patent Experimentalism. Virginia Law Review, 101(1): 65-128.

21 Burke A, and Frazer S (2012). Self-employment: the role of intellectual property right laws. Small Business Economics, 39(4): 819-833.

22 Cozzi G, and Galli S (2014). Sequential R&D and blocking patents in the dynamics of growth. Journal of Economic Growth, 19(2): 183-219.

23 323 U.S. 386 (1945).

24 Arora V, and Gadasalli S (2014). Competition Law and Intellectual Property Rights: The balancing act. Competition Law Reports, 2: 109-125.

25 Whish R (2008). Competition Law. Oxford University Press, USA.

In other words, the purpose of R&D by the follower is to catch up and surpass the leader, while the purpose of R&D by the leader is to escape the competition of the follower.[26] The market leaders in such scenario may resort to unfair practices by using their patents to create entry barriers for prospective players. Hence, the misuse of patents at a certain stage in the high technology industries cannot be denied. **However, the National IPR Policy, 2016 only outlines the positives that may be gained and not the strategies to counter the negative contingencies such as the above, which will come out in the future.** It only states that the Competition Commission of India (CCI) shall be taken up on assistance. But, this may prove a complicated strategy, especially at a time the CCI itself is in a state of uncertainty with regards to key sectors as displayed through contrary decisions in key sectors such as electronic commerce, telecommunications and other high technology industries.

At this juncture, it must also be stated that the present policy is more in alignment with the Lockean idea of 'original acquisition', according to which if a person has expended his labour, skill and time on an object over which no prior ownership exists, the material property rights vest with the person who has expended his labour and skill because an exercise of tracing the real owner would lead to no one except the person who has acquired ownership. Such an interpretation is also in alignment with similar idea propounded by Roscoe Pound from the sociological school of jurisprudence. But, it remains to be seen how far these theories help the policy overcome the following practical difficulties which have arisen.

Patents and Public Health

The National IPR Policy, 2016 will stumble upon one of the biggest roadblocks in its implementation. Essentially, the clash is between the right to enforce a firm's intellectual property and the socialistic ideals as given under the Indian constitution. At the heart of the matter, lies the following debate. Western multinational firms, engaged in the process of developing medicines, incur significant costs in R&D in making these drugs fit for retail consumption. The Active Pharmaceutical Ingredient (API), the main formula used in the preparation of drugs, confers on such firms the patents for the formulations used in the medicines. **On the other hand, in a country like India, where there is considerable lack of affordable medicine, many firms engaged in developing generic versions of these medicines, have sought to justify their practices on account of making affordable medicines a reality.** This practice of 'evergreening' of patents has been emphasized in *Novartis AG v Union of India.*[27]

The issue of compulsory licensing under the Patents Act, 1970 therefore comes to play. Under this concept, patent holders must license their patents compulsorily under the force of the applicable law, to make developing generic drugs a reality. The important consideration is such licensing must take place as a matter of necessity to meet public interest. The obligations of the Indian state as a welfare state under

---

26 Acemoglu D, and Akcigit U (2012). INTELLECTUAL PROPERTY RIGHTS POLICY, COMPETITION AND INNOVATION. Journal of the European Economic Association, 10(1): 1-42.

27 (2013) 6 SCC 1.

the Indian Constitution are further greatly enhanced by similar provisions under the National IPR Policy, 2016. **For instance, encouraging public funded R&D institutes to engage in developing affordable medicines, undertaking measures to counter attempts of treating generic drugs as spurious and reducing API imports and manufacturing APIs indigenously.** On account of the above, countries such as US and many European countries are up in arms against India's stringent IP laws, what are often termed as 'weak IP laws'.

The above debate again reignites the debate between Northern innovation and southern imitation as elaborated upon by many commentators. For instance, it has been documented that the major **issue for developing countries is, there is concern that consumer welfare may be adversely impacted by enhancing the monopoly powers of the innovators.**[28] On the other hand, advocates of stronger IPR have asserted with little evidence that stronger IPR will yield benefits by inducing multinational firms to engage in more technology transfer.[29] Such advocates, namely the western multinational firms always have the scope to rely on 'the **trickle down effect', which implies that protection given to companies with significant technological leads over their rivals also dynamically incentivizes companies with more limited technological leads.**[30]

This essentially implies that the API patent holders can always claim that the companies developing generic versions must expend more on R&D to catch up with their western counterparts, instead of tweaking API patent holding firms' innovations and claiming it to be patentable. **While, this argument may be tenable from an IP rights perspective, it is certainly not so when viewed from the prism of the socialistic principles as enshrined in the constitution.** Therefore, actions by countries like US, such as putting India in the Special-301 Report is a natural outcome of a failure to balance the aforesaid competing interests. The Special-301 Report is a comprehensive document which contains the name of the countries put on a watch list, which do not confirm to US standards of intellectual property. The Report is an annual one brought out by the United States Trade Representative (USTR).

Besides, the issue is not merely confined to conferment of patents upon western firms for drugs, but broader than that. **The life threatening diseases which the developing and the least developing countries suffer from are not much prominent and are therefore called by the international community as 'neglected diseases'.**[31] This again provides incentive for Indian companies to develop generic drugs so that affordability and awareness of such medicines can both be achieved

---

28 Branstetter L, Saggi K (2011). Intellectual Property Rights, Foreign Direct Investment And Industrial Development. The Economic Journal, 121(555): 1161-1191.

29 Branstetter LG, Fisman R, and Foley CF (2006). DO Stronger Intellectual Property Rights Increase Technology Transfer? Empirical Evidence From U.S Firm–Level Panel Data. The Quarterly Journal of Economics, 121(1): 321-349.

30 Acemoglu D, and Akcigit U (2012). Intellectual Property Rights Policy, Competition and Innovation. Journal of the European Economic Association, 10(1): 1-42.

31 Agitha TG (2013). Global Governance for Facilitating Access to Medicines: Role of World Health Organization. Journal of Intellectual Property Rights, 18: 589-595.

and implemented on a mass scale. To counter western firms' arguments, India has always affirmed its stand that as long as India is in compliance with the TRIPS and other related treaties which India has ratified, it does not need to be in compliance with other countries' IP law demands.

The TRIPS Agreement does not set down a single and universal IPR system that the members have to follow, they are free to adopt a regime that is stricter than the one required by TRIPS Agreement.[32] Article 8 further endorses the priority which must be given to the right of public health. Besides the TRIPS Agreement, **India is also a part of the Doha Declaration on the TRIPS Agreement and Public Health, 2001**, which has endorsed right to public health as independent from IP rights. A number of international treaties and conventions affirm the right to public health. For instance, the Universal Declaration of Human Rights, 1948, International Covenant on Civil and Political Rights, 1966, Convention on the Elimination of all forms of Discrimination Against Women, 1979, International Covenant on Economic, Social, and Cultural Rights, 1966.

At the domestic front, the Indian judiciary has also been at the forefront of advocating right to public access of life saving drugs and right to health as part of right to life under Article 21 of the Indian constitution. Judgments such as *State of Punjab v Mohinder Singh Chawla*[33], *People's Union for Democratic Rights v Union of India*[34], *Consumer Education and Research Centre v Union of India*[35], *All India Drug Action Network v Union of India*[36], along with the landmark judgment in *Novartis AG v Union of India*[37] are few important ones which have made the aforesaid idea a part of India's intellectual property law jurisprudence. In the Novartis case, the apex court upheld the constitutionality of section 3(d) of the Patents Act, 1970, which forbids patent protection for minor improvements on a patented invention.

Keeping the social realities in mind, the apex court upheld the provision and held that the drug, Glivec, manufactured by Novartis, a Swiss based company, had already provided the manufacturers with sufficient price for the research on that drug and there was no necessity for patent protection towards further incremental innovation. On the executive front, it is the continuous endeavor of the Union Health Ministry and authorities such as the National Pharmaceutical Pricing Authority (NPPA) to ensure the growth of the Indian generic drugs industry. Else, an important constitutional obligation may not be discharged.

---

32 Guennif S, and Lalitha N (2007). TRIPS Plus Agreements and Issues in Access to Medicines in Developing Countries. Journal of Intellectual Property rights, 12: 471-479.

33 (1997) 2 SCC 83.

34 AIR 1982 SC 1473.

35 AIR 1995 SC 922.

36 (2011) 14 SCC 479.

37 (2013) 6 SCC 1.

Lack of Recognition for Emerging Trends in International IP Jurisprudence

On the face of it, the policy aims to set a noble goal to grant IP protection and make the masses aware about the importance of IP in national development. It also needs no mention that it is imperative that the policy must be in sync with domestic and international developments, not only in the field of IP, but also areas where IP is increasingly interacting. Else, assuming the policy to be futuristic in character will be an exercise in futility. A thorough introspection of the policy will reveal that it's a mixed bag as far as the objectives it sets out to achieve. Provisions such as linkage of the policy with India's startup plan, the digital India drive, smart cities mission, Standard Essential Patents (SEPs) and competition law, usage of IP for financing are testimony to the agenda for integrating major policies with the IPR policy. Having said that, there are certain flaws.

Firstly, there is increasing evidence of digital piracy and IP infringement through cyberspace, but a reading of the policy does not bring out any concrete strategy to counter such practices. Whereas the Information technology Act, 2000 and the extant IP laws are in place, India's emergence as a hotspot for such practices is a cause for concern. At this juncture, one must understand that the policy is supposed to lay down a broad roadmap for the respective legislations to implement it, and not elaborate on every detailed aspect of the laws. But, **there exists a difference between the laying down of a blueprint and a mere passing reference of emerging trends in IP jurisprudence**. For the sake of convenience, the author has divided the integration of the emerging IP trends with the policy into the aforesaid categories. On a closer observation, one can find that there is no explicit strategy to counter infringement of IP on cyberspace and the only reference is to cyber security and IP.

Secondly, technologies such as AI and block chain find no mention under the policy. There is only a small reference to integration of IP with any future related areas as and when the need arises. In the opinion of the author, this can set a dangerous precedent as there is emerging literature which provides for complicated implications when these technologies interact with IP. For instance, thousands of block chain projects have sprouted all over the world, attracting billions of dollars in investment. These companies are now hiring aggressively in core development, research, developer relations, marketing and finance.[38]

But, the policy does not make a reference to usage of block chain with regards to IP, despite clear evidence in literature that they can be used for enforcement of smart contracts such as licensing agreements, and the like. Similarly, **AI has also produced interesting questions from the copyright perspective, as explained in the introduction, but AI hardly finds mention in the policy.** AI, for instance, has raised questions with regards to ownership of work and application of the fair use doctrine under copyright law.

---

38 Saha R (2018). Cryptic Chain, The Telegraph 8 May.

Regulatory Dilemmas: Domestic and International

Though the aforesaid problems also emanate from the policy, the author has not included them under this sub heading because the above are implementation issues more based on attitudinal and ideological assumptions and inferences, and are wrong at the fundamental level. However, **this part shall deal with implementation issues of certain provisions, which though noble, can cause headaches in the absence of adequate infrastructure, or lack of clarity, among other things.** Such regulatory dilemmas can be classified at the domestic and international level.

At the domestic level, the National IPR Policy has certain contentious provisions. Though the policy at a number of levels demarcates appropriate collaboration among the relevant stakeholders, it lacks clarity in certain areas. For instance, **the policy envisages IP awareness at the rural level, but does not lay down a blueprint of how the goal is sought to be achieved.** Similarly, for generating IP awareness, a requirement for adopting IP in school curriculum has been proposed, and engaging celebrities and road shows for IP promotion has been given recognition. However, the author views this as a flawed agenda.

Firstly, knowledge about IP creation is not a perquisite at the school curriculum level. What **students actually need is the ability of analytical thinking** as opposed to rote learning. Further, in a country, where the school dropout rates are high, the method of teaching requires changes, for which the method of '**unlearning' has to be adopted. Unlearning is a process where all or most knowledge acquired is considered obsolete and requires up gradation or change altogether.**[39]

Secondly, the policy envisages organization of IP road shows and involvement of celebrity personalities for awareness. The idea again though noble, lacks a practical approach because **there needs to develop an entrepreneur culture**, which can truly claim national development. Though such culture has started, a lot more needs to be done. However, **IP road shows and celebrity involvement can at best provide lip service for promoting IP as a major development goal.** Another major regulatory hurdle is usage of CSR funds for innovation. After the mandatory CSR regime for companies qualifying under section 135 of the Companies Act, 2013, the Ministry of Corporate Affairs (MCA) has constantly issued clarifications. **But, it is also true, that at the time of writing, India faces a lack of qualified CSR professionals.**[40] This raises eyebrows over the implementation because even if funds were to be allocated, tardy monitoring can impede their proper utilization.

The policy prescribes that there should be regular IP audits and stimulating large firms with R&D capabilities to create and protect IPR. This idea seems farfetched. Firstly, **IP audits have not been explained by way of a definition** which can lead to

---

39 Ryan AP (2018). Learn to Unlearn. The Hindu, 10 Feb, http://www.thehindu.com/education/learn-to-unlearn/article22713689.ece accessed on 08 May.

40 Corporate Social Responsibility In National Priority Areas: Education, Healthcare and Skill Employment, http://iica.in/images/1.per cent 20 Summary per cent 20- per cent 20CSR per cent 20GAP per cent 20 Analysis per cent 20- per cent 20 Education, per cent 20 Health, per cent 20SKILLS.pdf, accessed on 07 May, 2018.

questions over the meaning of the term. Secondly, the **dependence on large firms' R&D capabilities assumes that there is 'perfect competition' among firms, an idea which is utopian even under international competition law** jurisprudence. Large firms with expansive R&D will, and as illustrated in preceding sections, have engaged in unfair practices.

Even though there is a passing reference to competition law, this particular provision nullifies to a considerable extent the understanding of linkages between IP and competition law. **The policy by assuming that large firms will only use their R&D to create and protect IP culture provides a simplistic view for IP implementation.** The policy also stresses upon using best practices for filing and maintenance of records by the CGPDTM. But there is **no reference to even an illustrative list of which practices constitute internationally accepted best practices leaving scope for ambiguity**. The policy encourages setting up of IPR Chairs in higher educational institutions. Sadly, there is evidence to suggest funding issues and lack of proper monitoring of such chairs to stimulate research activities in the field of IP.[41]

One of the prominent concerns which can arise is with regards to punishments for IP infringements. Though, India has laws dealing with specific IP kinds, just like other laws, these too suffer from lack of proper implementation. The many instances of economic crimes recently and the inability of sectoral regulators to prevent them is a testimony to the casual approach adopted. The lack of an ex-ante approach towards prosecution of economic offences, can compel one to arrive at the conclusion that **if a government tends to be corrupt, or does not prosecute ordinary crimes within its own country effectively, it is likely that prosecution of IPR violations within its borders is also lax.**[42] These, coupled with the understaffing seen amongst the courts and the well known problem of case pendency further compound the problem.

At the international level, the following regulatory dilemmas can impede implementation of the policy. Firstly, the policy sets the objective of **effective negotiation of international treaties which lay emphasis on IP, and usage of international forum to develop binding international instruments.** Recent literature presents a rather gloomy outlook because when it comes to the monitoring of implementation of economic agreements and treaties. Investment by way of technology transfer is now included under international trade and investment agreements such as Free Trade Agreements (FTAs) and Comprehensive Economic Partnership Agreements (CEPAs), of whose IP is an integral part.

A preliminary assessment of the FTAs/CEPAs indicates that India has not been able to sufficiently leverage these agreements to increase its presence in

---

41 MHRD IPR Chairs- The Anarchy and Hollow Attempt at Development of IPR in India, https://spicyip.com/2015/02/mhrd-ipr-chairs-the-anarchy-and-hollow-attempt-at-development-of-ipr-in-india.html, accessed 08 May, 2018.

42 Chiang EP (2004). Determinants of Cross-Border Intellectual Property Rights Enforcement: The Role of Trade Sanctions. Southern Economic Journal, 71(2): 424-440.

the market of its partners.[43] Similarly, poor implementation of the South Asian Free Trade Agreement (SAFTA) is the principal cause of slow growth in the intra-regional trade within the SAARC region.[44] Hence, **provisions relating to IPR based products under the policy stand to lose out as inefficient monitoring of trade and investment agreements may affect flow of exports to other countries.**

Besides the above, **the Trans Pacific Partnership (TPP)** as a free trade agreement has the potential to raise serious questions about IP implementation not only amongst the signatory countries, but also **countries like India as it could suffer market share losses in certain categories of exports.**[45] Key IP specific provisions include creating an environment for **high technology exports, criminal penalties for trade secret theft, enhancing the fair use exception** for copyright law, among others. However, the TPP breaks new ground by **addressing cross-border chains of counterfeit and pirated goods, including activities that threaten health and safety.**[46]

This provision addressing counterfeit and spurious goods **can be used effectively against India's generic drugs industry**, something which the present policy also seeks to counter. However, with a strong lobby in the US clamoring for insertion of such a clause, it is likely to be a hard bargain for India in two ways. Firstly, **Indian pharmaceutical exports may suffer and secondly, availability of cheap drugs effectively may be derailed**. The policy envisages transfer of clean energy from developed to developing countries to comply with India's UNFCCC obligations. But, considering the raging debate over the Intended Nationally Determined Contributions (INDCs) between the developed and the developing nations, India's bargain for clean energy may not be that easy.

In light of the above implementation issues discussed, it is safe to presume that the subjectivities involved in IP regulation, protection and promotion requires collaboration among stakeholders at multiple levels. The inconsistencies of IP regulation therefore operate primarily at two levels. **Firstly, at the level of countries, it becomes next to impossible to implement an agenda that is conducive for every country's commercial interests because of varied levels of economic growth. The second inconsistency acts as a corollary to the first, because in a developing economy, the hard bargain is not only towards securing the country's commercial interests, but also securing the right to access public health of its citizens.**

Therefore, if essential medicines are caught up in a battle of patents, the accessibility of these drugs becomes expensive for such developing economies. This is precisely why the Nobel Prize winning economist Joseph Stiglitz has vehemently

---

43 Dhar B, and Chalapati Rao KS (2014). India's Current Account Deficit: Causes and Cures. Economic and Political Weekly, XLIX(21): 41-45.

44 Negi A (2016). India's Export Relations with SAARC Nations. Pratiyogita Darpan, 87-89.

45 Singh SK (2016). Recent Innovation in Regional Groupings: Trans-Pacific Partnership (TPP). How is it important to India?. Pratiyogita Darpan, 81-83.

46 Rogowsky R (2016). Intellectual Property in the Trans-Pacific Partnership. The Brown Journal of World Affairs, 22(2): 123-136.

opposed the TPP. In other words, managing the tradeoffs between producers and consumers is particularly complex with regards to intellectual property.[47] Because of the aforesaid implementation issues, **policy makers face the dilemma of having to decide how much and what type of IPR laws to enact and likewise how much resource to devote to support their enforcement.**[48]

Therefore, India cannot be an exception to such a dilemma. However, as far as the reading of the policy goes, **due to its perceived lack of clarity as explained earlier, the policy may not necessarily incorporate all strategies** for an effective IP enforcement regime. This is in line with the criticism which India has received because of its **Foreign Trade Policy (FTP) 2015-20** because it **proposes integration with policies Make in India and Digital India but there is no clear roadmap for such integration** and offers a bird's eye view and continues to be India's main challenge for India's trade regime.[49] Similarly, India's National IPR Policy, 2016 proposes IP as a tool for national development strategy, and also proposes integrating IP with Make in India, Startup India and Digital India, but **apart from a generic statement as to collaboration among stakeholders, there is no concrete agenda specifying the methodology of the integration. This can be termed as one of the major drawbacks of the policy.**

Conclusions

As India strives to move forward as a knowledge and innovation economy, the country's National IPR Policy, 2016 must also reflect this attitudinal shift in formulating rules for an effective IP regime. But, India may be prevented from achieving this goal if certain errors are not rectified as highlighted above. Further, it must also be realized that turning IP into a holistic national development strategy requires changes at multiple levels such as streamlining CSR practices for utilizing IP innovation funds, framing a national education policy which focuses more on analytical thinking, undertaking efforts to implement changes in teaching methodologies, ensure effecting monitoring of international economic agreements which specify IP exports and commercialization as an objective.

This should be a top priority as India very recently ratified the Trade Facilitation Agreement (TFA), which aims to reduce procedural hassles at borders and contribute to domestic and global GDP. **Akin to the idea of 'new institutional economics' as propounded by the renowned economist Douglas North, the institutional framework to ensure the coordination mentioned above must be continuously upgraded.** This can therefore propel India to secure higher rankings in the global competition index and the other such indexes which measure India on a number of innovation parameters.

---

47 Shadlen KC, Schrank A, and Kurtz MJ (2005). The Political Economy of Intellectual Property Protection: The Case of Software. International Studies Quarterly, 49(1): 45-71.

48 Burke A, and Frazer S (2012). Self-employment: the role of intellectual property right laws. Small Business Economics, 39(4): 819-833.

49 Singh SK (2016). India's Foreign Trade Policy of 2015-20. Pratiyogita Darpan, 95-96.

But, considering the challenges due to a constant inability to balance right to public health and IP for innovators and the inherent flawed assumptions which have formed the basis for the policy, it may be a herculean task for the government to truly take the policy to its logical conclusion. Considering the developments in the manufacturing industry, the automation processes undertaken in the different industries, and the new policies such as Make in India, Digital India and Startup India which are in a nascent stage, maintaining IP as a priority during each stage of integration of such policies is going to be realistically difficult. **The fundamental problem will be to balance the rent seeking behavior of the market players in the innovation economy with the socialistic demands of the Indian constitution.**

What must also be remembered is that, the policy must also devise a strategy to obliterate the practical difficulties in implementation, because India's present IP laws, future amendments, and future laws will always be modeled on this policy. For a robust IPR policy, it is imperative that IP laws and the IP enforcement mechanisms must be in place. Hence, the legislation should be free from ambiguity to the fullest extent possible, the executive must implement the laws timely and efficiently, and lastly, the judiciary must endorse a pragmatic approach keeping in mind the social realities, as displayed through the Supreme Court judgments in case of patents and the right to public health. Hence, **for an effective IPR regime, what is required is a proactive step rather than a reactionary outcome every time any implementation difficulty comes up from the policy**. In the end, it might be pointed out, that the framing of the IPR Policy is a step in the right direction, but is a mixed bag of sorts when termed as a substantial development. In light of the above, the following suggestions can be made:

- ✰ The policy envisages usage of CSR funds for innovation. The Ministry of Corporate Affairs (MCA) being the parent regulator must bring about relevant rules for linkages between IP and CSR. Similar provision must be brought about under the Companies Act, 2013.
- ✰ The commerce ministry has set up a task force for proper monitoring of compliance with trade agreements. Non adherence to binding obligations under the trade agreements must be reviewed consistently and on top priority.
- ✰ Instead of setting up of special commercial courts, which are already lacking manpower, more staffing of existing adjudicatory forums must be undertaken to facilitate speedy disposal of cases.
- ✰ The policy must be amended to incorporate explanations to certain vague terms, such as international best practices, IP audits, and the like. Further, the policy must incorporate emerging technologies such as AI and block chain, IP infringement through cyber space, into its realm. Further, the policy must seek to be implemented in a phase wise manner, for which appropriate timelines must be set and provisions regarding these which are absent now, must be incorporated.

Chapter 5

India and Global Pharma Patents Norms

Arvind Sankar[1] and Rohith Venkatesan[2]

National Law University, Odisha, 753015
e-mail: [1]17bba013@nluo.ac.in, [2]17ba080@nluo.ac.in

ABSTRACT

This chapter seeks to address the issue concerning India's compliance with modern day pharmaceutical patent regime. The issue has been discussed in light of India's role in the global pharmaceutical market, specifically the impact on the populace dependant on generic drugs. India being the pharmacy of the world, these conventions threaten supply to both the domestic and global market. Despite strong criticism from large MNCs and developed countries, India so far has stood by its stance, *i.e.* in the protection of the masses. This has been discussed thoroughly with the example of the adoption of TRIPS agreement and Doha Declaration. Since the TRIPS agreement played an important role in the formation of WTO, India was in a position to 'take it or leave it' to be a part of WTO. This lead to the amendment of the Indian Patent Act. Many amendments to the Act took place along with the addition of section 3 (d), concerning the 'test of patentability' of pharmaceutical drugs. The central debate between the welfare state and incentivised innovation has come to judgement in the famous Novartis Case. While activists for the former argued that the section 3(d) of the Indian Patent Act was intended to protect public health, MNCs on the other hand vehemently attempted to set a precedent in Indian Law in favour of Pharmaceutical companies. It is hard to take a balanced view in same as a decision in favour of the latter could mean the end of all types of generic drugs in India for both consumption and export, meanwhile, if the decision favours domestic industry, then MNCs would be disincentivised to operate in India. Hence the question arises, "should the public health be held ransom by a certain group of people or companies?".

Introduction

In the past decades, the nations of the world and international organizations have increased focus on the universalization of laws pertaining to intellectual property. However this has not been without dissenting opinions form developing nations like India who primarily depend on the production of generic drugs at massive scale to meet the demands of the ever-growing population. They fear that with the induction of strong patent laws as advocated by developed nations like USA, the native drug manufacturers will die out leading to exorbitant drug prices. Although during the initial phases India was pressured and strong armed into adopted the TRIPS agreement it effectual use of the gestation period is remarkable. The strategy followed by India to follow through with the adoption process is an example for other developing nations struggling with the adoption of TRIPS. The chapter has been divided into 4 parts to analyse the impact of 'Global Pharma Conventions' on India. Part I deals with the Development of Indian Pharmaceutical Industry, in light of its History from pre-colonial era. Part II of the chapter revolves around the Legal Aspects pertaining to the topic in discussion namely, section 3 (d) of Indian Patents Act, Section 27 of TRIPS, *etc.* Subsequent to part II, part III of the chapter addresses the issues pertaining to section 3 (d) and the implication of the same. Part III is followed through by conclusion to the discussion and solutions to the questions and problem that have arisen.

Development of Indian Pharmaceutical Industry

The first ever patent law was passed in 1856 during the British colonial rule. The act, which was based on the British Patent Law of 1852, granted 'exclusive privileges' to the inventors for a period of 14 years. The act was later repealed since it was enacted without the approval of the British Crown. Later, a string of new acts and amendments were brought forth which culminated in the enactment of the Inventions and Designs Act of 1888[1]. This, again, was replaced by the Indian Patents and Designs Act 1911[2], which remained in force till 1970. All the while, the pharmaceutical industry remained in its infancy with no scope for progress. Under the colonial rule, the British enacted laws to cater the needs of its own pharmaceutical industry. It allowed foreign companies to have complete control over the production of their patented drugs in India. Thus, the domestic drug industry remained stagnant up until independence.

India during its independence, being one of the poorest countries, was presented with many challenges. With its abysmal state of the domestic pharmaceutical industry, it became increasingly problematic for the country to provide affordable healthcare service.[3] To solve this issue, the government appointed the Tek Chand Committee to restructure the patent regime to bring it in alignment to the country's needs. The committee issued a report suggesting the government to bring a number of amendments to the Indian Patents and Designs Act. The committee managed to trigger the enactment of a new bill, however it lapsed along with the dissolution of the parliament.

---

1 Janice Mueller (2007), The Tiger Awakens: The Tumultuous Transformation of India's Patent System and the Rise of Indian Pharmaceutical Innovation, 68 U. PITT. L. REV. 491, 514–15

2 KALYAN C. KANKANALA *et al.* (2010), INDIAN PATENT LAW AND PRACTICE 1.

3 Supra note 1.

The next government constituted a committee under the chairmanship of Rajagopala Ayyangar.[4] The Ayyangar Committee built its report on top of the Tek Chand Committee's report, and presented it with a more persuasive reasoning and empirical data. The Ayyangar Committee emphasized on the need for a higher threshold and a narrow scope for patentability of pharmaceutical drugs. The committee also observed that majority of the patents was held by foreign companies while a substantial number of these were not even worked in India. Medicines were also becoming unaffordable due to the hold on supply of drugs foreign patent holders had. Thus, the Ayyangar Committee advocated the abolition patenting of pharmaceutical products. These recommendations were subsequently adopted in the Indian Patents Act, 1970.

As per Section 5 of the Indian Patents Act 1970, patents could only be claimed for processes and not for pharmaceutical products. The distinction provides greater flexibility to the generic manufacturers to create affordable versions of the same product through different processes, opening up opportunity for 'reverse engineering'. It allowed the Indian companies to copy pharmaceutical products whilst they were patented in other foreign countries. The abundant workforce and highly competitive environment enabled the Indian pharmaceutical Industry to become adept at reworking the compositions of drugs manufactured by other companies.

Thus, the burgeoning growth of the domestic pharmaceutical industry seen during this period could be accredited to 1970 act. The industry became known for its supply of affordable generic drugs. It was able to churn out countless generic drugs, making India a world leader in terms of manufacturing of medication. The affordability of these drugs not only enabled India to serve its own populace, but also made India the' pharmacy of the developing world'.[5]

However, this success did not come with its share of criticism. The US, along with other developed countries which sought to include IP under the ambit of trade within the framework of General Agreement on Tariffs and Trade (GATT) negotiations, did not welcome this change. The US government introduced changes to the Trade and Tariffs Act of 1974 which allowed the imposition on trade sanctions against countries which had 'weak' IP laws, which mainly included developing countries. South Korea and Brazil fell victims to such sanctions, despite showing resistance. This loss of support and threat of trade sanctions yielded India's acceptance to the inclusion of IP rights within the framework of Uruguay Round Negotiations. Subsequently TRIPS was adopted and India became one of its signatory. The TRIPS agreement, as Shamnad Basheer[6] put it, was coerced upon

---

4 N Rajagopala Ayyangar, Report on the Revision of the Patents Law (September 1959) 60.

5 Eg Simon Reid-Henry and Hans Lofgren, 'Pharmaceutical Companies Putting Health of the World's Poor at Risk' The Guardian (26 July 2012) <www.theguardian.com/global-development/poverty-matters/2012/jul/26/pharmaceutical-companies-health-worlds-poor-risk> accessed 25 April 2018.

6 Shamnad Basheer (2018): Trumping TRIPS: Indian patent proficiency and the evolution of an evergreening enigma, Oxford University Commonwealth Law Journal, DOI: 10.1080/14729342.2018.1455479.

the poor and the developing countries by the stronger developed countries to suit their national and industrial interest, rather than the developmental priorities of the developing countries.

Legal Aspect

WTO, TRIPS and Product Patents

With the culmination of *Uruguay Round of the General Agreement on Tariffs and Trade (GATT)*[7], two very important things happened; firstly it was the basis for the establishment of World Trade Organization (WTO)on January 1, 1995, and secondly, the 'Trade-Related Aspects of Intellectual Property Rights (TRIPS)was formulated. India one of the signatories to the WTO was obliged to ratify the TRIPS agreement too. Any country pursuing an easy access to the international market spaces created by WTO was required to adopt the IP law as authorized by TRIPS. The led to TRIPS being regarded as the most crucial and comprehensive document for the globalization of intellectual property laws.

The TRIPS agreement sought to set a **high minimum standard** on a number of forms of Intellectual Property. The question of whether or not to adopt the TRIPS agreement was a battle to choose between protecting the interests of few "big pharmas" and the welfare of public fought between developed and developing nations. While the former pressed for the adoption of the agreement in order to strengthen the Intellectual Property Rights, whose current condition of infringement according to them was 'Trade Destroying'; the latter feared the induction of such Patent Laws. Developing countries argued against the strengthening of Patent Laws in accordance with TRIPS, saying that it would increase the costs of manufacturing drugs with lesser and lesser producers available for the same and consequently the end of generic drugs in the respective country. This was the major reason why India was initially reluctant to sign the agreement.

India's Adoption of TRIPS – Reshaping Worldview on TRIPS for Developing Nations

India in its adoption of the TRIPS agreement was very novel so as to secure the interests of the masses. According to section 65.2[8] of the agreement **Developing Nations** were allowed a period of 10 years as **Transition Period,** so as to implement most provisions of the agreement (some needed to be implemented immediately). India had until the 1st of January 2005, in order to amend its patent law in line with the agreement, in the areas of Pharmaceuticals and Agriculture.

India adopted the TRIPS agreement in 3 Phases:

1. In 1999, The exclusive marketing right and mailbox requirement

In line with Article 70 (9) of the TRIPS agreement – 'mailbox requirement', it required patent applicants to submit their applications with the patent office that

---

7 https://www.wto.org/english/thewto_e/whatis_e/tif_e/fact5_e.htm Accessed on 30 April 2018.

8 https://www.wto.org/english/docs_e/legal_e/27-trips.pdf Accessed on 1 May 2018.

would be held for examination until 2005. No application would be approved till then. In this way India ensured that no single manufacturer or producer of drugs unjustly enriched from this dark phase of transition in Indian PharmaPatent history.

Exclusive marketing rights (EMRs) are rights similar patent rights. It is a restricted right to market the drug within the territory of India. It vests with the applicant the exclusive right to sell and distribute the concerned product. It is different from patent, in was that patent offers the right to the manufacturer also. Since the right to manufacture is of little value without the consequent right to market and distribute, it seemed as an attractive alternative to offer in place of patents. It was at this very time that the European Union and the United States challenged India's failure to implement the obligations prescribed by WTO. Hence the 'EMR' was a weak and loosing case before the WTO.

Hence only little of the EMR applications were granted (4 of 17).[9] Subsequently by this time India was halfway in crafting the adoption of the nuances of TRIPS, evidence to the same being the 2005 Amendment to the Patents Act with the addition of section 3(d).

2. Patents (Amendment) Act of 2002

It ensured the further integration of the Indian Patent Act with the guidelines offered by TRIPS with the extension of patent terms to **20 years**.

3. Patent (Amendment) Act, 2005

It was more commonly referred to as the New Patent Act of 2005, as the changes it brought struck as a surprise to not only the WTO members but also the MNCs and the masses. Despite the fact that it was within this act that 'product patents' were formally introduced and made legally available, it was more highlighted for the addition of **Section 3(d)** to the Patent Act. Hence in all terms to say this Amendment was most controversial both nationally and internationally.

In light of the adoption of TRIPS marked by the inclusion of controversial s. 3(d), India was looked upon by the then developing nations of the world. In response to then rising concerns over 'bilateral investment protection agreements' as a hurdle to the effectuation of TRIPS in line with public interest, India urged the governments to *"respect the letter and spirit of the Doha Declaration on TRIPS and Public Health"*.

India also recommended that the governments *"adopt and implement legislation that facilitates the issuance of compulsory licenses"*.

Compulsory licensing is when a producer apart from the one who has received the patent is allowed to produce the patented drug by the order of the government without the consent of the patent owner. India inducted the same under section 84 of the Indian Patent Act, 1970. It provides that 'compulsory license' for a patented drug may be issued 3 years after the patent was issued for the drug, if the drug isn't yet available in the market at an affordable price[10].

---

9 Supra Note 6.

10 https://www.firstpost.com/world/india-at-wto-takes-strong-stand-to-save-generic-drugs-industry-calls-for-transparent-health-assessment-of-trade-deals-3102716.html Accessed on 4 May 2018.

Section 3 (d) of the New Patent Act

So during the era of new patent regimes as India moved from process to product patents, it made requisite changes in the respective legal provisos. Firstly it scraped off section 5 of the Patent Act of 1970 in its 2005 Amendment – which expressly prohibited the patenting of products. In the next step which was innovative to some and controversy to most, India added section 3 (d) to the Patents Act. It was formulated to act as a tough drug patent filter so as to pave way for only high quality pharmaceutical innovations to obtain patent rights. To supplement the provision in securing the interests of the public, the act also retained the 'compulsory licensing' terms from the previous regime. This would guarantee manufacturers of generic drugs to continue supply of drugs at an affordable price. The Section 3 (d) of the Act provides that:

What are not inventions. -The following are not inventions within the meaning of this Act,-

[(d) the mere discovery of a new form of a known substance which does not result in the enhancement of the known efficacy of that substance or the mere discovery of any new property or new use for a known substance or of the mere use of a known process, machine or apparatus unless such known process results in a new product or employs at least one new reactant.

Explanation. -For the purposes of this clause, salts, esters, ethers, polymorphs, metabolites, pure form, particle size, isomers, mixtures of isomers, complexes, combinations and other derivatives of known substance shall be considered to be the same substance, unless they differ significantly in properties with regard to efficacy;][11]

Scope of the Section

The 2005 amendment to the act makes clear the difference between 'invention' and 'discovery'. It clearly states that any knowledge already existing cannot be granted a patent. The amendment provides for 3 conditions on whose fulfilment a product patent may be granted as a certain 'novelty standard':

1. Non-obviousness
2. Inventive step
3. Industrial Applicability.

'Inventive Step' has been carefully worded as 'enhanced efficacy' in the section 3(d) leaving its definition and purview in doubt.[12] More about 'enhanced efficacy' will be explain in further sections of this chapter.

---

11 https://indiankanoon.org/doc/1845556/ Accessed on 13 April 2018.

12 http://www.mondaq.com/india/x/581560/Patent/Section+3d+of+the+Patents+Act+interpretation+continues+to+remain+subjective Accessed on 7 May 2018.

Interpretations of Section 3 (d)

From the above explanation only a broad idea may be formulated about the scope of the section. The real question is the one subject to most controversy and criticism, it is the scope of the phrase 'enhanced efficacy', used in the section. To build up to the meaning and purview of 'enhanced efficacy' we must first analyse the interpretations of the more definitive parts of the section.

1. *Mere Discovery of a New Property of a Known Substance*

A substance may have more properties than known to man. Over time man uncovers new properties of the substances he has already been using. Even still such new properties have already existed beforesuch discovery. Hence merely discovering new properties of substances already in existence doesn't amount to 'innovation' and hence doesn't qualify for patent protection.

E.g. Paracetamol having antipyretic property is often used in treatment of high fever. Further the discovery of its analgesic property doesn't qualify it for patent protection.

2. *Mere Discovery of any New Use of a Know Substance*

The property of a substance is what attributes to its function/use. Overtime with the discovery of new properties, new uses of the substance is uncovered respectively. But since such use already existed prior to its discovery it is not 'innovative' hence not patentable.

E.g. Aspirin was initially used as an analgesic (*i.e.* provide relief from physical pain). The discovery of a new use of Aspirin in the 'treatment of Cardiovascular Disease' is not patentable.

3. *Mere Use of Known Process*

The use of a process that is already known is not patentable. However;

Exception: unless the process results in the formation of a new product or involves a new reactant.

In other words only those existing process may be patented that either results in the formation of a new product or involves the use of a new reactant in the formation of the same/old product.

E.g. Discovery of a new method to manufacture Aspirin is patentable.

4. *Mere Discovery of a New Form of a Known Substance*

If a new form a substance already in existence is discovered, *e.g.* polymorphs, isomers, mixtures of isomers, *etc.* it is not patentable. The new form may be similar in function to the original substance. However,

Exception: if the discovery of the new form of a substance enhances the efficacy of the original substance then it can be patented.

This part of the section has brought the most controversy to it since its induction. Furthermore about the controversy will be discussed in the further sections of the chapter.

Aim of Section 3 (d)

As discussed earlier section 3 (d) was instituted with idea of limiting the scope of patent protection that which was demanded as a part of TRIPS agreement by the WTO.[13] The goals it was sought to fulfil were;

a) *Stop Evergreening of Patents*

Evergreening is the method adopted by manufacturers to extend the period of their patents simply by making slight or minor modifications in the existing drug to brand them as a new innovation.[14] Evergreening is usually done by applying for patents on variations (against the original product) like: - new dosages, new forms of release, new combinations, *etc.* Consider the following illustration;

An innovator firm named XYZ which formulates a chemical strain to cure a particular disease. XYZ files for patent for the new strain on May, 2005. On approval of the application by the patent office a patent will be formulated providing protection for the following 20 years. If on May 2012, XYZ files for another application before the patent office for a slight change (not affecting the efficiency) in the previously patented drug. If it were so approved then the patent protection period of the drug will now extend to 2032 in contrast to the initial time expiring on 2025. This will in turn delay the generic drug for the same product to be delayed from entering the market on which much of the populace is dependent on.

To prevent the misuse of Evergreening among manufacturers, section 3 (d) has set a very high standard for patent qualification. As evident from the section - Mere Discovery of a new property of a Known Substance, Mere Discovery of any new use of a Know Substance, Mere use of Known Processes and/or Mere Discovery of new form of Known Substance aren't patentable unless it can show in an increase in efficacy.

b) *Protects interests of Indian Pharmaceutical Companies*

Unlike common perception the addition of section 3 (d) to the patent act was also done with the intention to protect the Indian Pharmaceutical companies. It is so because the foreign manufacturers who have obtained a patent for a particular drug cannot apply for secondary patents by making a slight modification (by substituting a compound) to the original patented drug, in accordance with section 3 (d) of the Patents Act. Consequently Indian companies can manufacture copies of the foreign drug by using substitutes of compounds used in the original drug. Due to the absence of any patent for the substitute compound by the foreign companies, Indian Companies cannot be held for patent infringement. The only option then available for foreign manufacturers is filing a 'Markus-type claim' that includes patent protection for substitute compounds used in the manufacturing of similar drug.

---

13 https://legalconclave.com/blog/significance-of-section-3d-of-indian-patent-act/ Accessed on 3 May 2018

14 https://www.thehindubusinessline.com/opinion/is-section-3-d-of-patents-act-good-for-innovation-yes/article22996192.ece Accessed on 3 May 2018

The section 3 (d) hence has been very cleverly crafted to secure the interests of Indian Pharmaceutical companies while abiding by the restrictions laid down by the TRIPS.[15]

Compliance Issues

One of the main Novartis's[16] contentions was that section 3(d) was not in compliance with TRIPS Agreement. There has been a lot of speculation as to the view WTO would have taken had Novartis appealed. However, many scholars believe that WTO would not have ruled it in Novartis's favour mainly due to the flexibility Article 27 provides. Article 27 of TRIPS states the criteria to decide whether a product is patentable; *viz.* novelty, inventive step and industrial application. But, a strict definition to each of these terms is lacking in the agreement, leaving enough room for countries to have their own interpretation. In this case, India utilized this leeway to cater to its own needs by setting a higher bar of patentability for pharmaceutical drugs. Section 3(d) requires the product to exhibit 'enhancement of the known efficacy' for it to be patentable. The Supreme Court also reiterated similar points on compliance of Indian patent laws with TRIPS in Novartis case despite lacking jurisdiction to rule in such matters. Former WIPO director, Nuno Pires de Carvalho, also expressed a similar opinion.[17] He stated that each WTO member can individually define the term invention for the purpose of patentability, and therefore India is not violating TRIPS by merely not included technical creations under inventions. However, he showed concern over the interpretation of the term 'efficacy'. Shamnad Basheer[18] too cautioned that compliance of 3(d) with TRIPS would in-turn depend upon the degree of the term 'efficacy'. The scope of the said term will not only determine its compliance with TRIPS, but also make it clear as to what is patentable under Indian patent law, which the Supreme Court fialed to do in the Novatis case. The court felt it was unnecessary to define the term and instead let the interpretation taken depending upon the facts and circumstance of the case.

Some scholars[19], however, argued that section 3(d) blatantly violates the TRIPS agreement. They argue that section 3(d) is an additional barrier which a product must go through as a patentability test and the flexibility from Article 27 only acts as an excuse for such violations. It was argued that the medical efficacy of the drug was not remotely connected to 'inventive step', when compared to US's strict definition of the same. Moreover, some scholars felt that the Supreme court was biased towards the public and thus delivered a judgement which may violate the spirit of Article 27 to promote free and fair trade. However, it should be noted that these arguments are based upon strict interpretation of Article 27 read along

15 Supra Note 13.

16 Novartis A.G vs Union of India.

17 Linda Lee (2008). Trials and TRIPS-ulations: Indian Patent Law and Novartis AG v. Union of India, 23 BERKELEY TECH. L.J. 281, 299.

18 Supra Note 6.

19 Dorothy Du (2014). Novartis Ag v. Union of India: "Evergreening," Trips, and "Enhanced Efficacy" Under Section 3(d), 21 J. Intell. Prop. L. 223.

with the US's laws, since TRIPS is majorly follows US's IP law model. In any case, both sides complain about the lack of a strict definition for the term 'efficacy'. The Novartis case served as an opportunity to define the same, however, the court refused to give it a strict definition, failing to resolve the issue.

US Opposition to Section 3 (d)

The United States has flagged India under the 'priority watch list' unfair market access and insufficient patent protection since 1998. The US personnel engaged in the IPR protection consider the state of Indian Laws as – 'serious intellectual property violation'.

The addition of section 3 (d)during the 2005 Amendment to the Patents Act of 1970 only elevated the matter. It was so because concerns arose for the US Pharmaceuticals who are now prohibited patents in the Indian market unless their incremental innovation had therapeutic efficiency enhancement.

Consequent to such beliefs, the US imposed a unilateral step to pressurise the countries on the priority watch list. In the process the USIBC (US India Business School) formulated a report in 2009 whose outcome held that the section 3 (d) of the Patents Act would in ultimate analysis disrupt the Foreign Direct Investment coming to India.

Enhanced Efficacy

The lack of a proper definition to 'enhanced efficacy' has challenged the pharmaceutical patent law regime in India. The lack of such definition leaves the industry with legal ambiguity as to which inventions are patentable.

Though the ruling in the Novartis case had beneficial implication to the developing countries, it left this issue unanswered. The Supreme Court interpreted the term 'enhanced efficacy' as 'therapeutic enhancement' or 'enhancement of its medical efficacy', giving it a narrower scope. The court stated that the test of efficacy in cases of medicines can mean 'therapeutic efficacy'.[20] This meant that Gleevec, which displayed better properties such as solubility and bioavailability, could not be patented as the drug did not demonstrate an increase in its curative or restorative aspects, but merely added auxiliary benefits. However, the court noted that bioavailability can satisfy the condition of 'significant enhancement of its efficacy', provided there was empirical data suggesting the same. [21]

Nevertheless, despite taking a strict and narrow interpretation of section 3(d), the court refused give a clear cut definition and left enough ambiguity to MNCs and domestic industry to pursue patents for their invention without having a bright line distinction of its patentability. It also failed to provide the criteria needed to define which drug was therapeutically superior when compared with other. Thus,

---

20 Supra Note 8.

21 SHAMNAD BASHEER, THE "GLIVEC" PATENT SAGA: A 3-D PERSPECTIVE ON INDIAN PATENT POLICY AND TRIPS COMPLIANCE, available at www.atrip.org/Content/Essays/Shamnad per cent 20Basheer per cent 20Glivec per cent 20Patent per cent 20Saga.doc

the court did not bring clarity to the earlier legal obscurity in what Basheer called a 'missed opportunity'.[22]

Section 3(d) with this interpretation successfully achieved its primary objective, *i.e.* the prevention of ever greening. However, the narrow interpretation also risks blocking of genuinely innovative products since it is very difficult to prove its enhanced efficacy at the time of its patent application. Empirical evidence for its efficacy would require the company to run clinical trials, which may potential expose the product, and also cost the company handsomely. Also, the clinical data they derive from the trials could be termed as 'prior art' and eventually reject the application. Thus, pharmaceutical companies were discouraged to function within the country since they could capitalize on their invention, even if they were genuinely innovative.[23]

Despite the implications of not having 'efficacy' defined, the court suggested that it may not be necessary to give it a definition and each case should be decided upon the facts and circumstances of each case. Moreover, a strict definition to the same is very difficult to make because it could be easily construed to one side of the debate. The implications of defining the term are discussed below.

Implications of Section 3 (d)

As explained so far section 3 (d) of the Patents Act is a slide carefully balanced between two opposing ends – on one side a patent regime in favour of MNCs, possibly having more leeway for the Evergreening of drugs and on the other a generic drug supporting regime that sets the highest of standards for the application and selection of patents, possibly carrying along with a clause for easy 'compulsory licensing'. The section and its interpretation (as to its effect) are quite balanced on the phrase 'enhanced efficacy'. Due to lack of any definition or scope of 'enhanced efficacy' being mentioned anywhere throughout, the section has been repeatedly interpreted in favour and for the benefit of the general public. The likely implication of the same being; rejection of patent applications with no or less 'novelty' and allowing the manufacturing of generic drugs in most favourable instances. This has been reiterated in the *Novartis*Case, which ruled in favour of the public at large.[24]

One may hardly question such approach by government bodies and courts after considering the socio-economic conditions of Indian populace. Generic drugs will be no doubt essential to the survival of the Indian low and middle-income population. Hence one may even go to the extent of reading Article 21 – Right to Life and Personal Liberty, into the interpretation of section 3 (d) of the patent act, as to the definition of 'enhanced efficacy'.

But as a mixed economy the government must keep in mind the interests of the general public as well as manufacturers (of drugs and other pharmaceuticals). Hence

---

22 Supra Note 6.

23 Supra Note 21.

24 Shalini A. and Rekha C. (2016). Section 3(d): Implications and Key Concerns for Pharmaceutical Sector. Journal of Intellectual Property Rights 21 pp 16-26.

both must be seen as stakeholders to the implication of implementing section 3 (d) in the New Patent Regime. Since section 3 (d) has been open-endedly construed it has theprospective of toppling over to either of the opposing sides, thereby affecting the interests of the other.

Broad Interpretation of Section 3 (d)

If the interpretation of section 3 (d) especially that of 'enhanced efficacy' as mentioned earlier would be broader and would provide more leeway for the Evergreening of patents, thenthe scenario would be such that patents would be provided to companies for every modification that they make that enhances efficacy even slightly. This would in turn imply that the manufacturers of generic drugs in India would no longer have the right to produce substituted compounds as they would be protected in the abundance of patents that would be granted. This means that only few 'Big Pharmas', especially foreign MNCs will have a dominance in the Indian Pharmaceutical market, thereby causing the prices of drugs to rise exorbitantly. Hence a broad interpretation of section 3 (d) would eventually lead to the end of generic drugs which coupled with the lack of proper public health care system would mean the drastic fall in the health and survival of the populace.[25]

Narrow Interpretation of Section 3 (d)

A narrow interpretation of section 3 (d) as most view implies more stringent standards for the selection/approval of patent applications. This would mean only those product patents even those of 'Big Pharmas' that qualify high standards of 'efficacy' are patentable. This would mean that Indian Pharmaceutical Industry will become disincentivised for these MNCs. In the short run this in turn would mean that local manufacturers will be capable of manufacturing generic drugs for over a range of diseases and ailments as compared to before.[26]

However in the long run this may take one of the two possible courses:

1. *Increase in Innovation*

With the exit of foreign MNCs form the Indian Pharmaceutical Industry, the local industry would face reduced competition and hence more investment may go into its own R&D than simply 'reengineering' patented drugs. Hence in the long run India may see a boom in the innovation among native manufacturers.

2. *Domination by Indian MNCs*

It may also be possible in one course of actions that with the exit of foreign MNCs from Indian Pharmaceutical Industry, the local manufacturers who have 'reengineered' patented drugs so far would slowly die out, because of lack of access to the patented drugs manufactured and sold in US and other countries. This would leave the Pharmaceutical market with just the few major MNCs of Indian origin like Ranbaxy, Cipla, *etc.* which might possibly dominate the market.

---

25 *Ibid.*

26 *Ibid.*

Nevertheless it is the majority opinion that the section 3 (d) must be construed in the narrower sense so as to secure the interests of the public at large by keeping generic drugs in production.

Analysis of Health Care Systems across the World

The clever law making during 1970s is definitely laudable; however it should not be used as an excuse to not develop a proper health-care system. Today, nearly 4 decades after 1970 law which made the domestic pharmaceutical industry thrive, the public still pay 72 per cent of their medical expenses incurred from purchase of drugs from their own pockets.[27] Meanwhile, only 17 per cent in the US and around 15 per cent in Europe constitutes to direct out of pocket expenditure on drugs.[28] This is can be attributed to the health care schemes prevalent in such developed countries. Since the government run insurance schemes constitute a very large number of their citizens, the health care providers, including pharmaceuticals, are forced to yield to the prices set by the government. The government schemes cover so many people that the government can demand lower prices from the health care providers. If the provider refuses to lower the prices, the provider will lose out on a huge share of its customers who are covered under the said scheme. Thus, health care providers are forced yield to the government demands. It should also be mentioned that the majority of the money allocated to health care by the government goes to compensation for the expenditure incurred by its citizens, unlike India where infrastructure is also given importance to.

Such a structure for health care is absent in India. There is no single insurance system which covers a vast number of people to give it sufficient bargaining power to reduce its prices. With many private insurers popping up, the bargaining power of each insurer only diminishes. This, in turn, lets the health care providers have complete control over the prices on the treatment and prescription drugs. The insurers only obtain a limited scope for providing a claim and thus make the ultimate patient bear the brunt of the medical expenditure. Despite making the drugs affordable, a lack of a health care system is only likely to cause further detriment in the future, which the US is facing right now. The health care providers have nearly quadrupled the price of their drugs in response to the decrease in the bargaining power of the insurers. And this is likely to happen if India still approaches this issue by manipulating the criterion for the patentability of the drug.

Conclusion and Suggestion

Providing affordable drugs to its citizens is of a real concern. India, so far, has managed to provide satisfactory health care service through free-riding from medicines created by foreign MNCs, to which extent it has received a fair share of criticism. However, as mentioned earlier, this should be used as an excuse to not develop its health care system.

---

27 https://timesofindia.indiatimes.com/india/Indians-pay-78-of-medical-expenses-from-their-own-pocket/articleshow/7270363.cms

28 https://www.oecd.org/els/health-systems/Health-at-a-Glance-Europe-2016-CHARTSET.pdf Accessed on 1 May 2018.

One way of letting the interest of foreign pharmaceutical companies and those of the public to co-exist will be use incremental changes to the drug as a marketing tool. Any additions made to the original drug should be used as a USP to that particular brand for a very short amount of time. This way, the foreign companies will be able to reap benefits of their invention for the said time. This will keep the MNCs incentivized to invent within India, and help the domestic industry to grow and incentivizes them to invest on R&D as well. It would help the foreign companies to have some return on investment while the domestic pharmaceutical industry continues to work on cheaper versions of the same drug and also, when the company grows may be able to directly challenge the foreign company in terms of innovation. The short span of the available right in this set up will also force the industry to speed up the innovation process, making the industry much more dynamic and fruitful to the public as a whole.

Coming to the primary discussion of this chapter 'India and Global Pharma Patent Conventions' we understand that major changes that took place in the patent law pertaining to Pharmaceuticals was primarily because of the rising pressure from countries like US and EU and organizations dominated by them like the WTO. However India took it upon itself to adduce requisite changes in the adoption process and guidelines keeping in mind the general populace. In this manner it reshaped the world view on the TRIPS agreement acting as an inspiration for developing countries especially with the addition of section 3 (d) to its Patent Law.

If India really wishes to grow scientifically and technologically while keeping in mind the needs of the public, it must work towards better protection of intellectual property as better IP protection directly corresponds to more R&D investments and in turn more innovation.

Chapter 6

Stem Cell Research: An Emerging Sector and its Challenges

Chandrika

Dept. of Laws, Panjab University, Chandigarh, 160014
e-mail: chandrikasingh88@gmail.com

ABSTRACT

Health is a significant factor to analyse the human development which is the basic ingredient of economic and social development of a country. Since time immemorial health is considered as an important aspect and thus, the independent India approached the public as the right holder and imposed the state with the duty of providing primary health for all. With the advancements in science and technology, regenerative medicine and stem cells research has come to rescue the patients suffering from debilitating diseases. Scientists hope to be able to use stem cells to find treatments for spinal cord injuries, cancer, diabetes and diseases such as Alzheimer's and Parkinson's but as they say every advancement comes with a sacrifice, this area of biotechnology needs to be taken care of before it comes to bedside. The clinical application of stem cells and its outcome is not yet clear and hence their potential use need to be ascertained by evidence before accepting them as safe and effective treatment. Stem cell research is basically a field full of various challenges like destruction of human embryos to create human embryonic stem (hES) cell lines, potential for introducing commodification in human tissues and organs, menace of reproductive cloning including the risk of exploitation of individuals particularly the one belonging to the underprivileged groups. Allied socio-ethical problems consist of premature use of stem cells for therapy (unproven therapy) putting patients in health and financial risks, of voluntary and informed consent, donor risks, rights of donors and beneficiaries, affordability of expensive treatments, accessibility, commodification and lack of awareness in people. Also comes, the other international problems like it is difficult to catch- hold the particulars of licensing agreements between grant applicants and patent holders in absence of strict, definite regulations and laws. Stem cell tourism and fear of negative health consequences require extraordinary awareness amongst ethicists and medical practitioners. Need of the hour is to ponder upon the various related issues in the backdrop of present regulatory framework, to critically analyse it to check for loopholes and come up with feasible solutions to curtail and limit the negative effects of this research.

Keywords: *Stem cell research, Debilitating disease, Health, Regenerative medicine, Commodification.*

Introduction

Economic and social development of a country is only possible when health is given prime importance and forms a major part of the policies for human development. With the advent in science and technology, overall health has significantly improved over times. After independence, Indian Constitution imposed the state with the duty of providing primary health for all. Much advancement can be seen in regenerative medicine and stem cells research that has come to rescue the patients suffering from debilitating diseases. In future regenerative medicine and stem cell research can become a boon to the patients suffering from various skin diseases and acid attack victims as well.

Now, stem cell science is moving into the clinical sphere at a fast pace. No field of human scientific inquiry displays the global diversity of ethical, cultural, and religious heritage as much as stem cell research.[1] It is important to highlight that before such stem cell products, treatments come to bed side, the efficacy of all these need to be tested. Like every scientific research, Stem cell research is also surrounded by various challenges. Some of them are destruction of human embryos to create human embryonic stem (hES) cell lines, potential for introducing commodification in human tissues and organs, menace of reproductive cloning including the risk of exploitation of individuals particularly the one belonging to the underprivileged groups. There are other social and ethical problems that consist of premature use of stem cells for therapy (unproven therapy) putting patients in health and financial risks, of voluntary and informed consent, donor risks, rights of donors and beneficiaries, affordability of expensive treatments, accessibility, commodification and lack of awareness in people. Other international problems with respect to licensing agreements, patent holders also occur in deficiency of strict, definite regulations and laws.

The stem cell research shows potential in nature and that's why it is urgent need of the hour to shape and regulate it. There are various concerns, apprehensions, threats which are posed by it but not tackled effectively. Present situation of India speaks that here a common Indian is enormously bamboozled by farthest assumptions, hypothesis and baffling terminologies used by stem cell scientists, false and mischievous claims of biotechnological companies in the backdrop of continuing clash between religion and science in this sacred nation.

Meaning and Concept of Stem Cells

---

1 Furcht L and Hoffman W (2011). The Stem Cell Dilemma: The Scientific Breakthroughs, Ethical Concerns. Skyhorse New York. pp. 225.

Stem cells are the basic cells of every tissue and organ of a human body which carry two significant characteristics that discriminate them from other types of cells; first they are unspecialized cells that renew themselves for long periods through cell division and second that under certain physiologic or experimental conditions, they can be induced to become cells with special functions such as the beating cells of the heart muscle or the insulin producing cells of the pancreas.[2] There are two primary types of stem cells *i.e.* **Embryonic Stem Cells** and **Adult Stem Cells,** which have different functions and characteristics mentioned below;

a) **Embryonic stem cells** are obtained from a variety of species which includes humans as well and are described as *pluripotent* which means that they can generate all the different types of cells in the body and can be obtained from the blastocyst which is a nascent stage of growth consisting of a mostly hollow ball of just about 150-200 cells barely discernible to the bare eye.[3] The ability of these cells to generate all of the cell types of the body is why they offer such potential for scientific and medical purposes and why they are of great interest in the research community.[4]

b) **Adult Stem Cells:** These are Tissue-specific stem cells, which are sometimes referred to as "somatic" stem cells, are already somewhat specialized and can produce some or all of the mature cell types found within the particular tissue or organ in which they reside.[5]

The other major source of human Embryonic Stem cells involves a technique in which the nucleus of an adult cell from the patient's own body is transferred into an unfertilized egg from another source to generate Embryonic Stem cells and is known as **Somatic Cell Nuclear Transfer (SCNT).**[6] In humans, Somatic Cell Nuclear Transfer (SCNT) was envisioned as a means of generating personalized embryonic stem cells from patients' somatic cells, which could be used to study disease mechanisms and ultimately for cell-based therapies.[7]

In 1962, John Gurdon reported that his laboratory had generated tadpoles from unfertilized eggs that had received a nucleus from the intestinal cells of adult frogs.[8] Another success in birth of *Dolly*, the first mammal generated by somatic cloning demonstrated that even differentiated cells contain all of the genetic information

---

2 Stem Cell Information: National Health Institute, http://stemcells.nih.gov/staticresources/info/basics/StemCellBasics.pdf, accessed on 04 Apr 2018.

3 Stem Cell Facts: International Society For Stem Cell Research, http://www.isscr.org/docs/default-source/isscr-publications/isscr_11_stemcellfactbrch_fnl.pdf, accessed on 03 Apr 2018.

4 Mark Noble, 'Stem Cells: Their Potential for Treating PD', http://www.pdf.org/en/spring05_Stem_Cells, accessed on 04 Apr 2018.

5 Supra note 3.

6 Ibid.

7 Tachibana (2013). Human Embryonic Stem Cells Derived by Somatic Cell Nuclear Transfer, Cell', http://dx.doi.org/10.1016/j.cell.2013.05.006, accessed on 05 May 2018.

8 Yamanaka S. Induced Pluripotent Stem Cells: Past, Present and Future. http://www.sciencedirect.com/science/article/pii/S1934590912002378, accessed on 01 May 2018.

required for the development of entire organisms and oocytes contain factors that can reprogram somatic cell nuclei.[9]

Relation between Stem Cells and Major Diseases

Human Embryonic Stem Cell (HESC) research offers much hope for alleviating the human suffering brought on by the ravages of disease and injury.[10]

Scientists hope to be able to use stem cells to find treatments for spinal cord injuries, cancer, diabetes and diseases such as Alzheimer's and Parkinson's.[11] Bone Marrow Transplant (BMT) is used for cancers such as leukaemia, where it allows the marrow to receive fresh and healthy cells, which then multiply and give rise to the different types of blood that are necessary for life.[12]

Stem cell research into heart disease has also shown wonderful results and the goal seems to eventually replace all of the damaged heart tissue with healthy cells as some of the initial research in laboratory animals such as mice has suggested that when adult stem cells derived from non-heart tissues are transplanted into a damaged heart, the cells grow healthy heart muscle cells.[13] Stem cell therapy has been proposed as a means to replace and regenerate functional cardiac muscle, rather than just prevent further damage following a heart attack.[14]

Stem cell transplantation in spinal cord injury patients has shown encouraging results as it is reported that transplanting autologous enriched mononuclear bone marrow stem cells (CD34) in Spinal Cord Injury (SCI) patients brought good results of clinical safety through open surgery transplantation.[15]

People who are diagnosed with type I diabetes have abnormal insulin regulation and the pancreatic cells that would normally produce insulin are destroyed by the sufferer's own immune system.[16] Research is now suggesting that it may be feasible to control stem cell differentiation so that stem cells are guided in the laboratory to

---

9 *Ibid.*

10 Siegel A. Ethics of Stem Cell Research: The Stanford Encyclopedia of Philosophy, http://plato.stanford.edu/archives/spr2013/entries/stem-cells/, accessed on 30 Apr 2018.

11 Baynes T. U.S. High Court Won't Review Federal Embryonic Stem Cell Funds, http://www.reuters.com/article/2013/01/07/us-usa-court-stemcell-idUSBRE9060IQ20130107, accessed on 05 May 2018.

12 Murnaghan I. Major Diseases and Stem Cells, http://www.explorestemcells.co.uk/majordiseasesstemcells.html accessed on 15 Apr 2018.

13 Goldthwaite C A. Mending a Broken Heart: Stem Cells and Cardiac Repair, https://stemcells.nih.gov/info/Regenerative_Medicine/2006Chapter6.htm retrieved on 2017-07-06.

14 Schwartz P H and Bryant P J (2008). Therapeutic Uses of Stem Cells. In: Monroe K R (ed) Fundamentals of the Stem Cell Debate, The Scientific, Religious, Ethical and political Issues, 1st ed., 37-59 at 45.

15 Paspala S A B. Neural Stem Cells and Supporting Cells - The New Therapeutic Tools tor The Treatment of Spinal Cord Injury. Indian Journal of Medical Research 130 (2009), 379-391, at 385.

generate specialised cells capable of producing insulin.[17] Beta-cell replacement is a potential therapy that might reverse rather than simply palliate both -type 1, type 2 diabetes and also that pancreas transplantation is effective, improving quality if not duration of life in people with type-1 diabetes.[18]

A recent study with embryonic stem cells found that transplanted cells were able to function and release dopamine, relieving the symptoms of Parkinson's disease.[19] The Dean of Harward University Faculty of medicine claimed that stem cell therapies have potential to do for chronic diseases what antibiotics did for infectious diseases' and hopes that current research will lead to 'Penicillin for Parkinsons'.[20] Regarding Human stem cell therapy, scientists are developing a number of strategies for producing dopamine neurons from human stem cells in the laboratory for transplantation into humans with Parkinson's disease and the successful generation of an unlimited supply of dopamine neurons could make neuro-transplantation widely available for Parkinson's patients at some point in the future.[21]

As the occurrence of numerous serious diseases increase, the pressure and anxiety similarly increases to discover cures and treatment techniques. Stem cells offer the potential to noticeably trim down human suffering from disease but as of yet, the research is still in the primitive stages of providing safe and successful treatment.

Controversies aligned to Stem Cell Research

Like many innovations, stem cell research has been a source of major ethical, legal, and social controversy since the first successful culturing of human Embryonic Stem Cells in the laboratory in 1998 by Dr. Jamie Thomson who directed the group that reported the first isolation of Embryonic Stem cell lines from a non-human primate in 1995, work that led his group to the first successful isolation of human embryonic stem cell lines in 1998.[22] Stem cell biology can be useful in vibrant fields of biomedical research that includes drug development, toxicity testing, developmental biology, disease modelling, tissue engineering *etc.*[23]

---

16 In-Depth Report on Diabetes- Type 1, http://www.nytimes.com/health/guides/disease/type-1-diabetes/print.html, accessed on 01 April 2018.

17 Hussain M A and Theise N D. Stem-Cell Therapy For Diabetes Mellitus. http://w.neiltheise.com/pdfs/LancetDM.pdf, accessed on 04 May 2018.

18 Meier J J, 'The Potential for Stem Cell Therapy in Diabetes. http://bhushanlab.med.ucla.edu/downloads/publication7.pdf,accessed on 05 Apr 2018.

19 http://stemcells.nih.gov/staticresources/info/basics/StemCellBasics.pdf,accessed on 05 May 2018.

20 Korobkin R(2007). Stem Cell Century: Law and Policy for a Breakthrough Technology. Yale University Press, London. Pp 3.

21 Lund University. Breakthrough in production of dopamine neurons for Parkinson's disease. https://www.sciencedaily.com/releases/2016/10/161028085830.htm, accessed on 02 May 2018.

22 http://discovery.wisc.edu/home/morgridge/research/regenerative-biology/leadership/leadership-home.cmsx,accessed on 02 May 2018.

Internationally also, there are various legal difficulties related to intellectual property rights like patents and licensing of stem cells, contractual rights of parties, the imposition of restrictions and limitations by patent holders for stem cells availability and their usage along with the fact that it is difficult to catch- hold the particulars of licensing agreements between grant applicants and patent holders in absence of strict, definite regulations and laws.

A legal action arose which involves licensing, patent, and intellectual property right issues relative to stem cell research in *WARF* v. *Geron* wherein 1999, Geron Corp. obtained an exclusive license from the Wisconsin Alumni Research Foundation (WARF) for human embryonic stem cell technology developed by Dr. Thomson of the University of Wisconsin.[24] The license grants Geron exclusive commercial rights to develop six types of human cells, *e.g.*, nerve cells, heart and liver cells, derived from stem cells; however later, Geron attempted to exercise its option on commercial rights to additional 12 cell types but Foundation countered that the option had expired and on August 13, 2001, the foundation filed a lawsuit in U. S. District Court in Madison, Wisconsin asking the court to declare Geron's exercise of the option invalid.[25] Geron has asked the court to decide the dispute by discerning the meaning of the agreement without a trial.[26] In September 2001, National Institute of Health (NIH) began discussions with Wisconsin Alumni Research Foundation (WARF) concerning access by federally-funded researchers to human embryonic stem cells.[27] Secretary Thompson announced that an agreement has been reached with Wisconsin Alumni Research Foundation (WARF) that allows federal researchers access.[28]

Therefore, stem cell research involves patents and like issues which need to be catered for the future problems and to mitigate the litigations and various legal actions. An appropriate Intellectual Property Rights protection may be considered on the merits of each case and if the Intellectual Property Rights is commercially exploited, a proportion of the benefits shall be returned to the community, which has directly or indirectly contributed to the product.[29] "Community" includes all potential beneficiaries such as patient and research groups.[30]

23 Supra note 7.

24 Civ. No. 01-C-459-C (D. Wis. Aug. 2001).

25 *Ibid.*

26 Duffy D T. Background and Legal Issues Related to Stem Cell Research. CRS Report For Congress, http://www.law.umaryland.edu/marshall/crsreports/crsdocuments/RS21044.pdf, accessed on 02 May 2018.

27 *Ibid.*

28 *Ibid.*

29 Supra note 7.

30 *Ibid.*

Pro-choice and Pro-life Controversy

The question as to when human life begins is deeply controversial and closely connected to debates over abortion and its laws. The Supreme Court in 1973, in the case of *Roe* v. *Wade*, declared most existing state abortion laws unconstitutional where this decision ruled out any legislative interference in the first trimester of pregnancy and put limits on what restrictions could be passed on abortions in later stages of pregnancy.[31] "Pro-life" and "pro-choice" evolved as the most common self-chosen names of the two movements, one to outlaw most abortion and the other to eliminate most legislative restrictions on abortions.[32]

It is not disputed that embryos have the potential to become human beings; if implanted into a woman's uterus at the appropriate hormonal phase, an embryo could implant, develop into a fetus, and become a live-born child.[33]

The 2005 National Academies' Guidelines for Human Embryonic Stem Cell Research laid out standards for responsible and ethical conduct in a controversial field of research that largely lacked federal funding or oversight and guidelines helped this important field of research to develop within a framework of defensible, self-imposed rules.[34]

Social Aspects of Stem Cells

The study with respect to human Embryonic Stem Cell (hESC) show the importance of rules and regulations, laws and ethics at early stages of a science and explain how flawlessly they can encourage, facilitate, or retard the development of science and technology at nascent stage. It is important that while conducting research on human subjects which involves derivation and extraction of stem cells and tissues from human embryos and foetuses, basic fundamental rights, human rights, dignity, and fundamental tenets of beneficence, non- malfeasance, fairness, non arbitrariness, justice and autonomy should be adhered to.

Canadian AIDS Society v. *Ontario* is the case which is informative with respect to limits on prior consents and unforeseeable future research and went on, to balance an individual's right to privacy with public health interests, holding that public health could prevail over individual rights in some circumstances.[35]

There is another social aspect which is related with the commercialisation of biological materials. Special care needs to be taken when cells are obtained from

---

31 410 U.S. 113.

32 http://womenshistory.about.com/od/abortionuslegal/a/abortion.htm, accessed on 02 May 2018.

33 Lo B. Ethical Issues in Stem Cell Research. Endocrine Review, 30(3): 204–213, http://press.endocrine.org/doi/abs/10.1210/er.2008-0031, accessed on 03 Apr 2018.

34 Final Report of The National Academies' Human Embryonic Stem Cell Research Advisory Committee and 2010 Amendments to The National Academies' Guidelines for Human Embryonic Stem Cell Research, http://www.buffalo.edu/content/www/wnystem/hescguidelines/_jcr_content/par/download/file.res/NASguidelines2010.pdf, accessed on 01 May 2018.

35 (1995) 25 O.R. (3d) 388 (Gen. Div.)

embryos and foetuses as donation of gametes and embryos raise special ethical and moral concerns and it becomes necessary to ensure that the donors are not exploited and commoditized because of the considerable commercial value of research on stem cells/lines and their applications.

With regard to the great social importance and ethical acceptance of cord blood stem cell research, original legal status of the cord blood was analyzed with the result that the cord blood belongs to the child, and thus the child can claim certain personal rights regarding the cord blood.[36] It is important to mention that since the newborn itself is not able to take part in legal transactions, it is the moral duty of its parents to ensure that its personal and financial concerns are protected for the future, as they are its legal representatives. Because of the paretal custody they must ensure that the cord blood related rights are protected. They have to give their consent to the donation of the cord blood as well as to the collection of personal data of the child.[37] Maternity clinics and cord blood banks need this permission and those blood banks that stock up on cord blood stem cell preparations for indefinite recipients have to obtain an additional authorization because these preparations are prefabricated drugs.[38]

According to some studies, certain types of stem cells found in cord blood may even possess some of the pluripotential capacities of embryonic stem cells, which would make their application virtually limitless.[39] As the Royal College of Obstetricians and Gynaecologists (RCOG) report states, future non haematopoietic use of cord blood stem cells may be "still speculative", but the scientific literature provides clear evidence that with sufficient effort and resources devoted to research, cord blood may prove to be one of the most important tools in the specialty of stem cell therapy.[40]

Also, Assisted Reproductive Treatments provide an opportunity for infertile couples to realize their right to procreate, have a family. Because of present-day scientific limits, creation of surplus embryos is often required for successful treatment, and because this creation also cannot be shown to harm a non-consenting third party, parents are morally permitted to create these surplus embryos.[41]

Recent findings by a group of scientists from the Kyoto University Institute for Integrated Cell-Material Sciences (iCeMS) have taken the scientific world by storm,

---

36 Dohmen D, Cord Blood Stem Cells: Legal Basics and Problems. http://www.ncbi.nlm.nih.gov/pubmed/15205820, accessed on 02 May 2018.

37 *Ibid.*

38 *Ibid.*

39 Chan S. Cord Blood Banking: What Are The Real Issues https://www.ncbi.nlm.nih.gov/pmc/articles/PMC2563294/, accessed on 03 May 2018.

40 *Ibid.*

41 Dolin G. A Defense of Embryonic Stem Cell Research. International Law Journal 84:1203,(2009), 1203-1257 at 1222. http://ilj.law.indiana.edu/articles/84/84_4_Dolin.pdf, accessed on 02 May 2018.

by announcing a stem cell discovery made that will allow gay people to create their own eggs that could be used in a surrogate birth.[42]

It can be seen that this can result in a fortunate thing for older women that wish to have children later in life, women with infertility issues, such as inability to create viable eggs or who suffer from miscarriage or for whatever other reasons as bio-engineered eggs made from stem cells could be created and refined to eliminate these problems, giving affected women hope. This discovery could also lead to gay men in same-sex relationships having the ability to create an offspring completely from just the two donors' DNA; skin cells from one of the men could be used to create the egg and sperm, or sperm created from the skin cells of the other man can be used to fertilize the egg in-vitro, leaving only the surrogate uterus for implantation on the table.[43] With the advent in the field of stem cells, scientists have completed Neanderthal genome sequence.[44]

A question arises as to the threats which this can pose to health of surrogate mothers as there is still a murky situation which raises other thorny and allied questions like how can assistors, donors, surrogates be cosseted and protected from society based discrimination and prejudice? There is a doubt about these technologies perpetuating the bio-medicalization of human bodies or promoting reproductive autonomy to women through surrogacy. Is an embryo a human life and is it morally just to cull some embryos as they are not fit to be implanted in a womb? Who should decide that Assisted Reproductive Techniques (ARTs) are harmful or helpful to women – A theologist, clinician, doctor, social worker, lawyer, and patient, National Governments or International Authorities? It is also significant to make out as to how and to what level these technologies are influencing Family as a social institution.

Finally, should the use of these technologies by gay couples be encouraged as a part of national and international debate on the legitimacy of gay family forms, including marriage?[45]

Stem Cell: Indian View

The National Guidelines for Stem Cell Research 2013 and 2017 prohibit stem cell therapy and apparently regard its application which is for any other purpose and

---

42 Donahue J. Stem Cells Discovery Will Allow Gay Men to Create Eggs for Surrogate Birth. http://guardianlv.com/2012/10/jd-stem-cell-discovery-will-allow-gay-men-to-create-their-own-eggs-for-surrogate-birth/,accessed on 05 Apr 2018.

43 Richardson H. Biological Babies For Same-Sex Parents: A Possibility After Stem Cell Breakthrough. http://www.newsweek.com/biological-babies-same-sex-parents-possibility-after-stem-cell-breakthrough-309453, accessed on 02 May 2018.

44 Lallanila M. Could a surrogate mother deliver a Neanderthal baby. http://www.mnn.com/green-tech/research-innovations/stories/could-a-surrogate-mother-deliver-a-neanderthal-baby,accessed on 10 Apr 2018.

45 Carmeli D B. Assisting reproduction, Testing Genes. http://www.marciainhorn.com/olwp/wp-content/uploads/docs/inhorn-chapter-assisting-reproduction-tesing-genees.pdf accessed on 09 Apr 2018.

outside the ambit of clinical trial as unethical in the country. National Guidelines for Stem Cell Research (2013) and guidelines of 2017 too have retained the earlier classification of stem cell research into three categories, namely Permitted, Restricted and Prohibited categories; an additional layer of oversight, besides the Institutional Ethics Committee (IEC), in the form of Institutional Committee for Stem Cell Research (IC-SCR) and National Apex Committee for Stem Cell Research and Therapy (NAC-SCRT) has been introduced.

One major recommendation of the Committee was to omit the word **Therapy** from the title of the Guidelines which was implemented and this has been done to emphasize the fact that stem cells are still not a part of standard of care; hence there can be no guidelines for therapy until efficacy is proven.[46] It has been made clear in these Guidelines that any stem cell use in patients, other than that for hematopoietic stem cell reconstitution for approved indications, is investigational at present.[47]

It is visible that these 2013 and 2017 guidelines are intended to cover only stem cell research, both basic and translational, and not therapy. Despite various doubts about the compliance of guidelines, there is still a hope that this clear definition will serve to curb the malpractice of stem cell "therapy" being offered as a new tool for curing incurable diseases.

Regulatory system of clinical trials of stem cell transplantation is still in development as there are currently different mechanisms to regulate clinical translation, variable criteria are used by oversight bodies for protection for human subjects and the ability to regulate practice of medicine separate from research.[48] There are the new Department of Biotechnology (DBT) draft guidelines on stem cell research, and the Central Drugs Standard Control Organization (CDSCO) draft on compensation towards injury due to participation in clinical research that are responses to several questions that face us today.[49]Depending on the research topic, projects will be approved nationally or institutionally; research will be categorized into permissive, restricted, and prohibitive areas for research, and all projects will have to register nationally.[50] India's guidelines are relatively permissive when compared to other countries.

---

46 http://www.drugtodayonline.com/institutions/670-icmr-issues-fresh-guidelines-for-stem-cell-research.html accessed on 12 Apr 2018.

47 Dhar A. Centre issues new guidelines to check malpractice in stem cell treatment. http://www.thehindu.com/todays-paper/tp-national/centre-issues-new-guidelines-to-check-malpractice-in-stem-cell-treatment/article5718133.ece accessed on 09 Apr 2018.

48 Stem Cell Therapies in Clinical Trials. Workshop on Best Practices and the Need for Harmonization, http://www.cell.com/cell-stem-cell/pdf/S1934-5909 per cent 2810 per cent 2900447-9.pdf, accessed on 02 Apr 2018.

49 Draft Guidelines on Formula to determine the quantum of compensation in case of Clinical Trial related Injury, http://www.cdsco.nic.in/forms/list.aspx?lid=1585 and Id=1,accessed on 02 Apr 2018.

50 Lander B. Harnessing Stem Cells for Health Needs in India. Cell Stem Cell 3(2008), 11-15, at 14, http://www.sciencedirect.com/science/article/pii/S1934590908002944,accessed on 02 Apr 2018.

The value of human embryonic life highlights the controversy surrounding human Embryonic Stem Cell (HESC) research as various competing views are prevalent about this; however the scope of ethical issues in non-human Embryonic Stem Cell (HESC) research is broader than the question of the ethics of destroying human embryos. It is visible that the scientific expansion and use of stem cell therapies in India come out to be currently taking place in a largely unregulated manner. It seems that very less exercise has been done to check how workable the Indian stem cell governance is in practice as it gives the impression that government has been unable to ensure that ethically problematic stem cell practices are still being followed by varied clinics, private hospitals, and like institutions. These critical issues have not been dealt comprehensively at all, which have large-scale implications in future.

However, many Indians see optimism in the air that such guidelines' existence will promote researchers to carry on working in the area of stem cells while simultaneously preventing unethical Research and Development. For now it is uncertain to make out how successful the guidelines' implementation will be, with India's poor track record at monitoring In Vitro Fertility clinics and enforcing its guidelines for biomedical research using human subjects. With hospitals, fertility centers and clinics already initiating and carrying on stem cell-based trials and experimental procedures, the Indian government needs to proactively take a stricter action. If it fails to do so, a poor stem cell regulatory framework may become a significant hindrance to the field's development, particularly in relation to international collaborations and commercial links.

There are additional predicaments like whether researchers who exploit but do not derive human Embryonic Stem Cell (HESCs) are complicit in the destruction of embryos or not; whether there is a moral difference between creating embryos for research purposes and creating them for reproductive ends or not; and the justifiability of cloning human embryos to produce human Embryonic Stem Cell (HESCs), along with the ethics of creating human/non-human chimeras.

In view of author, commoditization of human tissues and cells, risk of exploitation of individuals particularly the one belonging to the underprivileged groups, challenges pertaining to human germ-line engineering and reproductive cloning are some cantankerous subjects which need to be catered for by a strict law in India. Premature use of stem cells for therapy before attaining sufficient data on their safety and effectiveness is also creating an unprecedented quandary related to therapeutic profligacy.

According to the guidelines, any stem cell use in patients is to be done within the purview of an approved and monitored clinical trial with the intent to advance science and medicine, and not offering it as therapy for the *'National Guidelines for Stem Cell Research 2013'* and *'National Guidelines for Stem Cell Research 2017'*, issued recently by the Union health ministry, has omitted the word 'Therapy' from the title of the Guidelines to emphasize the fact that stem cells are still not a part of standard of care and hence there can be no guidelines for therapy until its efficacy is proven.

In recent years, India has emerged as one of the leading centres for stem cell-based research and therapy. In view of author, as a place of aboriginal science, a variety of clinics in India are offering for the most part unproven therapy which puts desperate patients at health and financial risks. Unregulated growing market for private banking of cord blood, the desperate patients and parents are paying hefty amounts for an unproven therapy. As Stem cell research is also related to controversial issue of surrogacy, the human Embryonic Stem Cell research on human surrogate mothers also involves ethical and legal issues as it affects surrogate mother's health. Government and regulatory authorities' efforts have so far proved ineffective in preventing the rapid growth of various private hospitals, clinics and private cord blood banking firms that make unproven claims of success using stem cells as there is no legislation so far pertaining to the issue and the awareness level concerning the products and its benefits are still near to the ground. These factors show how complicated the trajectory of innovation can be. The research in this field, therefore, needs to be regulated in order to strike a balance.

It is also pertinent to figure out that will it be possible for India to extend personal autonomy of Lesbian Gays Bisexuals Transgenders (LGBTs) in relation to surrogacy and those who obtain parenthoob by such means as their rights are still to be decided and since it involves ethical and legal issues, it will ignite the debate over Lesbian Gays Bisexuals Transgender (LGBT's) rights in India.

Conclusion

It is important to highlight the significant socio-ethical issues raised by the scientific development, use of stem cells in India and related regulatory guidelines and frameworks to deal with challenges it put in the course. It has a direct significance to researchers, scientists, clinicians, biotech companies, various regulators and policymakers in both India and other countries. Need of the hour is to ponder upon the various related issues in the backdrop of present regulatory framework, to critically analyse it to check for loopholes and come up with feasible solutions to curtail and limit the negative effects of this research.

As India has no laws to regulate and oversee different stem cell activities, and for that many clinicians are free to conduct illegal experiments, unregulated trials without any check. Sometimes they blame the incapacity of the Department of Biotechnology-Indian Council of Medical Research Guidelines for unregulated stem cell activities since these have no statutory power. A regulatory Framework in the form of a legislation governing the field instead of the existing guidelines is a need of the hour for the proper growth of stem cell research and applications in India. The guiding philosophy should be to promote scientific and ethical stem cell research in a balance way while preventing premature commercialization and potential exploitation of vulnerable patients. Every scientific research should be regulated in order to curb the menace and threats posed by it.

Similarly, Stem Cell research experiences show the significance of rules and regulations, laws and ethics at early stages of a science. A very well regulated field perfectly can promote, facilitate, or speed up the development of science and technology at blossoming stage. Merely by framing and revising any guideline for such important area of scientific research wouldn't be sufficient, because guidelines are recommended best practices that aim to set standards in the future for this research.

In India patchwork of various regulations discourages the investors, various biomedical companies and researchers, scientists, who are eventually moving to other countries leading to much brain-drain and funds-drain. Introduction of legislation would not only keep a check on rogue scientists but would also provide protection to vulnerable patients. It has become important to focus on effects of lack of legislation because this gap or legal vacuum succumbs the patients who are misled, scammed by such fraudsters. Though the field of stem cell research is still infantile and virgin, the mounting global interest in stem cell research mandates the enactment of a sturdy, effective and penalising legislation and oversight. The need of hour is a rigorous legislation which can efficiently deal with the area of stem cell research and industry both.

Also the legislation and guidelines must be founded on full and sound scientific and ethical evaluation of the techniques involve because hasty, rushed policies and enactments that are neither well thought through nor suitable for managing and regulating the field can have potentially harmful consequences. It implies that it is very well understood that lack in a well planned legislation and beneficial policies can hinder the growth of a nation. It is very important to cater for the mechanisms for accommodating alteration within the regulatory organization. In this fast growing era of technology it is important to anticipate changes within future, in order to build a strong framework. The constant deficiency of legislation jeopardise the scope of growth and development of the research with no lawful, fair, ethical or public oversight. Dfvb The legislation must provide for the penalty clauses where different acts are dealt with different punishments. The deterrent effect of such provisions will definitely curb the unusual surge in medical malpractices. It is believed that later on it will become a way of life and can be a help to generate a tradition of compliance of laws, rules and regulations by stem cell research and related institutes.

Another effort can be made with respect to public awareness as it is significant to make public aware and well illuminated on this subject. It is also important that detailed information is propagated so that it becomes easier for them to take independent and favourable decisions.

Indian Council of Medical Research, the Department Of Biotechnology and the Department of Science And Technology are governmental agenciesthat are dealing with stem cell research. It would definitely be legitimate that a solo agency grant funds and keeps an eye on all stem cell and clinical investigations in the country and has authority to punish defaulters.

The issues allied to stem cell research and industry offers various ethical and social issues which need to be undertaken for the welfare of society. It is a scientific development having much potential for improving human health, so research in this field must be regulated with special attention to these issues.

Chapter 7

Genetically Modified Crops: Issues and Challenges in Context of India

Ipsita Kaushik

Department of Law, Gauhati University, Assam 781013
e-mail: ipsita.kaushik.3@gmail.com

ABSTRACT

Genetic engineering and its application in agriculture has become one of the most debated fields of biotechnology. A conflict is going on between the supporters and opponents of the Genetically Modified Crops. Genetically Modified Crops have been facing various controversies in the field of environment, religion, ethics, labelling, health etc. But at the same time one cannot deny the outstanding potential of genetic engineering to increase the efficacy of crops by which the whole world can be fed. Genetically Modified Crops are such crops whose genes are modified in the laboratory in order to enhance desired traits or to improve its resistance and nutrition level. Genetic engineering can reduce the maturation time of the plant, increase nutrients, yields, and stress tolerance, and can create a plant that can withstand diseases, and heavier applications of pesticides and herbicides. In India, field trial of genetically modified crops has been facing serious prejudices. Apart from that the patentability of biotechnology inventions and ethics involved in patenting such inventions is repeatedly questioned. Granting of monopoly rights on inventions involving living being in pursuant of TRIPS agreement is also facing serious criticism. In one hand, biotechnology being an expensive technological application that collaborate human ingenuity with natural biological processes deserves protection to encourage further research and development. But on the other hand, monopoly rights over living organism have been considered as immoral and unethical. In India Patent Act 1970 has been amended in 1999, 2002 and 2005, to make it fully compliant to TRIPS agreement. Under Indian Patent Act patentable subject-matter includes Genetically Engineered Microorganisms (GEMs) that are characterized by- novelty, inventive step and industrial applicability.

Moreover, proper regulation of use and application of GMC is paramount to reduce global hunger without endangering environment and biodiversity. In India there is no specific legislation which particularly deals with G.M.C. It is the combination of various legislations which are made applicable according to the need of the case. The existing legal system and the patent laws are not effective enough to protect and regulate the biotechnology inventions. A responsible management of biotechnology is a prerequisite to achieve desired goals and it requires sound regulations for bio- safety and food safety wherever transgenic crops are to be developed and released.

Keywords: *Biotechnology, Genetic Engineering, Patent, Genetically Modified Organism, TRIPs*

Introduction

Today's contemporary world is technological world. Technology has become the part and parcel of an individual's life from dawn to dusk. Technology simply means the application of knowledge or information to deal with the practical problems. One of the most unexpected unimagined and debated, technological revolution of present era is "Biotechnology". Biotechnology means any technique that uses loving organisms or parts of organisms to make or modify products, improve plants or animals, develop microorganism for intended uses[1]. It was beyond the imagination and expectation of anyone that the natural biological process of plants, animals and human beings could by manipulated through human intervention. Some of the examples of modern biotechnology are tissue culture, genetic engineering, recombinant DNA techniques, mutagenesis, drugs, antibiotics, monoclonal antibodies, antipyretics, analgesics, breeding, cloning *etc.* Biotechnology plays a significant role in the modern day to day life. Modern biotechnology provides unprecedented products and technologies to combat debilitating and rare diseases, improves crop insect resistance, enhances crop herbicide tolerance and facilitates the use of more environmentally sustainable farming practices. [2]

It is well established that Biotechnology is currently one of the most important expressions of technological progress. It embraces all technologies that use molecular and cellular biology for solving problems linked to agriculture and food, as well as human health. Medical biotechnology has application both in diagnosis and in producing new drugs. Biotechnologies applied to agriculture are used for producing and modifying plants, animals, and micro-organisms. Plants and animals have been modified for the benefits of humankind for hundreds of years using conventional

---

1 Shukla U.K *et al.* (2010). Intellectual property Right: A Prospective Approach towards Conservation of Biodiversity and Promotion of Biotechnology. In: Kumar Aravind, and Das Govind (ed.) Biodiversity, Biotechnology and Traditional Knowledge: Understanding Intellectual Property Rights, 1st edn. Narosa Publishing House, New Delhi, pp 191-196.

2 Sreenivasulu N.S., and Raju C.B (2001). Biotechnology and Patent Law: Patenting Living Beings. Manupatra, Noida.

methods such as grafting and selective breeding; biotechnology has now introduced an unprecedented qualitative change by enabling human beings to transfer genes from one species to another.[3]Living beings body naturally produces certain proteins, enzymes and antibodies to fight against diseases and attacks of virus.

Genes inside the body gets activated to resists and to fight against diseases or virus attacks by expressing certain protein or antibody or enzyme. Through biotechnology it is possible to isolate specific genes coding for such antibodies and proteins in order to produce the same commercially on large scale. Isolated genes could be incorporated into any microorganism say bacteria to produce the protein or antibody that the gene is coding for. The resulted protein or enzyme or antibody could be made use of in producing medicines and cures to diseases.[4]

One of the most debated offshoots of biotechnology is genetically modified crops (G.M.C). G.M.Cs can be defined as those crops, which are produced by introducing some new genes and organism into the natural genes through the process of genetic engineering, in order to obtain desired distinguishing features and nutritional content. Genetically Modified Crops have been developed by using input traits (*e.g.* resistance to insect pests and plant disease) output traits (*e.g.* delayed fruit ripening, better taste, nutritious, elimination of saturated fats in cooking oil, elimination of allergens, better delivery of necessary nutrients) agronomic traits (*e.g.* resistance to drought, salinity, acidity, flood *etc.* and increase in crop yield).[5]

Intellectual Property is a cluster of legally recognised rights associated with innovations and creativity, results from creative efforts from mind and intellect. Biotechnology industries also claim Intellectual property protection for their inventions as it takes a decade or more periods to develop a technology and perhaps one invention in thousand becomes a successful commercial product and process. The protection of IP provides incentive for biotechnology industry to invest time and money in research and development, which is driving force for unprecedented benefits in the quality of human life that biotechnology, is expected to bring. Such benefits may not be so forthcoming without the underlying profit motivation afforded by IP protection.[6]

Since biotechnology concerns life or living beings, it gives rise to certain questions. The patentability of Genetically Modified Crops and ethics involved in patenting such inventions is repeatedly questioned. But at the same time one cannot deny the role that GMC could play to reduce the hunger of the world. Therefore it is necessary to evaluate the positive and negative effects of GMC and protection should

---

3 Saraswat Darpan (2010). Biotech Patents and Questions of Patentability in India and Abroad. In: Kumar Aravind, and Das Govind (ed.) Biodiversity, Biotechnology and Traditional Knowledge: Understanding Intellectual Property Rights, 1st edn. Narosa Publishing House, New Delhi, pp 99-104.

4 Smith J. (1996). Biotechnology. Cambridge University Press, United Kingdom.

5 Gahukar R.T (2003). Issues Relating to the Patentability of Biotechnological Subject Matter in Indian Agriculture. Journal of Intellectual Property Right, 8: 9-10.

6 Supra Note 3, at 100.

also be provided to the inventors to encourage more research and development in the field of Biotechnology.

Biotechnology has changed the entire scenario of the world; the collaboration of human ingenuity with natural biological processes has yielded great results.

Section-1

Genetically Modified Crops

Meaning of Genetically Modified Organisms (GMOs)

All living organisms, from viruses to human beings, are made up of cells, with a nucleus at the centre, which contains a unique set of instructions regarding their size, strength and other qualities. These instructions are found on a long molecule called DNA (Deoxyribonucleic Acid), which is divided into small sections called genes. It is the sequencing of genes on DNA that determines an organism's characteristics. Very simple organisms such as bacteria may have fewer genes than the more complicated ones. In simple terms, the complete set of genetic material of an organism, *i.e.*, the entire DNA contained in an organism, is called a genome. The process of isolating gene from the genome of one organism and inserting the same into the genome of another organism is known as Genetic Engineering. In nature, exchange of genes happens only between compatible or closely related species. However, the modern technique of genetic engineering facilitates the removal of group of genes from one species and insertion into another, there being no need for compatibility.

Genetic modification involves altering an organism's DNA. This can be done by altering an existing section of DNA, or by adding a new gene altogether. A gene is a code that governs how we appear and what characteristics we have. When a scientist genetically modifies a plant, they insert a foreign gene in the plant's own genes. The result is that the plant receives the characteristics held within the genetic code. Thus with genetic modification it is possible to transfer genes from one species to another and to get the desired result. Using new technologies, scientists are now able to pinpoint the specific gene responsible for a particular trait and then extract or add that gene to a specific plant.[7] Genetically modified organisms (GMOs), are organisms made for agricultural or industrial or medical purpose into which one or several genes arraying for desirable traits through the process of genetic engineering.[8]

The world population is increasing day by day and it is expected to be double in the coming future. As a result, ensuring an adequate food supply has become a challenge and the Genetically Modified Crops are the effective solution to this problem. According to the scientists, GMCs can act as a means to provide the

---

7 Chopra Paras, and Kamma Akhil. Genetically Modified Crops in India. http: //www.deskuenvis.nic.in/pdf/gm.pdf., accessed on 24 Dec. 2017.

8 Kawamura Satoko (2011). GMO Trade in the Context of TRIPS: From the Perspective of an Autopoietic System Analysis. Ritsumeikan International Affairs, 10: 243-268.

growing population with continuous food supply with nutritional value. GMCs can be defined as variety developed by transforming the genes through utilization of techniques of genetic engineering. GMC are such crops whose genes are modified in the laboratory in order to enhance desired traits or to improve its resistance and nutrition level. As per the scientists, such crops are cost-effective for farmers, as they cut down the use of pesticides, insecticides and are drought tolerant.[9] As per the scientists, such crops are cost-effective for farmers, as they cut down the use of pesticides, insecticides and are drought tolerant. But there are some environmental activists, religious organisations, public interest group, who vehemently criticises the GMC. So, there are two sides to the GMCs *i.e.*, their advantages and disadvantages; around which the important issues related to health, environment, legal control and labelling of GMCs revolves. It was in 1990s that the GMCs were launched in the market and the first GMC that was commercially grown tomato puree (called *Flavr Savr*). Currently, a number of food crops such as soya bean, corn, cotton, tomatoes, Hawaiian papaya, potatoes, rapeseed (canola), sugarcane, sugar beet, field corn as well as sweet corn and rice have been genetically modified to enhance either their yield, or size, or durability, *etc.*[10]

Genetically Modified Crops and India

In India experiments have been carried out and GM crops like Golden Rice which is rich in protein have been used. But unfortunately the GM business is owned by top multinational companies and Agri-business is only for vested interest. In India, the first commercially grown GMC was the BT Cotton. The Maharashtra Hybrids Seed Company (Mahyco) jointly with the US seed company Monsanto developed the genetically modified Bt Cotton to tackle the bollworm problem that had devastated cotton crops in the past, by introducing into the cotton seed a gene of the common soil microbe called *Bacillus Thuringiensis* that encoded an insecticidal protein lethal to the bollworm (hence the name Bt. Cotton). In 2002, Bt Cotton became the first and only transgenic crop approved by the Genetic Engineering Approval Committee (GEAC) for commercial cultivation in six States namely, Andhra Pradesh, Gujarat, Karnataka, Madhya Pradesh, Maharashtra and Tamil Nadu. It has been further extended to Punjab and Haryana. The Bt Cotton seeds were marketed by the Monsanto-Mahyco joint venture. Though the public opinion has been divided on this issue, the Government has indicated satisfactory performance of the Bt Cotton. It has been claimed as the 'Bt Cotton Revolution' with transgenic cotton being grown in 90 per cent of the cotton growing areas, increasing yields by as much as 50 per cent in certain regions. However, the critics, especially various civil society groups have contested this claim. It has been argued that Bt Cotton cultivation has resulted in adverse economics for farmers, highly priced seeds, changed

9 Sharma V.K (2011). Genetically Modified Food and Consumers Interest: Some Legal and Ethical Issues, RGNUL Law Review, 1: 332-333.

10 Paarlberg Robert L (2001). The Politics of Precaution Genetically Modified Crops in Developing Countries. Johns Hopkins University Press, Baltimore and London.

pest ecology in cotton fields, increased incidence of diseases (requiring more pesticides to control these), unpredictable crop performance and more resources being used by farmers as part of their risk insurance mechanisms (use of more irrigation, fertilizers, *etc.*). There have been reports of adverse impact on soils, human health (allergic symptoms) as well as toxicity in animals grazing on the Bt Cotton fields. There have also been reports of large scale contamination and rapid proliferation of various illegal varieties. Another Genetically Modified Crops that generated great debate in India is BT Brinjal. Bt Brinjal is a transgenic Brinjal created out of inserting a gene [Cry1Ac] from the soil bacterium *Bacillus Thuringiensis* into Brinjal.[11] Bt Brinjal is being developed in India by the Maharashtra Hybrid Seeds Company (Mahyco). It has many advantages as the promoters say that Bt Brinjal will be beneficial to small farmers because it is insect resistant, increases yields, is more cost-effective and will have minimal environmental impact. But there are many disadvantages related to the production and use of Bt Brinjal relate to its possible adverse impact on human health and bio-safety, livelihoods and biodiversity.[12]

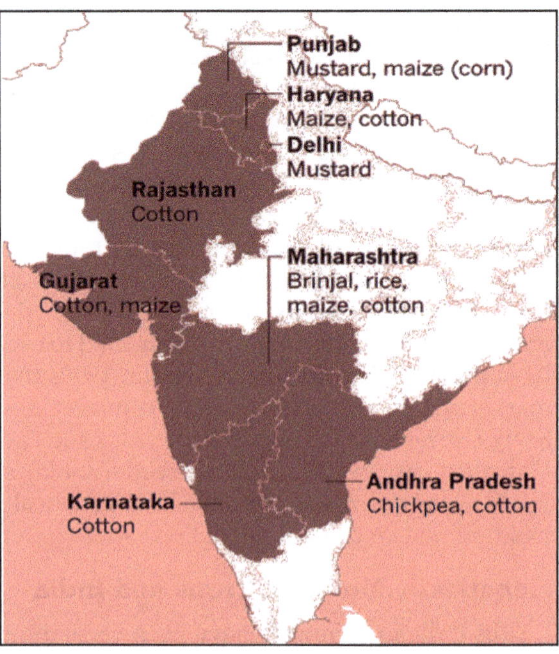

Figure 7.1: Indian States where GEAC Approval Field Trial.

When Bt Brinjal was sought to be introduced in the market a few years ago, it led to a controversy. However, on February 9, 2010, the Ministry of Environment and Forests imposed a moratorium on Bt Brinjal. In the absence of scientific consensus and opposition from state governments and others, the ministry decided to impose a moratorium on the commercialisation of Bt Brinjal until all concerns expressed by the public, NGOs, scientists and the state government were addressed adequately. Clearance of Bt Brinjal as a commercial crop by Genetic Engineering Approval Committee (GEAC) in October 2009 and then its ban by government of India in February 2010, becomes a point of debate whether Bt Brinjal should be

11 Sahai Suman (2010). Potential of agricultural genetic engineering for food security in India: Research on transgenic food crops. http: //genecampaign.org/wp-content/uploads/2014/07/Potential_Of_Agricultural_Genetic_Engineering_For_Food_Security_In_India.pdf. Accessed on 24 Dec, 2017.

12 Whitman Deborah B (2000). Genetically Modified Foods: Harmful or Helpful. https: //www.sandiegounified.org/schools/sites/default/files_link/schools/files/Domain/8628/GMO.pdf., Accessed on 24Dec. 2017.

commercialized or not. However the Minister of State for Environment and Forests, responding to strong views rose both for and against the introduction of the Bt Brinjal, has called for public consultations across the country before taking a final decision on this issue. Companies with any seeds of Bt Brinjal will have to register the details with the government, and the National Bureau of Plant Genetic Resources (NBPGR) was made responsible for storage of all the Bt Brinjal seeds in India.[13]Now the controversial field trial of genetically modified crops such as mustard, maize, cotton, brijal, and rice is going on some of the states in the country such as Rajasthan, Maharashtra, Gujarat, Delhi, Haryana, Punjab, Andhra Pradesh *etc.*[14]

Advantages of Genetically Modified Crops

There is a great debate on the subject of genetically modified foods, or GMCs. For some, genetically modified food is boon because the modifications allow crops to become resistant to drought and infestations, letting more people have more regular meals. Others look at genetically modified foods as a dangerous proposition. Because GMC food has adverse health affect from allergic reactions to potential intestinal damage, many people wish to avoid GMC foods because it causes the changes in internal cell structure, abnormal tumour growth, and unexpected deaths. So it can be said that GMC has both pros and cons. various advantages of GMC are as follows-

a) **Enhance quality and taste:** Genetically modified crops are rich in quality and taste. Through the modification of foods, the flavours can be enhanced. Peppers can become spicier or sweeter. Corn can become sweeter. Difficult flavours can become more palatable with the help of genetic engineering.[15]

b) **More resistant:** Plants and animals that have been genetically modified can become more resistant to the unexpected problems of disease. Genetically modified foods are more resistant and stay ripe for longer so they can be shipped long distances or kept on shop shelves for longer periods. GMCs are inbuilt resilience to diseases, viruses, insects and herbicides and therefore require lesser pesticides. These reasons make them supposedly environmental friendly. GM crops can be made resistant to pests, so pesticides do not need to be sprayed on them. This is also better on the environment.

c) **More nutrition benefits:** GMC foods can have vitamins and minerals added to them through genetic modifications to provide greater nutritive benefits to those who eat them. Some foods can be genetically modifies to contain higher amounts of important vitamins and minerals. Vitamin A deficiencies cause blindness. In Africa, 500,000 go blind each year. If rice

---

13 Harriss John, and Stewart Drew (2015). Science, Politics, and the Framing of Modern Agricultural Technologies. In: Herring Ronald J. (ed.) The Oxford Hand Book of Food, Politics, And Society, 1st edn. Oxford University Press, United Kingdom, pp 56-58.

14 Kumar Sanjay (2015). India eases stance on GM crop trials. https: //www.nature.com/news/india-eases-stance-on-gm-crop-trials-1.17529, Accessed on 26 Dec. 2017.

15 Elena Grigore M. *et al.* (2017). Approved Genetically Engineered Foods: Types, Properties and Economic Concerns. In: Holban Alina Maria, and Grumezescu Alexandru Mihai (ed.) Genetically Engineered Food, 1st Edition, Academic Press, USA, pp 89-93.

can be modified to contain more vitamin A, the amount of people going blind will decrease.[16]

d) **Reduces hunger:** GMC could potentially solve hunger. Many people agree that there is not enough food in the world to feed everybody. As genetically modified foods increase the yields of crops, more food is produced by farmers.

e) **Tolerance to herbicide:** Cultivation of many crops requires the removal of weeds that grow along with it. Weeding is a time-consuming and costly process, therefore farmers resort to the use of herbicides. Often they use multiple herbicides, increasing costs, causing harm to crops and environment, and having harmful after-effects for consumers. Genetic engineering ensures that a crop is made tolerant to one particular herbicide. By using this herbicide, crops can be protected from the need to use several herbicides resulting in reduced costs and reduced health risks.[17]

f) **Tolerance to drought and salinity:** Drought and salty ground water have wasted several areas of land. These uncultivable lands now need to be used due to the growing population and lack of agricultural lands. By creating drought-resistant crops and plants that can grow in grounds with high salinity, we can overcome the problem of waste lands and convert them into cultivable lands. [18]

Controversies Relating to GMC

Genetically modified food controversies are disputes relating to the use of foods and crops derived from genetically modified crops instead of conventional crops, and other uses of genetic engineering in food production. The dispute involves consumers, farmers, biotechnology companies, governmental regulators, non-governmental organizations, and scientists. Key areas of controversies revolves around Environmental Aspects, Labelling of Genetically Modified Foods, Ethical and Religious Aspects, Human health aspect *etc.* Controversies can be discussed here under:

1. GMC and Environmental Aspect

The production of GMCs poses great environmental risks, mainly, to plants and birds. One of the most prominent risks is increased weediness. The pollens of GMCs spread to non-GMCs in nearby plants, through the process of cross

16 Walker Shawn (2016). Beeting the Controversy. https: //www.scribd.com/document/364719201/gmo-crops-research-paper, Accessed on 25 Dec. 2017.

17 Kowalski Stanley (2007). Rational Risk/Benefits Analysis of Genetically Modified Crops.Journal of Intellectual Property Rights.12: 92-103.

18 Qaim Matin (2010). The Benefits of Genetically Modified Crops—and the Costs of Inefficient Regulation.http: //www.rff.org/blog/2010/benefits-genetically-modified-crops-and-costs-inefficient-regulation, Accessed on 25 Dec. 2017.

pollination. This process of cross pollination may allow the spread of traits such as herbicide resistance from GMCs to non-target plants, resulting of latter crops into weeds or super weeds. Mainly due to the advent of herbicide resistance super weed, which is created due to the accidental transfer of genes from GMC crops to the surrounding weeds, as a result more powerful and larger amount of herbicide is required to destroy the super weed. Another risk is that, BT toxin used in GMC crops can kill not target caterpillar and butterflies such as monarch.[19] The another risk in respect of negative impact of GMC on environment is that there are possibilities that insects become resistant to BT or other GMCs, as happened in case of BT Cotton resulting into low yield. A research at the Scottish Crop Research Institute showed that potatoes that have been engineered to be resistant to insect pests could also harm beneficial insects which would further disturb the food chain and thus would hamper the biodiversity.[20] Once a GMC is introduced in the environment, even if for trials, it has the capacity to multiply and spread uncontrollably and as a result the entire crops species can become genetically modified. Contamination from GMCs is perhaps the biggest threat as far as biodiversity and food security is concerned.[21]

2. GMC and Health Aspect

In case of GMCs, there is introduction of foreign gene which may cause harmful impact on health, not only of the human being but also of other living creatures. The study has revealed that GMC poses a serious health risks in the area of toxicology, allergy and immune function, reproductive health and metabolic, physiologic and genetic health. GM crops do have the potentiality to cause allergenic reactions, more so than conventional crops. In Australia, for example, GM peas were found to cause allergenic reactions in mice[22]. GM peas also made the mice more sensitive to other food allergies.The studies conducted on the affects of GMCs in animals reveals that GMCs result in swelling in lungs, blood clotting in stomach and intestine and declining fertility. There is 80 per cent similarity of human genome with genome of rat. The experiment on rats shows the toxic affect of GMFs on food canal, lungs and kidneys. So, this reveals that GMC would have negative impact n the health of human being as well. Various studies conducted by scientists have revealed that there is a large number of adverse effects associated with GMCs, namely, reduced organ weight, reduced growth, reduced fertility, compromised immune function, inflammation, mutations, allergic reactions, new diseases, and reduced nutrient content of food, cancer and premature death. Thus, GMFs adversely affects the immune system of human body. Some people could develop sensitivity to such

---

19 Luke Anderson (2000).Genetic Engineering, Food and Our Environment. Resurgence Books, United Kingdom.

20 Supra Note 10, at 19-21.

21 Mahgoub Salah E. O (2015). Genetically Modified Foods: Basics, Applications, and Controversy. CRC Press Taylor and Francis group.

22 Smith Jeffrey (2003). Seeds of Deception: Exposing Industry and Government Lies about the Safety of the Genetically Engineered Foods You're Eating. Yes! Book Publication, Fairfield, Iowa.

foods gradually after being exposed to it over a period of time, whereas others might have an acute allergic reaction after eating a minute amount.[23]

3. Labelling of Genetically Modified Crops

Labelling of GMC is a controversial issue not only in India but also worldwide. India proudly claims to the biggest democratic country of the world. But, if the BRAI Bill[24], 2013, is passed, it will be the grave violation of the democratic structure of the country; because the Bill has a provision to keep the information relating GMCs secret on the ground of it being "confidential commercial information" superseding the right to information of the consumer. Labelling of GMCs is not made mandatory under the Bill, which in turn violates the "Right to information" of the consumer. No literate consumer would like to have any food without knowing the contents or ingredient in the food. Moreover, as it is evident that, there are health and environmental risk associated with the GMC, in such a situation, the labelling of GM food in India has become very much essential. In other countries, the governments have either banned or have ensured adequate choice for their citizens on GMFs. The European Union, China, Brazil, Japan, Australia, Russia are some of the examples where the government have made the labelling of GMFs mandatory[25]. However, in India recently, a gazette notification came from the *Ministry of Consumer Affairs* which makes it mandatory for packaged foods using GMCs as ingredients to carry labelling from 1 January 2013. The efficiency of this notification remains a question to be answered. The notification stipulates that "Every package containing the genetically modified food shall bear at the top of its principal display panel the words "GM". It will help the consumer to be informed about the intake of such foods.[26]

4. GMC and Rights of the Consumer

It is the right of every consumer to be well informed about the food they are eating. They have the right to be assured about the quality of the food they are consuming. Biotechnology Regulatory Authority of India (BRAI) Bill, 2013, if passed, will result into food dictatorship of multinationals companies and at the same time abridges the citizen's right to speech and expression guaranteed under Article 19 (1) (a) of the Constitution of India, 1950. Right to speech and expression contains the right to information of the consumer about the food being consumed, right to public participation *etc.* But BRAI Bill has a provision to keep the information secrete asked on the ground of it being "confidential commercial information" superseding the right to information of the consumer. India being a democratic

---

23 Sloan A.E, and Powers M.E (1986). A Perspective on Popular Perspectives of Adverse Reactions to Foods. Journal of Allergy and Clinical Immunology, 78: 127-133.

24 Biotechnology Regulation Authority of India Bill (BRAI).

25 Caswell Julie A (2000). Labeling Policy For GMOs: To Each His Own?. Journal of AgroBiotechnology Management and Economics, 3: 53-57.

26 Azevedo Sophia (2015). Labeling GMO Foods. https: //www.scribd.com/doc/293489592/research-paper. Accessed on 25Dec. 2017.

country, the consumer must be informed of the food they are going to consume.[27] Thus, consumers want to participate in the process of safety standards and do not want to be dictated about the food intake. It is the right of consumers to be informed about what they are buying and eating; as they do not want to endanger their health by consuming foods about which sufficient data is not available.

5. Ethical and Religious Aspect

In contemporary era, the main motive of multinational companies working in the field of agriculture and biotechnology is to reap monetary benefits at any cost. Due to which they adopt every possible practice to make huge profits, altogether ignoring the ethics and religion of the consumers. The genetic engineering is abused to such an extent that, genes of animals, birds and fishes are being transferred into vegetarian food material to enhance their quality and characteristics. For the persons, who are vegetarians, the manufacturing and sale of such products without appropriate information is not only unethical but illegal as well.[28]

Section-2

Regulation of Genetically Modified Crops in India

Legislative Framework

In India, there is no particular legislation to regulate and govern the field of biotechnology in the food and farming sector. The legislative framework for governing this sector is the culmination of various enactments such as -The Environment Protection Act, 1986; the Patents Act, 1970; the Biodiversity Act, 2002; the Seeds Act, 1966, the Drugs and Cosmetic Act, 1940 *etc.*, depending upon the requirement of the case. It is the combination of various legislations, rules and regulations, which are made applicable according to the need of the case.

1. Environment (Protection) Act, 1986

The legal foundation for the Indian biotechnology system can be found in some of the provisions of the Environment (Protection) Act, 1986; namely - Section 6 which enables the Government of India to enact rules on procedures, safeguards, prohibitions and restrictions for the handling of hazardous substance; Section 8 imposes a prohibition on the person from handling any substances considered to be hazardous under this Act except safeguards and procedures have been complied to; and Section 25 places responsibilities on the central government of stipulating the rules regarding the procedures and safeguard for handling hazardous substances.[29]

---

27 GreenPeace. The Biotechnology Regulatory Authority of India (BRAI) Bill 2011 – The Bill to end the right to safe food!. http: //www.greenpeace.org/india/Global/india/report/brai per cent 20 per cent 20critique.pdf, Accessed on 25 Dec. 2017.

28 Indian Council of Medical Research (2004). Regulatory Regimen for Genetically Modified Foods the Way Ahead. http: //icmr.nic.in/reg_regimen.pdf, Accessed on 25 Dec. 2017.

29 Ramanna Anitha. India's Policy on Genetically Modified Crops. Asia Research Center Working Paper 15.http: //www.lse.ac.uk/asiaResearchCentre/_files/ARCWP15-Ramanna.pdf., Accessed on 25 Dec.2017.

2. Consumer Protection Act, 1986

The central objective of this Act is to protect and promote consumer's right in the market. Consumer's rights include but not limited to right to be shielded from the marketing of potentially hazardous good, right to be informed about the quality, quantity, purity, standards and price of goods, and right of consumer education. Under this Act, all movable properties with the exception of actionable claim and money bills are considered as good.[30] Therefore, genetically modified organisms based products are goods under this Act. Fraudulent and bogus claims aimed at deceiving consumer by misrepresenting goods and services fall within the ambit of Consumer Protection Act 1986.[31] Therefore marketing of GMO without the label indicating grade and composition, especially when the legal requirement to label the GMOs exists, is an unfair trade practice prohibited by this Act.

3. Biosafety Rules 1989

In exercise of the powers conferred by sections 6, 8 and 25 of the Environment (Protection) Act, 1986 and the concern to protect the environment, nature and health lead to the promulgation of 1989 Biosafety Rules by Ministry of Environment and Forests.[32] The Biosafety rules apply to the products made from genetically engineered microorganism and other gene technologies and regulate their manufacture, storage and import. These rules also cover the pre release facet of genetically modified organism, namely their research and development besides the large scale application and trial. Hazardous organisms which are not genetically modified are also regulated by these rules. Rule 8 mandates the requirement of approval of regulatory authorities prior the discharge or even the production of Genetically Modified Organism or cells. Rule 9 of this statue is foremost in significance which prohibits deliberate or unintentional release of genetically engineered organisms/ hazardous microorganisms or cells, even for the purpose of experiment, barring a situation where it has been approved as a "special case" by appropriate authority.[33]

4. National Seed Policy 2002

The Seed Policy 2002 issued by Ministry of Agriculture, Government of India contains a separate section (No. 6) on transgenic plant varieties. It has been stated that all genetically engineered crops/varieties will be tested for Environment and Biosafety before their commercial release as per the regulations on guidelines of the

---

30 The Act adopts the definition of "Good" from Section 2 (7) of Sale of Goods Act, 1930 (Act 3 of 1930).

31 Bhattacharya Sanjukta (2013). Indian Response to Genetically Modified Food and Labelling. file: ///C: /Users/hp/Downloads/SSRN-id2228786.pdf, Accessed on 25 Dec 2017.

32 Choudhary Bhagirath *et al.* (2004). Regulatory options for genetically modified crops in India. Plant Biotechnology Journal,12: 135-146.

33 Jha Bhuvan Bhaskar, and Shankar Ashutosh (2017). Evaluating the Law on Regulation of Genetically Modified Crops in India. Jamia Law Review,2: 119-121.

EPA, 1986. Seeds of transgenic plant varieties for research purposes will be imported only through the National Bureau of Plant Genetic Resources (NBPGR) as per the EPA, 1986. Required infrastructure will be developed for testing, identification and evaluation of transgenic planting material.[34]

5. Food Safety and Standards Act, 2006

As far as legal control on GMCs in India is concerned, the Food Safety and Standards Act, 2006 is the only laws which define and provide certain provisions to regulate the production, distribution, sale or import of Genetically Modified foods. Section 22 of the Act lays down: "No person shall manufacture, distribute, sell or import any novel food, genetically modified articles of food, irradiated food, organic food, food for special dietary uses, functional food, neutraceuticals, health supplements, proprietary food and other articles of food which the Central Government may notify in this behalf." Section 22(2) also defines "Genetically engineered or modified food" means food and food ingredients composed of or containing genetically modified or engineered organisms obtained through modern biotechnology, or food and food ingredients produced from but not containing genetically modified or engineered organisms obtained through modern biotechnology. This Act also provides for the explicit labeling of Genetically Modified Food.[35]

6. The Protection of Plant Varieties and Farmers Rights Act, 2001

The Protection of Plant Varieties and Farmers Rights Act, 2001 was enacted for the establishment of an effective system for protection of plant varieties, the rights of farmers and plant breeders and to encourage the development of new varieties of plants. The Act also aims to ensure the availability of high quality of seed and to facilitate the growth of seed industry.

7. The Biodiversity Act, 2002

The Biodiversity Act, 2002 and the Biological Diversity Rules aimed at implementing the Convention on biodiversity. This Act states that its goal is the conservation, sustainable utilization and equitable sharing of the benefits that result from genetic resources. In order to achieve its goals, the Act provides for access and benefit sharing mechanisms, including the disclosure of origin of the genetic material and incorporates conservation principles. For better understanding of the role of this Act it is necessary to understand definition of some terms. "Biological resources" under this Act means "biological resources" means plants, animals and micro-organisms or parts thereof, their genetic material and by-products (excluding value added products) with actual or potential use or value, but does not include

---

34 Ahuja Vibha, and Jotwani Geeta (2007). The Regulation of Genetically Modified Organisms in India. file: ///C: /Users/hp/Downloads/05-265-003[1].pdf., Accessed on 25 Dec.2017.

35 Food Safety and Standards Authority of India. Operationalising the Regulation of Genetically Modified Foods in India. http: //www.old.fssai.gov.in/Portals/0/Pdf/fssa_interim_regulation_on_Operatonalising_GM_Food_regulation_in_India.pdf., Accessed on 25 Dec 2017.

human genetic material.[36] "Commercial utilization" means end uses of biological resources for commercial use such as drugs, industrial enzymes, food flavours, fragrance, cosmetics, emulsifiers, oleoresins, colours, extracts and genes used for improving crops and livestock through genetic intervention[37]. The Act also created a new Institution by the name National Biodiversity Authority, whose prior approval has to obtain before using biological materials occurring in the country.

Regulatory Authorities of Genetically Modified Organisms

In India there are some regulatory authorities, which regulate and monitor the functioning of Genetically Modified Organisms in the country. They are:

1. Recombinant DNA Advisory Committee (RDAC)

This is constituted under the Department of Biotechnology, Ministry of Science and Technology, to recommend appropriate safety regulations in recombinant research, use and applications. The committee bears the responsibility of studying and reviewing the changes and developments made in the field of Biotechnology at national and international level. Consequently it renders apposite suggestions to enhance the safety regulation in the area of recombinant research and their applied utilities.[38]

2. Institutional Biosafety Committees (IBSC)

This committee is constituted under the Department of Biotechnology, Ministry of Science and Technology, to prepare site-specific plans for use of genetically engineered micro organisms. The duty of constituting IBSC lies with the institution which is conducting a research that includes the usage of even the smallest proportion of genetically modified organisms and even organism that are not natural to the local conditions. This committee needs to be comprised of the head of the parent institution directly invested in the research, the scientists hired by the institution for the genetic engineering of the organisms, at least one medical expert and one nominee of Department of Biotechnology. The parent institution is also required to prepare an up-to-date emergency procedure with the aid of IBSC which conforms to the guidelines of RCGM. It is also imbibed with the duty of providing copies of such a contingency plan and procedure to the District Level Committee and Genetic Engineering Approval Committee.[39]

3. Review Committee on Genetic Manipulation (RCGM)

This committee is constituted under the Department of Biotechnology, to monitor safety related aspects in respect of ongoing research projects and activities

---

36 Section 2 (c) of Biodiversity Act, 2002.

37 Section 2 (f) of Biodiversity Act, 2002. But this Section does not does not include conventional breeding or traditional practices in use in any agriculture, horticulture, poultry, dairy farming, animal husbandry or bee keeping.

38 Ahuja Vibha. An Update on Indian Biosafety Regulatory System. ilsirf.org/wp-content/uploads/sites/5/2016/06/V.Ahuja_.pdf., Accessed on 27 Dec 2017.

39 Supra Note 33, at 121-123.

involving genetically engineered organisms. It lays down procedures/regulations regarding research, production, sale, import and use of genetically engineered organisms with a view to ensure environment safety. This committee is concerned with the safety and precautionary aspects of research in genetic engineering. It also bears the responsibility of monitoring the products, field experiments, production, sale and shipment involving even a fraction of genetically engineered organisms and cells which are classified as so in schedule.

4. Genetic Engineering Approval Committee (GEAC)

The GEAC is a statutory body constituted under the Ministry of Environment and Forests (MoEF) and is empowered to approve or disapprove all large-scale use and environmental release of GM organisms. The GEAC is thus India's most powerful Biosafety policy gatekeeper. It is chaired by the additional secretary of MoEF and co-chaired by an expert nominee from the DBT, and it includes representatives from the DBT, the Ministry of Industrial Development, the Ministry of Science and Technology, and the Department of Ocean Development. The GEAC can authorize or prohibit, conditionally or unconditionally, the import, export, transport, manufacture, processing, use, or sale of any GM organism. [40]

5. State Biotechnology Coordination Committee (SBCC)

SBCC is constituted by the respective State Governments of India and acts as the state nodal agency monitoring and assessing the damage caused by the release of Genetically Modified Organism. SBCC in the States has the power to take punitive action in case of violations of safety after it has conducted an appropriate investigation. It has the additional power wherever necessary to inspect, investigate and control measures employed by industries and institutions in the handling of genetically engineered organisms.[41]

6. District Level Committee (DLC)

DLC is constituted in the districts wherever necessary under the District Collectors to monitor safety regulations in installations engaged in the use of genetically modified organisms and their applications in the environment. It is constituted in the districts where biotechnology projects are to be undertaken. Its authority is subject to SBCC. The committee's responsibility includes the checking of institution's compliance with the recombinant DNA guidelines and reporting the violations if any to SBCC and GEAC. It needs to co-ordinate the activities of concerned institution or industry to the effect that it becomes easier to contain emergency situations caused from accidental or even intentional discharge.

---

40 Supra Note 10, at 111-112.

41 Supra Note 38, at 13.

Section-3

Intellectual Property Rights and Genetically Modified Crops in India

"Trying to patent a human gene is like trying to patent a tree. You can patent a table that you build from a tree, but you cannot patent the tree itself"

William Haseltine-President, Human Genome Science

Intellectual Property Right Pertaining to Life Form

The life forms could not be patented before 1980. The decision of patenting life forms was initially influenced when in 1980 a US court allowed the patent in famous Chakraborty case.[42] Genetic engineer Ananda Mohan Chakrabarty, working for General Electric, had developed a bacterium capable of breaking down crude oil, which he proposed to use in treating oil spills. General Electric filed a patent application for the bacterium in the United States listing Chakrabarty as the inventor, but the application was rejected by a patent examiner, because under patent law at that time it was generally understood that living things were not patentable subject matter under Section 101 of Title 35 U.S.C.[43] The court ruled in favour of Chakrabarty, holding that: A live, human-made micro-organism is patentable subject matter. Respondent's micro-organism constitutes a "manufacture" or "composition of matter" within that statute. And this decision set the foot in the direction of towards the development of biotechnology throughout the world.[44]

A later patent issued for "Oncomouse" was another milestone in patenting of life form.[45]Among transgenic plants, herbicide resistant cotton, insect resistant tobacco and virus resistant potato have been patented. Bollworm resistant cotton has also been allowed patent protection. Transgenic plants and animals can be protected though patent claim in several countries including U.S.A, Japan, Europe, *etc.* In India after some debate, an agreement has been reached to accept the international practice of patenting life forms, if they fulfil the minimum requirements of invention that is novelty, non-obviousness and utility.[46]

According to Article 27(1) of Trade Related Aspects of Intellectual Property Rights, patent protection shall be available for any inventions, whether products or processes, in all fields of technology, provided that they are new, involve an inventive step and are capable of industrial application without any discrimination as to the place of invention, the field of technology and whether products are

---

42 Diamond v. Chakrabarty, 447 U.S. 303 (1980).

43 Stein Haley (2005). Intellectual Property and Genetically Modified Seeds: The United States, Trade, and the Developing World. North Western Journal of Technology and Intellectual Property, 3: 151.

44 Kevles Daniel J (1994). Ananda Chakrabarty Wins a Patent: Biotechnology, law, and Society 1972-1980. Historical studies in the physical and biological sciences. 25 (1): 111-35.

45 Harvard College v Canada (Commissioner of Patents) (2002) 4 SCR 45.

46 Supra Note 1, at 194.

imported or locally produced. This implies that the biotechnological inventions are patentable subject matter. Similarly, as per Article 27(3)(b) member countries may exclude from patentability plants and animals other than micro-organisms, and essentially biological processes for the production of plants or animals other than non-biological and microbiological processes.[47]

Protection of IP is very important in the field of biotechnology since biotech research is expensive, time consuming and results are uncertain. Patent gives an exclusive territorial right to the patentee to prevent others from making, using and selling a patented invention for a fixed period of time. Patent in biotechnology for micro-organism, vaccines, biological materials such as recombinant DNA, plasmids, processes of manufacturing such biological materials, provided they are produced by substantive human intervention, processes relating to micro-organisms or producing chemical substances using such micro-organisms.[48]

Biotech Patent and India

India is one of the first few countries to have its own patent law in place which was evolved on the basis of its socio and economic conditions. However after the advent of TRIPS, it becomes imperative for India to incorporate its essential provisions in its patent law. In the light of TRIPs laws, India has amended the Patent Act 1970, three times in a span of five years (that is between 1999 and 2005). The first amendment was made in 1999, then the second amendment in 2002 and the third amendment was brought about in December 2004, which came into force from 1st January 2005 to make patent act fully TRIPS compliant.[49]

The patenting of gene and DNA sequence is popular in USA, European Union and Japan. However patenting of gene and DNA sequences *per se* was not allowed in India until January 2005 but processes involving Recombinant DNA technology to produce protein involving a gene and DNA sequence was patentable subject matter. In 2005, however, by deleting Section 5 of Indian Patent Act 1970, the country significantly altered its patent regime in order to meet its obligations under TRIPS. The provision allowing only methods or processes of manufacture (as opposed to products) for certain classes of inventions to be patented was deleted, creating product patent protection in all fields of technology.[50] Patenting on DNA and gene sequence is a broad term which also includes genetically modified organism such as plant, animal, bacteria, fungi *etc.* Gene patenting is still a matter of concern to some, consider it as unethical because; gene are natural and therefore should not

---

47 Kawamura Satoko (2011). GMO Trade in the Context of TRIPS: From the Perspective of an Autopoietic System Analysis. Ritsumeikan International Affairs, 10: 252-253.

48 Supra Note 3, at 120.

49 Lakshmikumaran Malathi (2007). Patenting of Genetic Invention. Journal of Intellectual Property Right. 12: 50-52.

50 Bhattacharya Sujit (2007). Patenting in Biotechnology. DESIDOC Bulletin of Information Technology. 27: 31-39.

be owned by any individual or an organisation and gene are discoveries and not inventions and therefore not new. It is also argued that Gene isolation and cloning is such a well established technique that it no longer inventive to do it[51].

The *Dimminaco* case[52] opened the door of biotech patent in India. In 2002 Calcutta High Court made a historic judgment in this case which pertained to the patentability of 'living end-products of a biotechnological process'. Dimminaco A.G., a Swiss company, developed a live vaccine against Bursitis, an infectious poultry disease, and applied for patenting the process of its preparation. The Controller of Patents and Designs rejected the application on the bases of- end product containing a living material and its procedure of development being only a natural process. Conversely, on appeal, the Calcutta High Court concluded to accept the process of manufacturing as patentable, even if the end-product contained a living organism. This milestone decision paved way for the patentability of numerous such inventions containing living microorganisms. In Indian context, this ruling has helped flourish the Biotechnology Industry.

Naturally-occurring microorganisms are considered as discoveries and not inventions. These are therefore, not patentable in India. But patentable subject-matter includes Genetically Engineered Microorganisms (GEMs) that are characterized by- novelty, inventive step and industrial applicability. In order to get protection in microorganism, an inventor is required to deposit the strain of a microorganism in a recognised depository, which assigns a registration number to the deposited microorganism. This registration number needs to be quoted in the patent application dealing with the micro organism. There are many international depositories in different countries such as American Type Culture Collection (ATCC) and DSM *etc.* which are recognised under the Budapest Treaty. The Microbial Type Culture Collection (MTCC) at the institute of Microbial Technology (IMTEC), Chandigarh is the first Indian depository set up under the Budapest Treaty.[53]

In order to have better understanding of biotechnology patent in India it is necessary to evaluate patentable and non-patentable biological inventions. For a patent to be granted in India the invention should not be covered in the negative list in Section 3 of Patent Act.[54] According to Section 3 of Patent Act 1970, as amended in 2002 and 2005; following are not inventions within the meaning of this Act:

1. The living entities of natural origin such as animals, plants, in whole or parts thereof, plant varieties, seeds, species, genes and microorganisms are not patentable.

---

51 Kumar Jidesh. (2004). Biotechnology Patenting. Journal of Intellectual Property Right. 12: 475-476.

52 Dimminaco A.G. V. Controller of Patents And Designs and Others, IPLR 2002 July. 255.

53 Rai U.N, and Singh N.K (2010). Intellectual Property Right in Biodiversity Conservation, Biotechnology Transfer and Environmental Sustainability. In Kumar Aravind and Das Govind (ed). Biodiversity, Biotechnology and Traditional Knowledge: Understanding Intellectual Property Rights. 1st Edition, Narosa Publishing House, New Delhi.

54 Kumar K Suresh (2007).The Current Indian Patent Regime and the Scope of Protection in Agricultural Biotechnology: Some Issues and Considerations. Journal of Intellectual Property Right.12: 341-348.

2. Any process of manufacture or production relating to such living entities is also not patentable.
3. Any method of treatment such as medicinal, surgical, curative, prophylactic, diagnostic and therapeutic of animals or other treatments of similar nature are not patentable.
4. Any living entity of artificial origin such a transgenic animals and plants, any part thereof are not patentable.
5. Biological materials such as organs, tissues, cells, virus *etc.* and process of preparing thereof are not patentable under section 3(c).
6. Gene sequences, DNA sequences without having disclosed their functions are not patentable for lack of inventive step and industrial application.
7. Essentially biological processes for production of plants and animals such as method of crossing or breeding *etc.* are not patentable.
8. Any biological material and the method of making the same which is capable of causing serious prejudice to human, animal or plant lives or health or to the environment including the use of those would be contrary to public order and morality are not patentable, such as terminator gene technology.
9. The processes for cloning human beings or animals, processes for modifying the germ line, genetic identity of human beings or animals, use of human or animal embryos for any purpose are not patentable as they are against public order and morality.
10. Any invention which is in effect is traditional knowledge or which is an aggregation or duplication of known properties of traditionally known components is not patentable. [55]

However, various genetically engineered microorganisms for an array of specific uses, such as biodegrades, bio-stimulants, bio-protectants, *etc.* and the processes related to their application and use. The biological material such a recombinant DNA, plasmids and processes of manufacturing thereof are patentable provided they are produced by substantive human intervention. There are three basic requirements for an invention under Indian Patent Law. They are:

1. It should be new (Novelty)
2. It should involve an inventive step (Non-Obviousness)
3. It should be capable of industrial application

Novelty

Novelty is the first requirement that needs to be fulfilled. Section 2(1)(j) of the Indian Patent Act requires the invention to be new, that it must be different from "prior art". That is, it should not have been published anywhere in the world

55 Supra Note 3, at 118.

before the date of filing of the application. In addition, subject to certain exceptions provided in the Patent Acts of the countries concerned, it should not have been publically used or demonstrated before filing. This signifies that the work that requires patent protection should not form a part of public domain, prior to the filing of patent application.

The criterion of novelty with regard to genes and gene products is easily met, since they are considered chemical entities, and these can be patented in most patent offices, if they are purified and isolated from the form in which they occur in nature. In most countries, a claimed gene is considered novel if the claim covers the isolated and purified gene. The applicant must be able to prove that the existence of gene was not known and that he was the first to isolate it, characterise it and define its utility.

Non-obviousness

An Invention is non-obvious if that would not have been entirely obvious to a person skilled in the field to have created the invention taking into account the current state of knowledge in that field. Non obvious in the field of biotechnology patents is a fact-intensive determination where potential success in experimentation and new properties of the invention carry significant weight. An invention in biotechnology is obvious if the prior art provides motivation for the invention and enables one of the skill in the art to invent with "reasonable expectation of success".[56] In 1996, the Supreme Court in *Graham* v. *John Deere Co*[57] articulated four factors to determine non obviousness. The four factors include: (1) The scope and content of the prior art, (2) the difference between the prior art and the claimed invention, (3) the level of ordinary skill in the art; and (4) other secondary considerations. Secondary considerations may include commercial success; long felt but unsolved need; unexpected result; other's failure to solve the same problem.

Utility

In biotechnology patent also the inventions must have some utilities. The exclusive patent rights may be granted only where an appropriate level of concrete and practical use of the biotechnological invention is disclosed in the patent application. The examination guidelines for patent applications relating to inventions in the field of chemicals, pharmaceuticals and biotechnology states that gene sequence and DNA sequences are not patentable, if the functions and the utility of the genetic inventions are not disclosed.[58] A utility to support a claim for a DNA sequence must be specific, substantial, and credible.

Apart from these basic requirements, if any biological material is used in an invention, the source or geographical origin of such material is required to be mention in the specification.

---

56 In re O'Farrell, 853 F 2d 894.

57 383 US 1 (1996).

58 Annexure 1, Manual of Patent Practice and Procedure, Patent office (2005), India.

In respect to patent on genetically modified crops in India, the first name that comes for consideration is the Monsanto. Monsanto is an American multinational corporation known for its contribution to the field of genetically modified crops around the world. In India, Monsanto sells a genetically modified version of cotton seeds known as Bt Cotton and marketed as Bollgard and Bollgard-II through their Indian counterpart MMBL. BT cotton is claimed to contain an insecticidal protein, whose gene has been derived from a soil bacterium called Bacillus thuringiensis (Bt), making the seed resistant to bollworm attacks.[59] Monsanto was first granted a patent for the first version of their Bt cotton seed, Bollgard in the United States in 1992, which expired in 2012. In India, Monsanto tied up with Mahyco to import Bollgard. The Genetic Engineering Appraisal Committee (GEAC) gave Monsanto permission to commercially release Bollgard in 2002 and Bollgard II in 2006. Monsanto claimed that Bollgard II is resistant against American bollworm, pink bollworm and spotted bollworm. Through Indian Patent application no 1947/CHENP/2003, Monsanto was granted a patent (Patent No 232681) for the cottonseed on March 20, 2009 with effect from June 5, 2002. This has become possible since microbiological processes (such as methods of creating transgenic varieties) and microorganisms (such as new and inventive transgenes and their constructs) are patentable under the terms of the Indian Patents Act.[60]

But presently Monsanto is facing legal challenges on price at which Bt cotton seeds are sold to the public. The patentability of Monsanto's Bt cottonseeds, sold as Bollgard II is facing challenges at present as the cottonseeds are allegedly no longer function as claimed in its specification. The present issue has opened up the possibility that the patent may be revoked under Section 64(1) (g) of patent Act for being not useful.[61]

Conclusions and Suggestions

Genetic engineering and its application in agriculture especially in the context of India, where majority of population depends on agriculture as a mainstay for livelihood, involve too many questions. Genetically modified crops are those which have been altered genetically for several reasons. Those reasons might include reducing the maturation time of the plant, increasing nutrients, yields, and stress tolerance, and creating a plant that can withstand diseases, and heavier applications of pesticides and herbicides. A conflict is going on between the supporters and opponents of the Genetically Modified Crops.One cannot deny the fact that the population is growing in an alarming rate which need to be fed and the agricultural area is decreasing day by day. Genetic engineering has outstanding potential to increase the efficiency of crop and therefore, genetically modified crops can prove to be a boon in such situation. In combination with conventional technologies,

---

59 Arya Shishir, and Shrivastav Snehlata (2015, June 8). Bt cotton patent. The Times of India.

60 Basheer Shamnad (2016, October 4). The battle over Bt cotton.The Hindu.

61 Deshpande Vivek (2016, March 8). Monsanto patent under cloud as Bt cotton prone to pink bollworm. The Indian Express.

transgenic crops could not only boost global food production in a sustainable way but could also significantly contribute to increase the income of rural poor.[62] GM crops bring about environmental and health benefits. GM crops may also be suited for small scale farmers, because such seed technologies are scale neutral. But at the same time public concern is also growing about the health hazards such as cancers, nutritional problems, allergens, and environmental risks such as unintended transfer of genetic effects through cross-pollination to native plants, the unknown effects on other organisms *e.g.*, beneficial insects, soil microbes, and the loss of plant and animal biodiversity which GMCs carries with them. Moreover, no mandate for labelling of GMFs is a big concern amongst the consumers basically for those who are very much concern about their ethical and religious values.[63]

A responsible management of biotechnology is a prerequisite to achieve desired goals and it requires sound regulations for bio- safety and food safety wherever transgenic crops are to be developed and released. But safety measures should be based on science rather than opinion. However it is to be remembered that overregulation will also become a real threat for further development and use of GM crops. The costs of regulation in terms of foregone benefits may be large, especially for developing countries. This is not to say zero regulation would be desirable, but the trade-offs associated with regulation should be considered. In the public arena, the risks of GM crops seem to be overrated, while the benefits are underrated. Government has an important role to play in finding ways to maximise the net social benefits. More work is needed to quantify possible indirect effects of GM crops, including socio economic outcomes as well as environmental and health impacts.[64] Since many developing countries still lack the scientific and financial requirements, international cooperation could play an important role in building related capacities. The public discussion, however, often overemphasises the risks of transgenic crops, whether true or perceived, without taking sufficient account of the technology advantages. Risks should always be juxtaposed to the potential benefits and certain residual risks appear tolerable if they are offset by much higher benefit prospects. A completely risk- free technology does not exist. The application of transgenic crops now remains concentrated only in some richer countries. The main reasons for the developing countries' limited access to biotechnology are insufficient scientific and regulatory capacities, combined with the increasing privatisation of agricultural research and the international proliferation of IPRs.[65]

At international level in order to regulate inventions involving the use of GMOs, there are various treaties, conventions and protocols. Such as, The Budapest

---

62 Wu, Felicia and Butz, William P (2004). The Future of Genetically Modified Crops: Lessons From The Green Revolution.RAND Corporation, USA.

63 Qaim Matin (2009). The Economics of Genetically Modified Crops. Annual Review of Resource Economics, 1: 665-693.

64 Plahe Jagjit Kaur (2009). The Implications of India's Amended Patent Regime: sTRIPping Away Food Security and Farmers' Rights?.Third World Quarterly, 30: 1197-1213.

65 Qaim Matin (2001). Transgenic Crops and Developing Countries. Economic and Political Weekly, 36: 3064-3070.

Treaty on the International Recognition of the Deposit of Micro-organisms for the Purposes of Patent Procedure, 1977, The Convention on Biological Diversity, 1992, The Cartagena Protocol on Bio-safety, 2000, The Nagoya Protocol on Access to Genetic Resources and Equitable Sharing of Benefits, 2010, The World Trade Organization Agreements *etc.* In India, there is no specific legislation to regulate the issues related to Genetically Modified Organism. It is the combination of various legislations, rules and regulations, which are made applicable according to the need of the case. There is need for specific law to deal with this aspect of biotechnology and an independent authority to decide issues related to this aspect.

In India issues relating to genetically modified crops are not smooth but confusing. There is a need to stream line the same with necessary adjustment in existing laws. Arguments both for and against the cultivation and use of the GM crops are varied and there is a wide consensus that assessment should take place on a case-by-case basis before genetically modified food is brought to the market. These assessments should be done by Government or an independent credible regulatory authority or private agencies and these should not be driven by any commercial interests. Moreover, educating public opinion is also very important as food is always a sensitive cultural issue. Merely indicating whether a product is genetically modified or not, without providing any additional vital information, would not serve any purpose; rather information on its content and possible risks or benefits should be provided.

To sum up in the words of Food and Agriculture Organisation (FAO):

"Science cannot declare any technology completely risk free. Genetically engineered crops can reduce some environmental risks associated with conventional agriculture, but will also introduce new challenges that must be addressed. Society will have to decide when and where genetic engineering is safe enough".

References

Books

1. Herring Ronald J. (2015). The Oxford Hand Book of Food, Politics, And Society. Oxford University Press, United Kingdom.
2. Kumar Aravind, and Das Govind (2010). Biodiversity, Biotechnology and Traditional Knowledge: Understanding Intellectual Property Rights, Narosa Publishing House, New Delhi.
3. Luke Anderson(2000).Genetic Engineering, Food and Our Environment. Resurgence Books, United Kingdom.
4. Mahgoub Salah E. O (2015). Genetically Modified Foods: Basics, Applications, and Controversy. CRC Press Taylor and Francis group.
5. Paarlberg Robert L (2001). The Politics of Precaution Genetically Modified Crops in Developing Countries. Johns Hopkins University Press, Baltimore and London.

6. Smith J. (1996). Biotechnology. Cambridge University Press, United Kingdom.
7. Smith Jeffrey (2003). Seeds of Deception: Exposing Industry and Government Lies about the Safety of the Genetically Engineered Foods You're Eating. Yes! Book Publication, Fairfield, Iowa.
8. Sreenivasulu N.S., and Raju C.B (2001). Biotechnology and Patent Law: Patenting Living Beings. Manupatra, Noida.
9. Wu, Felicia and Butz, William P (2004). The Future Of Genetically Modified Crops: Lessons From The Green Revolution.RAND Corporation, USA.

CHAPTERS IN BOOK

1. Elena Grigore M. *et al.* (2017). Approved Genetically Engineered Foods: Types, Properties and Economic Concerns. In: Holban Alina Maria, and Grumezescu Alexandru Mihai(ed.) Genetically Engineered Food, 1st Edition, Academic Press, USA.
2. Harriss John, and Stewart Drew (2015). Science, Politics, and the Framing of Modern Agricultural Technologies. In: Herring Ronald J. (ed.) The Oxford Hand Book of Food, Politics, And Society, 1st edn. Oxford University Press, United Kingdom.
3. Rai U.N, and Singh N.K(2010). Intellectual Property Right in Biodiversity Conservation, Biotechnology Transfer and Environmental Sustainability. In Kumar Aravind and Das Govind (ed). Biodiversity, Biotechnology and Traditional Knowledge: Understanding Intellectual Property Rights. 1st Edition, Narosa Publishing House, New Delhi.
4. Saraswat Darpan (2010). Biotech Patents and Questions of Patentability in India and Abroad. In: Kumar Aravind, and Das Govind (ed.) Biodiversity, Biotechnology and Traditional Knowledge: Understanding Intellectual Property Rights, 1st edn. Narosa Publishing House, New Delhi.
5. Shukla U.K *et al.* (2010). Intellectual property Right: A Prospective Approach towards Conservation of Biodiversity and Promotion of Biotechnology. In: Kumar Aravind, and Das Govind (ed.) Biodiversity, Biotechnology and Traditional Knowledge: Understanding Intellectual Property Rights, 1st edn. Narosa Publishing House, New Delhi.

Articles

1. Bhattacharya Sujit (2007). Patenting in Biotechnology. DESIDOC Bulletin of Information Technology.Vol.27.
2. Caswell Julie A(2000). Labeling Policy For GMOs: To Each His Own?. Journal of AgroBiotechnology Management and Economics, Vol.3.
3. Choudhary Bhagirath *et al.* (2004). Regulatory options for genetically modified crops in India. Plant Biotechnology Journal, Vol.12.
4. Gahukar R.T (2003). Issues Relating to the Patentability of Biotechnological Subject Matter in Indian Agriculture. Journal of Intellectual Property Right, Vol.8.

5. Jha Bhuvan Bhaskar, and Shankar Ashutosh (2017). Evaluating the Law on Regulation of Genetically Modified Crops in India. Jamia Law Review, Vol.2.
6. Kawamura Satoko (2011). GMO Trade in the Context of TRIPS: From the Perspective of an Autopoietic System Analysis. Ritsumeikan International Affairs, Vol.10.
7. Kevles Daniel J(1994). Ananda Chakrabarty Wins a Patent: Biotechnology, law, and Society 1972-1980. Historical studies in the physical and biological sciences. Vol. 25 Issue 1.
8. Kowalski Stanley (2007). Rational Risk/Benefits Analysis of Genetically Modified Crops.Journal of Intellectual Property Rights, Vol.12.
9. Kumar Jidesh.(2004). Biotechnology Patenting. Journal of Intellectual Property Right. Vol.12.
10. Kumar K Suresh (2007).The Current Indian Patent Regime and the Scope of Protection in Agricultural Biotechnology: Some Issues and Considerations. Journal of Intellectual Property Right.Vol.12.
11. Lakshmikumaran Malathi (2007). Patenting of Genetic Invention. Journal of Intellectual Property Right.Vol.12.
12. Plahe Jagjit Kaur (2009). The Implications of India's Amended Patent Regime: sTRIPping Away Food Security and Farmers' Rights?.Third World Quarterly, Vol. 30.
13. Qaim Matin (2009). The Economics of Genetically Modified Crops. Annual Review of Resource Economics,Vol.1.
14. Qaim Matin(2001). Transgenic Crops and Developing Countries. Economic and Political Weekly, Vol.36.
15. Sharma V.K (2011). Genetically Modified Food and Consumers Interest: Some Legal and Ethical Issues, RGNUL Law Review, Vol.1.
16. Sloan A.E, and Powers M.E (1986). A Perspective on Popular Perspectives of Adverse Reactions to Foods. Journal of Allergy and Clinical Immunology, Vol.78.
17. Stein Haley(2005). Intellectual Property and Genetically Modified Seeds: The United States, Trade, and the Developing World. North Western Journal of Technology and Intellectual Property, Vol.3.

Internet Sources

1. Ahuja Vibha, and Jotwani Geeta (2007). The Regulation of Genetically Modified Organisms in India. file:///C:/Users/hp/Downloads/05-265-003[1].pdf.
2. Ahuja Vibha. An Update on Indian Biosafety Regulatory System. ilsirf.org/wp-content/uploads/sites/5/2016/06/V.Ahuja_.pdf.
3. Azevedo Sophia (2015). Labeling GMO Foods. https://www.scribd.com/doc/293489592/research-paper.

4. Bhattacharya Sanjukta (2013). Indian Response to Genetically Modified Food and Labelling. file:///C:/Users/hp/Downloads/SSRN-id2228786.pdf.

5. Chopra Paras, and Kamma Akhil. Genetically Modified Crops in India. http://www.deskuenvis.nic.in/pdf/gm.pdf.

6. Food Safety and Standards Authority of India. Operationalising the Regulation of Genetically Modified Foods in India. http://www.old.fssai.gov.in/Portals/0/Pdf/fssa_interim_regulation_on_Operatonalising_GM_Food_regulation_in_India.pdf.

7. GreenPeace. The Biotechnology Regulatory Authority of India (BRAI) Bill 2011 – The Bill to end the right to safe food!. http://www.greenpeace.org/india/Global/india/report/brai per cent 20 per cent 20critique.

8. Indian Council of Medical Research(2004). Regulatory Regimen for Genetically Modified Foods the Way Ahead. http://icmr.nic.in/reg_regimen.pdf.

9. Kumar Sanjay(2015). India eases stance on GM crop trials. https://www.nature.com/news/india-eases-stance-on-gm-crop-trials-1.17529.

10. Qaim Matin (2010). The Benefits of Genetically Modified Crops—and the Costs of Inefficient Regulation.http://www.rff.org/blog/2010/benefits-genetically-modified-crops-and-costs-inefficient-regulation.

11. Ramanna Anitha. India's Policy on Genetically Modified Crops. Asia Research Center Working Paper 15.http://www.lse.ac.uk/asiaResearchCentre/_files/ARCWP15-Ramanna.pdf.

12. Sahai Suman (2010). Potential of agricultural genetic engineering for food security in India: Research on transgenic food crops. http://genecampaign.org/wp-content/uploads/2014/07/Potential_Of_Agricultural_Genetic_Engineering_For_Food_Security_In_India.pdf

13. Whitman Deborah B (2000). Genetically Modified Foods: Harmful or Helpful. https://www.sandiegounified.org/schools/sites/default/files_link/schools/files/Domain/8628/GMO.pdf.

14. Walker Shawn(2016). Beet"ing the Controversy. https://www.scribd.com/document/364719201/gmo-crops-research-pape

News Paper Articles

1. Basheer Shamnad (2016, October 4). The battle over Bt cotton.The Hindu.

2. Deshpande Vivek (2016, March 8). Monsanto patent under cloud as Bt cotton prone to pink bollworm. The Indian Express.

3. Arya Shishir, and Shrivastav Snehlata (2015, June 8). Bt cotton patent. The Times of India.

Chapter 8

Patenting in IITs: An Empirical Study

Mayuree Sengupta

Intellectual Property Manager, Regional Centre for Biotechnology, Faridabad - 121 001 Haryana (NCR Delhi), India
e-mail: mayuree1sengupta@gmail.com

ABSTRACT

Intellectual property, if properly managed, is one of the greatest assets to leverage in a postindustrial society. A country like India, with her National IPR Policy aiming to incentivise and promote R&D with respect to intellectual property, needs to emphasise at the core place of learning i.e. the universities. The level of transfer of knowledge from universities and R&D institutions and its utilization for the creation of national wealth is sub optimal. However, the elite Indian Institute of Technology institutions have not only been involved in technology research but also invested in patenting and licensing endeavours. In the literature, several authors have analysed different aspects of IP but not delved into present topic of interest. This study aims to investigate the quintessential of IP narratives in IITs, with respect to various technological domains and also find successful examples of invention, patenting and commercialisation integration vide cases studies. The proposed chapter comprises a reflection on patent scenario in specifically the older IITs.

Objective of Study: (i) To examine the IP viz. patent landscape in the IITs and assess the patenting trends. (ii) To evaluate matters pertinent to commercialization of patents viz. licensing. (iii) To portray vide novel case studies the successful examples of invention, patenting and commercialisation integration.

Methodology: The study is based on a combination of primary and secondary research. The methodology adopted includes a detailed study from various sources. The primary sources of study mainly comprise technology, assignee and key-word dependent patent search and analysis, multi-jurisdictional patent office listed information along with licensing information. Secondary sources encompass regulations, existing laws and jurisprudence, industry white papers, relevant literature and other applicable resources and guides.

Research Gap: No germane references could be found in the literature although different facets of IP have been studied previously. No citation related to IP narratives in IITs could be ascertained.

Data Analysis: Data was analysed both qualitatively and quantitatively.

Keywords: *IITs, national IPR policy, patent, commercialization*

Introduction

Intellectual property[1], if properly managed, is one of the greatest assets to leverage in a post industrial society[2]. A country like India, with her National IPR Policy aiming to incentivise and promote R&D with respect to intellectual property, needs to emphasise at the core place of learning *i.e.* the universities. The level of transfer of knowledge from universities and R&D institutions and its utilization for the creation of national wealth is sub optimal. However, the elite Indian Institute of Technology institutions, autonomous public institutes of higher education that were declared as institutions of national importance, have not only been involved in technology research but also invested in patenting and licensing endeavours.

In the literature, several authors have analysed different aspects of IP but not delved into present topic of interest. This study aims to investigate the quintessential of IP narratives in IITs, with respect to various technological domains and also find successful examples of invention, patenting and commercialisation integration vide cases studies. The proposed paper comprises a reflection on patent scenario in the older IITs, specifically IIT Kharagpur, IIT Delhi, IIT Madras, and IIT Bombay.

Objective of Study

The study has the following objectives:

- To examine the IP *viz.* patent landscape in the IITs and assess the patenting trends.
- To evaluate matters pertinent to commercialization of patents *viz.* licensing
- To portray vide novel case studies the successful examples of invention, patenting and commercialisation integration.

Methodology

The study is based on a combination of primary and secondary research. The methodology adopted includes a detailed study from various sources. The primary sources of study mainly comprise technology, assignee and key-word dependent patent search and analysis, multi jurisdictional patent office listed information along with licensing information. Secondary sources encompass regulations, existing laws and jurisprudence, industry white papers, relevant literature and other applicable resources and guides.

---

1 Intellectual property refers to creations of the mind: inventions; literary and artistic works; and symbols, names and images used in commerce. Excerpt from WIPO document available at http://www.wipo.int/edocs/pubdocs/en/intproperty/450/wipo_pub_450.pdf, accessed 5th April 2018.

2 French sociologist Alain Touraine and American sociologist Daniel Bell were notable in coining and popularizing the term post industrial. It refers to the stage of society's development when the service sector generates more wealth than the manufacturing sector of the economy.

Research Gap

No germane references could be found in the literature although different facets of IP have been studied previously. No citation related to IP narratives in IITs could be ascertained.

Data Analysis

Data was analysed both qualitatively and quantitatively.

Innovation in IITs vis-à-vis Patent Landscape

The IITs albeit offering multi-disciplinary courses has its core firmly entrenched in technology and engineering domains. The innovations made in the laboratories are not let dormant but directed towards intellectual property protection and technology transfer vide licensing mechanisms finally leading to scale-up and commercial usage.

IIT Kharagpur

The oldest IIT in India, IIT Kharagpur has earned a moniker not only as a leading tech institute but has also been awarded for 'Top Academic Institute for Patents 2016' by Government of India. Credit for this recognition could be partly attributed to the novel '100 Days, 100 Patents' drive which IIT Kharagpur had initiated in 2012 to promote the spirit of research and patenting amongst its students. This drive majorly aimed at facilitating research practices on campus along with educating the students, professors and research scholars about Intellectual Property especially the process and merits of patenting. IPR activity is managed under the aegis of Intellectual Property Rights and Industrial Relations (IPR and IR) Cell which is responsible for the licensing and the transfer of technologies developed by researchers at the institute to the commercial sector.[3] The IPR policy, which is not available publicly, is reviewed internally and with stakeholders.

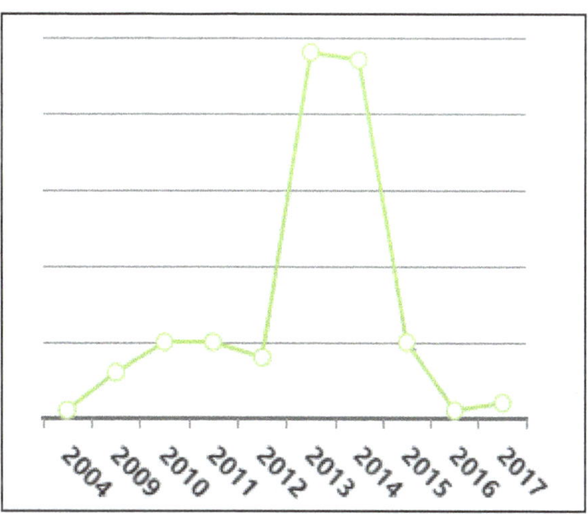

Figure 8.1: Patent Filing Pattern in IIT Kharagpur.

An applicant based search by author reveals that IIT Kharagpur has approximately 152 active applications and granted patents across jurisdictions.[4]

---

3 IIT Kharagpur IP Policy, http://www.iitkgp.ac.in/industry-ip-policy, accessed on 1 May, 2018.

4 This number includes PCT applications as national phase entry cannot be ascertained individually in all instances.

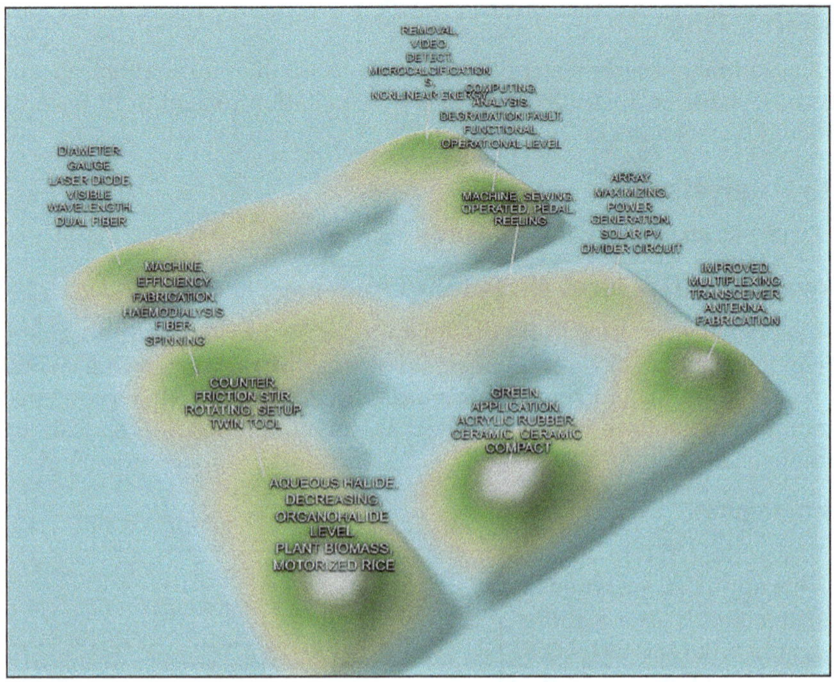

Figure 8.2: Prime Patent Landscape for IIT Kharagpur.

This number does not include unpublished, or abandoned or withdrawn patent applications or expired patents. Of these, 30 have been successfully passed through technology transfer stages and assigned to industry-academia partners. This is an accomplishment of 20 per cent successful licensing and can be considered as a start as per Indian standards. Of the total active applications, 34 belong to the genre of biological sciences, ranging from biotechnology and nanotechnology to food sciences. However, only a couple of these had been assigned to the Department of Biotechnology, Government of India. There is prima facie diminutive industry alliance available in public domain for biological science based innovations.

IIT Delhi

IIT Delhi not only has a rich innovation culture but also a distinctive bioincubator that supports and encourages innovation environment. With an IPR policy[5] guideline dating back to 1994, IIT Delhi's Foundation for Innovation and Technology Transfer (FITT) is responsible for evaluation of technology and also provides necessary administrative umbrella for IPR protection. It attempts to identify potential market and facilitate technology transfer so that the intellectual property created at the institute gets disseminated to the industry and end users through production and marketing. The stated objective purpose of processing commercialization by Indian Institute of Technology Delhi, which is a non-profit organization, is to

5 IIT Delhi IP Policy, http://ird.iitd.ac.in/policy/IPRPolicy-IITD.pdf, accessed on 1 May, 2018.

meet one of its stated objectives of disseminating the fruits of research and development for the benefit of public and society.

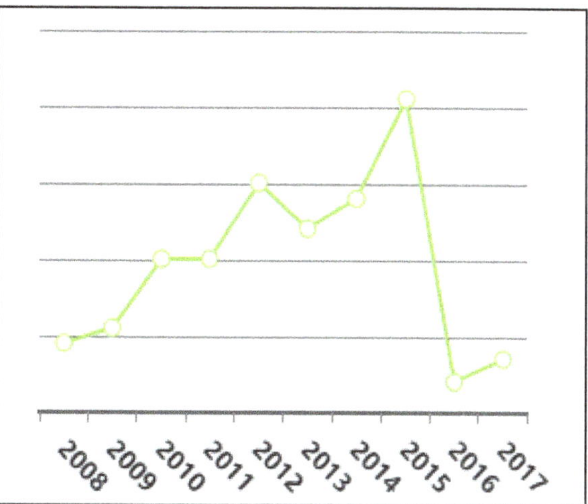

Figure 8.3: Patent Filing Pattern in IIT Delhi.

An applicant based search by author reveals that IIT Delhi has approximately 276 active applications and granted patents across jurisdictions.[6] This number does not include unpublished, or abandoned or withdrawn patent applications or expired patents. Of these, 63 have been successfully passed through technology transfer stages and assigned to industry-academia partners. This is an accomplishment of 23 per cent successful licensing and decent by Indian standards. Of the total active applications, 87 belong to the genre of biological sciences, ranging from biotechnology and nanotechnology to pharma and diagnostic kits. However, these had been jointly owned with IIT Limited, AIIMS; Department of Biotechnology, Government of India; Delhi University; Panacea Limited; Central Council for Research in Aurveda and Siddha, Resil Chemicals, DRDO, Amity University *etc.* There is no significant industry alliance prima facie available in public domain for biological science based innovations.

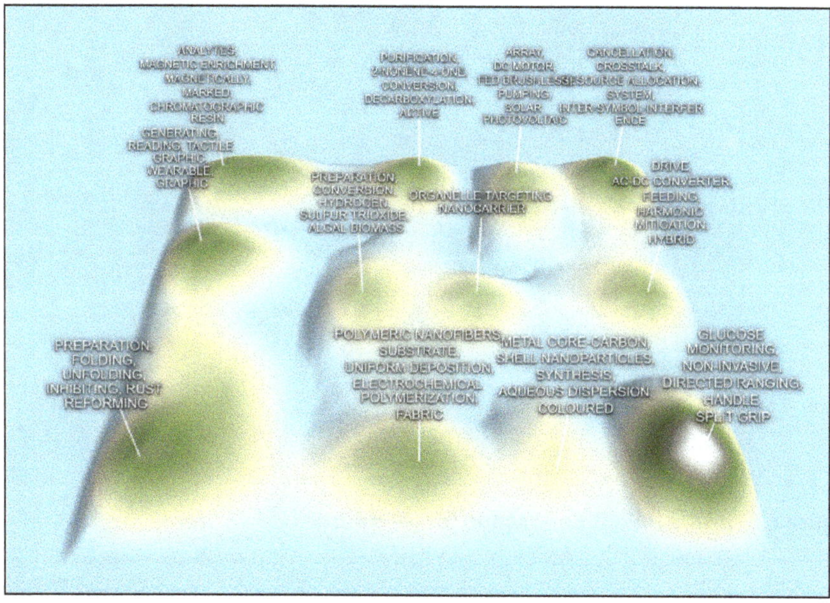

Figure 8.4: Prime Patent Landscape for IIT Delhi.

---

6 *Ibid* 3.

IIT Madras

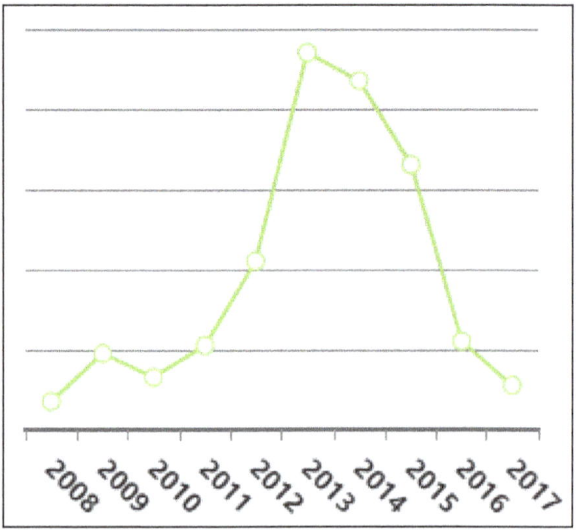

Centre for IC and SR is the nodal agency of IIT Madras for processing all IPR related matters.[7] The objective of the institute's IP Policy is to protect legitimate interests of faculty, scholars, students and the society, and to avoid conflict of interest scenarios. The patent cell of IC and SR is responsible for evaluating, protecting, marketing, licensing and managing the IP generated at the Institute.[8]

Figure 8.5: Patent Filing Pattern in IIT Madras.

An applicant based search by author reveals that IIT Madras has approximately 404 active applications and granted patents across jurisdictions.[9] This number does not include unpublished, or abandoned or withdrawn patent

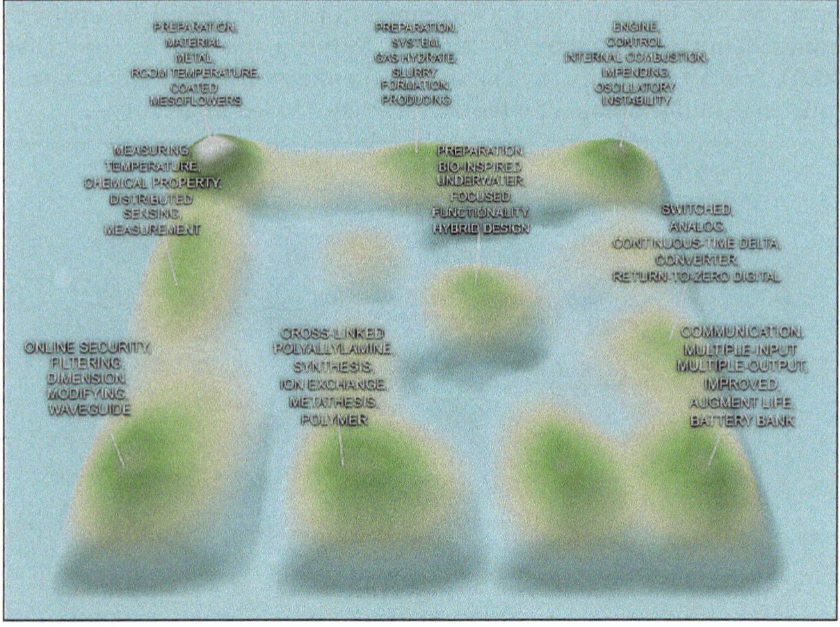

Figure 8.6: Prime Patent Landscape for IIT Madras.

7 IIT Madras IP Information, https://icsr.iitm.ac.in/admin/upload/forms/1428922150.pdf, accessed on 1 May, 2018.

8 IIT Madras IP Policy, https://icsris.iitm.ac.in/ipr/news/IPR per cent 20policy.pdf, accessed on 1 May, 2018.

9 *Ibid* 3.

applications or expired patents. Of these, 88 have been successfully passed through technology transfer stages and assigned to industry-academia partners. This is an accomplishment of 22 per cent successful licensing and similar to previous one. Of the total active applications, 69 belong to the genre of biological sciences, ranging from biotechnology and nanotechnology to pharma and diagnostic domain. However, these had been jointly owned with University of California, Aquamall Water Solutions Ltd, CSIR, Malladi Drugs and Pharmaceuticals Limited, Trivitro Healthcare Private Limited, Sundaram Medical Foundation, Purdue Research Foundation, Centre for Cellular and Molecular Platforms (C-CAMP). IIT Madras shows better and divergent industry alliance compared to others for biological science based innovations.

IIT Bombay

The IP Policy[10] of IIT Bombay, in vogue since 2003, entails recognition of the importance of innovations and assists in translating them into products, processes and services for both commercial benefits and achieving the widest public good. The IP Policy of IIT Bombay is segregated into two primary sub policies relating to inventions (relates to patent, design, layout, trademark, bio diversity and related rights) and expressions (for the Copyright and related rights).

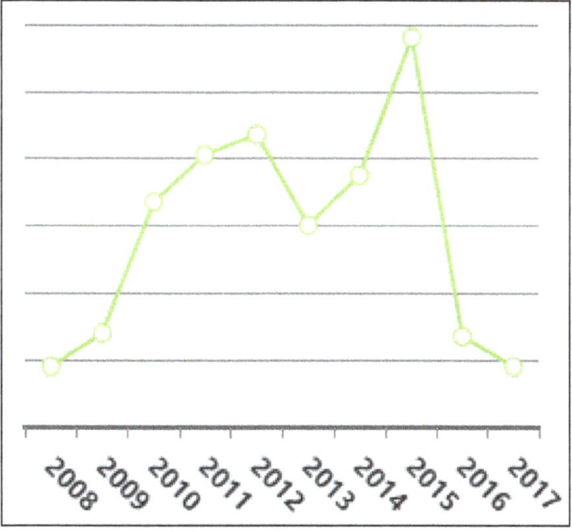

Figure 8.7: Patent Filing Pattern in IIT Bombay.

An applicant based search by author reveals that IIT Bombay has approximately 500 active applications and granted patents across jurisdictions.[11] This number does not include unpublished, or abandoned or withdrawn patent applications or expired patents. Of these, as per patent search results, 57 have been successfully passed through technology transfer stages and assigned to industry-academia partners. This is an accomplishment of 12 per cent successful licensing. Of the total active applications, 112 belong to the genre of biological sciences, ranging from biotechnology and nanotechnology to pharma and biofuels. However, these had been jointly owned with Nanyang Technological University, Embio Limited, Yeda Research And Development Co. Ltd., Ariel-University Research And Development Company Ltd., Tata Memorial Centre,

---

10 IIT Bombay IP Policy, https://www.ircc.iitb.ac.in/IRCC-Webpage/rnd/IITB_IP_Policy2012.jsp, accessed on 1 May, 2018.

11 *Ibid* 3.

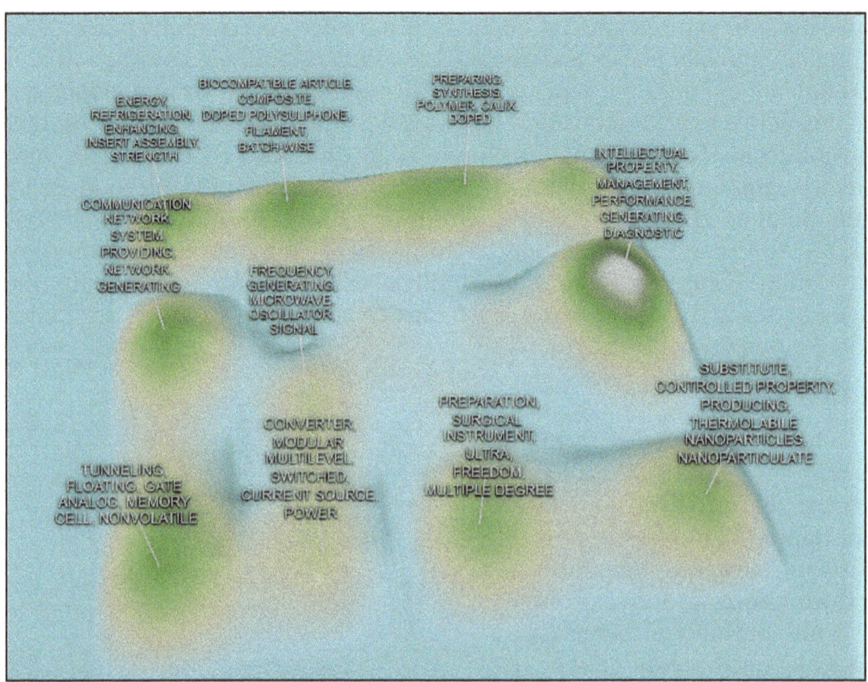

Figure 8.8: Prime Patent Landscape for IIT Bombay.

Colgate-Palmolive Company, Tata Consultancy Services Ltd., Indian Council Of Medical Research, Samsung Electronics Co. Ltd., National Institute Of Immunology, Department Of Biotechnology, Bigtec Private Limited, Tata Consulting Engineers Limited. IIT Bombay shows so far best and localised industry alliance compared to others for biological science based innovations.

Commercialization Case Studies

It is essential that any patentable invention be analyzed for its industrial relevance and commercial potential. There is nothing prima facie novel in conceptualizing innovations, applying for intellectual property protection and technology transfer for commercial production. However, the way this well known procedure is planned and implemented determines the effectiveness and triumph of the patent narrative. The following instances aptly depict that whichever be the route, adequately exploiting expensive innovation is requisite.

Water Treatment by Nanotechnology Patents Case

Professor T. Pradeep from the Department of Chemistry, Indian Institute of Technology, Madras was involved in water treatment research which was initially funded by the Nano Mission of the Central government. He then formed a company, InnoNano Research Private Limited, started as a start-up at IIT Madras Incubation Cell in 2008 and now an independent company. The product, water filter, Amrit (Arsenic and Metal Removal), is installed in 750 locations in West Bengal, Uttar

Pradesh, Bihar and Karnataka providing arsenic-free drinking water at nominal cost to nearly 500,000 people. It is based on gravity and functions without electricity or running water. The company signed agreement with Nanoholdings based in Connecticut, U.S. in 2016 wherein Nanoholdings would provide Indian team venture funding of $18 million to further develop its nanomaterials-based water technology.

The IIT Madras patents based on application of nanotechnology to water treatment that had been licensed to Nanoholdings number to 14 granted and/or pending Indian patent applications; 8 PCT applications and national phase entry in 16 countries.[12] Stakes at Inno Nano Incubator stand at IIT Madras funds amounting to Rs. 15 Lakh while Nanoholdings contributing Rs 5 crore. Licencing and royalty revenue is estimated at Rs. 1 crore. The valuation of the company is estimated at Rs. 250 crore where IIT Madras holds 5 per cent stake.

This is a robust example of invention, patenting and commercialisation integration that has been developed indigenously and received venture funding later on.

Alpha Amylase[13] and Biomethane[14] Production Patents Case

The novel process for developing α-Amylase technology developed by Professor Rintu Banerjee from Department of Agricultural and Food Engineering department of IIT Kharagpur[15] comprises production of enzyme that potentially boosts efficiency of cereals/grains based 1G ethanol production including some other promising industrial applications. Instead of following the age old practice of research and publication, a patent was applied for, followed by technology transfer vide agreement to M/S. IFB Agro Industries Limited, Kolkata on 29th November, 2017. The procedure was facilitated and mediated by sponsored research and industrial consultancy division.

Another technology that went from laboratory to industry after quintessential intellectual property protection was a process of biomethane production from lignite. ONGC Limited is co-applicant of the application, which is awaiting examination along with IIT Kharagpur. While the revenue or profit sharing particulars are not known, the protections of innovations vide IP and scaling up is the model procedure to be emulated for optimal exploitation of IP and garnering funds that can go back to research.

Sensor Patents Case

IIT Bombay is deeply invested in research and development of sensors with at least 12 active patent applications in the portfolio. The technology ambit is wide,

---

12 Intellectual Property Assets in IITM Innovation Ecosystem, http://alumni.iitm.ac.in/wp-content/uploads/2016/07/Intellectual-Property-Brochure.pdf, accessed on 1 May, 2018.

13 by *Bacillus amyloliquefaciens.*

14 From lignite by development of a novel anaerobic consortium.

15 Tech Tribune, Bi-annual Newsletter, Autumn 2018, IPR and IR Cell, IIT Kharagpur.

from sensor data sequence, biosensors for health monitoring to nano-in micro systems to glucose sensors to amino acid sensors. Of these, as per data available until April 2018, one technology transfer has taken place to Bigtec Private Limited and another to Tata Consultancy Services. IIT Bombay had also entered into a 'licence agreement' with Intellectual Ventures, an 'invention capital' company head-quartered in Washington D.C., for commercialization of its patents. Intellectual Ventures as a company focuses on building, buying, and partnering to generate invention related revenue. Way back in 2012, IIT Bombay earned Rs 72 lakh by licensing 28 solution reports to Intellectual Ventures for which different patent applications were filed. While it was confirmed that a MoU was in place between the parties, exact terms and conditions could not be ascertained as it does not fall within the purview of public domain.

Conclusion

An important indicator of industry-relevant research is the growth in the number of technologies which have been commercialised or transferred to user industries. IITs, as is evidenced through data, are not only leading research and development focused academic institutes in the country but also frontrunners in applying for patent protection. Albeit there are plenty of thriving examples of innovations reaching from laboratory to market passing through patent path, however the numbers are still far from reaching the peak potential. Specifically, the percentage of biotechnology and allied domain based inventions finding industrial partners is far lower than other sectors across all the IITs. This could also be attributed to intense costs and regulatory approval requirements exclusive to this sector. The common threads binding these IITs are: goodwill inherent in the brand name for obtaining sponsorship and research contracts, an appropriate IP Policy in place, a streamlined IP registration procedure and mechanism and a dedicated IP or technology transfer divisions engaged in technology transfer contrivance.

Chapter 9

Patenting of Biotechnological Products in India: Conflicting Issues and their Harmonization

Mona Purohit

Dept. of Legal Studies and Research, Barkatullah University, Bhopal, Madhya Pradesh 462026
e-mail: monahod@gmail.com

ABSTRACT

The patent provides owner with market exclusivity that creates increased profit for inventor. It also fosters dissemination of knowledge and further innovations. The legal protection became very sensitive and complex for the protection of biotechnological invention as it involve technical and ethical issues. The fast advance and biotechnological development is responsible for transforming and restructuring the older legal rules. To be more specific there are number of concepts that are in conflict with each other. Some of them are - Invention vs Discovery: how do you define a biotechnological advance clearly enough to be acceptable a discovery or an invention. Ethics vs Technicality: Biotechnology has attracted critics from religious and welfare groups concerning animals, that experiments on animals is unethical and should not be granted on living matter. Monopoly vs Community rights: The price of the product shoots up due to patent monopoly and they could take unfair commercial advantages that provide benefits to the individuals by sub serving the rights of community at large. Invention Done (Traditional Knowledge) vs. Invention Protected (Scientific proving of Patent law) like these there are number of conflicting issues that will be discussed in paper. Numbers of Challenges are before Indian patent system with regard to biotechnological products i.e.-How to protect the monopoly rights without harming or diming the community rights? How to prove that whether scientific work is a discovery or invention? Industrial application is another obstacle for securing patent for inventions in biotechnology.

The work aims to identify problems and challenges relating to biotechnological patent in India and tries to provide solution for Harmonization of the Conflicting issues in the related field. The basic understanding with regard to the issues how law attempts to stipulate an explanation for some of its contradictions will be dealt in the paper.

Keywords: *Biotechnological products, Conflicting Issues, Harmonization, Invention Done, Invention Protected.*

Introduction

Protection of Intellectual property rights is vital in the 21st century and the patent is also gaining attraction from the scientific community. Moreover, biotechnology is a prime area of patent protection. Trade Related Intellectual Property Rights (TRIPS) is raising awareness of intellectual property issues all over the world, as countries are under obligation to comply with the provision of TRIPS. Patenting encourages innovations and foster development but it is not free from blemishes. Patenting of Biotechnological products involves more sensitive issue as products includes living things too. Numbers of Challenges are before Indian patent system with regard to biotechnological products *i.e.*-How to protect the monopoly rights without harming or diming the community rights? How to prove that whether scientific work is a discovery or invention? Industrial application is another obstacle for securing the patent for inventions in biotechnology.

The patent provides the owner with the market exclusivity that creates increased profit for the inventor. It also fosters dissemination of knowledge and further innovations. The legal protection became very sensitive and complex for the protection of the biotechnological invention as it involves technical and ethical issues. The fast advance and biotechnological development are responsible for transforming and restructuring the older legal rules.

To be more specific there are a number of concepts that are in conflict with each other. Some of them are - Invention vs Discovery: how do you define a biotechnological advance clearly enough to be acceptable a discovery or an invention. Ethics vs Technicality: Biotechnology has attracted critics from religious and welfare groups concerning animals, that experiments on animals is unethical and should not

be granted on living matter. Monopoly vs Community rights: The price of the product shoots up due to patent monopoly and they could take unfair commercial advantages that provide benefits to the individuals by sub serving the rights of the community at large. Invention Done (Traditional Knowledge) vs. Invention Protected (Scientific proving of Patent law)

The paper aims to identify problems and challenges relating to a biotechnological patent in India and tries to provide a solution for Harmonization of the Conflicting issues in the related field. The basic understanding with regard to the issues how law attempts to stipulate an explanation for some of its contradictions are dealt in the paper.

The problems and challenges relating to a biotechnological patent in India are many. Some of the interests seem to be incompatible and need of harmonization of the Conflicting issues in the related field is felt. Work tries to understand and answer the issues that how law attempts to stipulate an explanation for some of its contradictions?

The aim of paten is of two fold it can be considered as "social contract" between the inventors and society. Patent is a financial reward to Inventors and for the investors, who invest for research and development. Law also imposes duty on inventors to disclose information of inventions for the benefit of the public good. This reflects that the ultimate object of patent protection is to maintain equilibrium and strike a balance between different interests of people. The purpose of patent system is to protect the interest of inventor as well as the interests of society. Whether the present patent laws are achieving this object? That is what discussed in this work.

Legal Regulation of Biotechnology

The biotechnology is highly innovative and is on a strong growth trajectory. The Biotechnological sector has immense growth potential and giving noteworthy contribution in innovative field. The sector is playing significant role in enhancing India's global profile and in the economies growth of the country. Indian Patent Act governs the legal regulation on patent of biological products. Section 3(j) of the Indian Patent Act provides that an essentially biological process is not an invention and patents shall not be granted for 'plants and animals in whole or any part thereof other than micro organisms but including seeds, varieties and species and essentially biological processes for production or propagation of plants and animals'. This section is modeled on article 27.3(b) of the TRIPS Agreement. Section 3(j) of the Patents Act deals with three broad classes, which are-Microorganisms, Essentially biological processes and Plants and animals.

TRIPS agreement excludes biological process for the protection of plants or animals as a patentable subject matter. Although, it allows the grant of patents for microorganisms, non-biological and microbiological processes. In the production of plants and animals, TRIPS provide an option to member states protecting new plant varieties by means of patent or sue generous system or both.

Patent Filing Trends

India stood amongst the top 12 biotechnology destinations in the world. It has the third-biggest biotechnology industry in Asia-Pacific. India's biotechnology industry is evolving rapidly and growing at a compound annual growth rate of 20 per cent.

Overall Patent filing in India has increased in the last few years. IN 2015 -16 biotechnology patent filing has decreased but again improved in 2016-17. The following data reflect the granted patent in the field of Biotechnology. Among other things, a reason may be more stringent criteria for patentability and grant of patents in the biotechnological domain.

Patent Granted during 2016-2017(Appendix-F1)[1]

Under Field of Invention Biotechnology year wise data:

- 2012-2013: 144

---

1 http://www.ipindia.nic.in/writereaddata/Portal/IPOAnnualReport/1_94_1_1_79_1_A nnual_Report-2016-17_English.pdf.

- 2013-2014: 220
- 2014-2015: 262
- 2015-2016: 185
- 2016-2017: 333

Increasing number of grant of patent protection does not denote smooth functioning of law enforcement. The more patent protection in the field of biotechnology brought more controversies. It is witnessed that grant of monopoly for biotechnological products adversely effecting and infringing other right like community rights, rights of tribal *etc.*

Any law posses saving clause that save it to be declare ultra-vires even in case of ancillary encroachment of other's rights. Some times these provisions are incorporated as exception, proviso *etc.* The exception and exemption in legal provision make law workable and feasible. A similar philosophy is also applicable for patent and particularly in the field of biotechnology. The obviousness of encroachment on others right is quit reflecting in paten rights. These conflicts are the focus of this work. A number of conflicting issues exist in patenting of biotechnological products in India but for this work, only four conflicting issues have been identified.

Conflicting Issues

The records shown that many of the new biotechnology products and processes have been developed in the private sector. The proprietary rights to these technologies might be exploit by private sector, which led to effect rights of poor. Many developing countries will be unable to access them, as private sector does not owe as much as moral responsibility as government owes for its citizens.

Another issue is intellectual property protection to living matters that is not morally acceptable.

This work is being done with a view to suggesting reforms in the existing Indian Patent system particularly relating to biotechnology. It is felt that the present Indian patent regime is more stringent than a Liberal system. Morality and public opinion are considered to be essential elements of Indian laws, so patent rights have to be tested on the basis of both the elements. Further, if there is a conflict between two concepts particularly when Indian laws protect both, which one shall prevail? To be more specific there are a number of concepts that are in conflict with each other. Some of them are as follows:

1. Invention Vs Discovery

Conceptually discovery and invention are different in scientific field. Moreover this difference becomes more significant in case of patent protection. Recognize something first time that already exists, no one found it before, is discovery and an invention is a process of creating something totally new with one's own intellect. An invention is completely new to the world. Discovery is merely making available what already in existence hence not patentable.

As we discussed an invention is patentable while a discovery is not. In the field of biotechnology, this well-settled rule is triggering differences. In the field of biotechnology, the dividing line between invention and discovery pose a challenge. With the broadened the range of potentially patentable subject matter it is becoming more difficult to determine the dividing line between these two.

The difficulty lies in defining the invention in a way that is legally acceptable. The whole basis of the patents system is monopoly rights that are granted for the full disclosure of what is new about the invention?, the disclosure to the public. Most of the biotechnological products are already exits in nature and to prove them invention are not an easy task. If it is invention than again a question arose -how do you define a biotechnological advance clearly enough to be acceptable, and ultimately in court? The controversy exists that whether the identification and separation by conventional methods of genes from well-known compound represent a discovery or an invention? How can genetically engineered known compounds can be claimed for acceptance?

Patents encourage the development of technologies and provide monopoly that does not serve the public interest so critics propose to abolish the patenting of all life-forms and their components.

Patents and Genetic Engineering

Legally, a patent is a monopoly granted for the use, manufacturing, and sale of an invention. An invention must meet the criteria of being novel, useful, and non-obvious for it to be patentable. Patent law provides a prerequisite for patenting of an invention that an invention must be new, useful and involve an inventive step. It means discovery can be a subject matter of Patent Protection.

In the field of biotechnology patenting of microorganisms, plants and animals have become increasingly common. Genetic engineering, DNA sequences has broadened the range of potentially patentable subject matter. The novelty that is the fundamental precepts of a patent is a challenge for patenting of genes and gene sequence. Novelty can't exist in case of genetic engineering or it is difficult to prove.

The growth in the patenting of gene sequences expanded exponentially and still looks set to continue. Critics argue, how naturally occurring genes isolated in a laboratory, mere discovery, can be patented? The gene patenting is justified on the ground that locating, isolating and describing biological matter involves substantial inventiveness. They claim that newly identified quality was also previously unknown to the world and are of industrial application. They possess all necessities to be an invention hence patentable

2. Ethics Vs Technicality

Ethics is concerned with questions of determining standard such as what is right or wrong? When is an act right or wrong? What is good or bad? The object of the patent is to promote and protect inventions. The emphasis of technology is on inventions and development, contrary to the ethics and moral values that demand humanitarian interests of society. The dilemma combines two differing ideas *i.e.*

ethics and technique. The harmonization of these two differing ideas is the biggest challenge before mankind, particularly legal luminaries.

In the 21st century, Biotechnology is signifying a considerable force in improving the quality of life of the people. Biotechnology is intimately tied to science and scientific knowledge and also closely tied to ethics. The relationship between biotechnology and ethics is controversial as considered conflicting. The ethical debate is some time for research on living things and if but could be justified on the ground of public god. If research was motivated by a common vision of benefit of the society it is the ethical thing to do. The efforts focused on the betterment of people are ethically laudable. Other controversies come at the sage of patent protection, which confirms monopoly on the individual where other ethical considerations need be considered.

Patenting of Biotechnological product has attracted critics from religious and welfare groups. They claimed that experiments on human or animals or any other living matter is unethical. Hence patent protection should not be granted on living matter. In this way they are suggesting that man does not have moral right to unreasonably exploit our mother nature.

Prof Gardner has put: "Our experience with animals suggests that there would be a very real danger of creating seriously handicapped individuals if anybody tries to implant cloned human embryos into the womb."

The nature of biotechnological inventions involves technical as well as ethical issues so the legal protection became very sensitive and complex for the protection of biotechnological inventions.

3. Monopoly Vs Community Rights

Much of the scholarly debate boils down to a difficulty how to maintain the balance between monopoly rights of the patent holder and social rights of a community.A problem worthwhile relating to patent is cost issues attached to the whole procedure of patenting. Obtaining patent is not cheap anywhere in the world. Even the simplest patent application with the necessary professional advice may cost a heavy price and for a complicated, difficult, biotechnology patent cost may be double or triple of it. As no universal rules regarding the costs are the available protection of patents is much more difficult than our imaginations. Hence, most inventions are of biotechnology have evolved and protected from the developed world. Few companies hold such patents and hence, their commercial applications are limited and commercial application of the technology, the product is often choked. In situations where a generic manufacturer has to license a number of patents from multiple patent holders, the price of the product shoots up and they could take unfair commercial advantages.

The developing nations are the worst sufferers of the monopoly practices that provide benefits to the individuals by subserving the rights of the community at large.

The object of the patent system is to encourage investors to disclose their inventions for the public good. In return for this, the investors are granted monopoly and authority to prevent others from using or practicing their invention. The patent rights create monopolies restricting benefits to the owners of this knowledge opposite to practice of TK to share benefit within the communities. Hence TK, which is transferred from generation to generation, needs continuous research and innovations to get patent protection.

To address the issue of collective rights and the individual rights under biotechnological patent should be harmonize in a balancing manner.

4. Invention Done (Traditional Knowledge) vs. Invention Protected (Scientific proving of Patent law)

The heading is self-explanatory that invention done are different from invention protected.An invention need not necessarily be protected as protection requires few techno-legal prerequisites. Proving of technicalities of these prerequisites is difficult task for a common man. Furthermore if it comes to knowledge of tribal person, it becomes more serious concern. Traditional knowledge (TK) is generally understood to mean the know-how, skills, innovations, and practices developed by indigenous peoples or local communities. Invention Protected denotes inventions that can be Scientifically be proved and get protected under Patent law.

A patent gives the holder the exclusive right to make or use the protected invention commercially. Patent protection has only territorial application and applies in a certain territory may be a country and valid for only a limited period of time, now generally be 20 years. The main purpose of the patent system is to promote technological innovation. It does this in two ways: by helping to ensure that inventors can get a fair commercial reward for their successful inventions, and also by ensuring that detailed information about inventions is recorded and published so that other people can learn from it. To qualify for patent protection, an inventor has to substantiate invention is new, inventive and of industrial use. Novelty can be assess by comparing invention with prior art search.

Let see the relation between Patents and traditional knowledge. Novelty, inventive step and prior to art are particularly important issue in this relationship. It is a challenge for indigenous peoples to accomplish and corroborate the patentability requirements of novelty and inventive step.

The prior art is known or disclosed facts, which were available in public domain before the date that the patent application was filed. It is considered as published work and is relevant to be getting patent on the invention. Another concern is over the traditional rights of the communities who has true authority on knowledge but unable to get protection due to legal bar. Many times Indigenous peoples have resisted for their intangible knowledge.

The protection of invention under the Indian patent system requires some technicalities, which have to be followed before obtaining patent monopoly but inspire of having the knowledge, indigenous people can't prove their invention by proving to know how. In this way, so-called regulatory authorities can reject inventions actually done.

'Scientific proving' and 'legal proofing' are the most difficult task for the traditional knowledge holders. Well-informed persons are easily obtaining a patent using the foundation laid by the traditional knowledge holders. This misuse is a global concern. The TRIPS Agreement has also some provide for limited application to the protection of Traditional Knowledge. The protection of geographical indications can be used to protect traditional knowledge.

Indian laws too include several provisions for protection of traditional knowledge but outside the realm of patents. To clarify it is pertinent to mention that Section 3(p) of the Act prevents patenting of "traditional knowledge or which is an aggregation or duplication of known properties of the traditionally known component or components"

Observation

The above-mentioned discussion reflects that conflicting issues are not altogether inconsistent but they are reconcilable. Reasonable restriction can be imposed on interest of any person to protect the interest of other or community at large. The traditional concept of priority of public interest over individual interest is not accepted in intellectual property rights protection. Usually in IPR system patent monopoly acquire weightage over public interest. Striking the right balance between the interests of real innovators and protected innovator is challenge for legal fraternity.

Contradictory theory of Monopoly (professionalism) Vs Community rights (public interest) the professionalism model attributes reward to the inventor and public interest model binds society together. The Community rights have brooder perspective. So harmonization can only be possible through a well-matured legal system. The tribal community should be educated and empowered to protect their TK. Government or non-government agencies should take initiatives to protect patent rights of tribal through existing legal mechanisms or take patents on the innovations made by them on the TK.

A fair balance between all the above discussed interests is possible if the scope of the claim of the patent are keep proportional to the opportunity to exploit the inventions by penurious.

Chapter 10

Status of IPR Education in Life Science Courses of Indian Universities

Neerja Shrivastava

Govt. College, Kota (Rajasthan), India 324001
e-mail: drnshrivastava@gmail.com

ABSTRACT

In India almost all university running life sciences courses including microbiology, biotechnology, botany,zoology. All these courses are related to innovation but when we analyze the statues of patent filling the number is very less. Students are not aware about IPR and its tool they also did not about patent law. patent filling procedure.Student are not know that they protect their intellectual property by law and can get monitory benefit. Present paper focuses on Status of IPR Education in Life Science Courses of Indian Universities The paper also discuses the need and suggestion for improvement of IPR education in Indian universities

Keywords: *Intellectual property rights, Life science, University.*

Introduction

Over the last decades the field of life sciences has raised to a major productive source of innovation related to technology. Along with this economic development, issues in intellectual property have become important to researchers of life sciences. The life science course which are currently running in various universities are not able to provide the basic information of IP and hands on experience in the management of patenting, copy right, trademark and other IPR tools,related issues and new job opportunities in the field of intellectual property rights. Students of Indian university and colleges did not know,How does knowledge of IPR in life sciences affect – my career? – academic research? – the society? They also did not know that there Inventions, scientific publications, research data, software, brands and designs can all be protected with intellectual property tools.

As we know that India is second biggest country in term of population. It is assumed that in coming years India has a largest number of young population and Indian Brain is very well known in world. Information technology,retail sector, computer technology and commodity sector are developed very fast. India has played a significant role in providing processing, designs and production of valuable commercial products utilizable to many area of the society as well as country (*e.g.*, agriculture, medical, health care, industry, environment *etc.*).Survey of various international agency indicates that in 10-15 years 30 per cent of American patents related to medicine will be end. And upcoming time is of Indian scientists. India has very good wealth of traditional knowledge. Various ethno-botanical surveys of the plants studied indicate that this wealth is going to be extinct at the present rate of utilization or over exploitation. So there is an urgent need that this traditional knowledge should be gathered and protected by legal way. Unfortunately, in India literacy status is not up to the mark and we are still behind in the field of education of masses. After independence the status of education is increased but we still need to go a long way ahead. And when we talk about education related to intellectual property rights and patent law, the status is very low. The information related to this area at grass-root level in very little, so there is urgent need that information related to IPR and Patent law should reach at village level because our strength is based on our rural areas. Their knowledge related to agriculture, medical use of plants, folk care uses of plants are very useful. Therefore, the cheap and innovative ideas of these people should be protected by intellectual property rights.

In the era E-World and globalization and emergence of modern science the legal characterization and treatment of trade related processes and products are popularly known and defined as Intellectual Property. In general the physical object such as land and household goods are the properties of a person. Every country has certain laws by which the rights and ownership on the property of a person is protected.

Need of IP Education

IPR is an umbrella protecting your creativity.

Through Knowledge of IPR You can

1. Protect your creativity or inventions
2. Get an economic return on funding invested in research and development
3. Get a reward or recognigetion as it is the fruit of your hard labour effort and time
4. Own your invention or creative works.
5. Create of an intellectual asset for licensing or selling

What happens if you did not have Knowledge of IPR

1. Somebody else might get right of your creativity or innovation.
2. Possibilities to license, sell or transfer technology will be hindered.
3. Somebody will take economic benefit of your invention.

4. You may lost reward or recognigetion which is the fruit of your hard labour effort and time

Overall the current awareness of IP is nit enough. As the use of electronic resources has developed in last decades,plagiarism has a important issue specially in the field of research. Indian universities and college has very idea about it. There isurgent need to educate our academicians and students about IP.

Current Status of IP

Annual report (2016-17) of the "The office of the controller general of patents, designs, trade marks and geographical indications India" indicates the present statues of patent filing by Indian universities (Table-1).As of February 2017, there are 789 universities, **37,204** colleges and 11,443 stand-alone institutions in India. According to AISHE- 2015 total enrolment in higher education has been estimated to be 34.6 million. This year, the Indian Institute of Technology (collectively) occupied the first position while, Amity university and Indian Institute of Science occupied second and third place respectively. Data indicates most of patent files from university or institute of metro city which indicates that we are not able to bring out our talent and inventers which are present in heart of our country that is in villages and in small town. These data indicates that we are far away from the our goal. Various study indicates that our traditional knowledge is not legally protected through IPR.Students are even did not know the trem IP,patent, copyright trademark,GI.Due to this ignorance India paid a lot our fight for Haldi and Basmati Patent is example of it.So if we want to protect our IP rights we should make aware our student which can only done by colleges and universities. In India,so far,very little work has been done on IP course development. When we look the syllabus of various university we can realize that only few universities included IPR studies.

Table 10.1: Top 10 Indian Applicants for Patents from Institutes and Universities

Sl.No.	*Name of Institutes/Universities*	*Applications Filed*
1	INDIAN INSTITUTE OF TECHNOLOGY (COLLECTIYE)	400
2	AMITY UNIYERSITY	106
3	INDIAN INSTITUTE OF SCIENCE	54
4	VELTECH HIGH/MULTI TECH DR. RR and DR.SR (COLLEGE AND UNIYERSITY	50
5	G.H. RAISONI COLLEGE OF ENGINEERING	49
6	BHARATH UNIYERSITY	45
7	CHANDIGARH GROUP OF COLLEGES	30
8	CHITKARA UNIVERSITY	29
9	HINDUSTAN INSTITUTE OF TECKNOLOGY and SCIENCE	28
10	NATIONAL INSTITUTE OF TECHNOLOGY(COLLECTIVE)	26

Source: The office of the controller general of patents, deisgns, trade marks and geographical indications, India, Annual Report, 2016-170.

In the emerging scenario,students of life science that would benefit from the intellectual property education is important. Keeping in view the needs of different branches of life sciences,well defined IP syllabus is require to be devised. In life science courses,some knowledge of IP will help in creating the scientific temper for innovation and innovation and innovative activities and how to reap the benefits of ones own creation among the students.

There is an urgent need that the knowledge related to IPR and Patent law should be given at earlier stage, starting from secondary classes.It is suggested that general information related to IPR and patent law should be incorporated,not only in the university/college syllabus but also in secondary school's syllabus.

We can't say that our policy makers are not aware of this problem. Many state's education boards have already recognized the importance of knowledge of IPR and Patent law. A number of indian universities and colleges have already incorporated the topics related to IPR and Patent law.

The Ministry of Commerce and Industry, Govt.of India is running an Intellectual Property Training Institute (IPTI) at Nagpur, it fulfils the following objectives:

- Research and Development
- IPR and Law Professionals
- Inventive activities and IPR related issues

The IPTI offers unique opportunity to gain first hand knowledge and training in patent and other IPRs at Nagpur.It is the only institute of its kind in our country set up by the Govt.of India.

The Table 10.2 gives a list of various universities/institutes promoting or providing such studies;

Table 10.2

Name of University/Institute	*Type of Course*
Amity Law School	PG Diploma in Intellectual Property Laws
Bioinformatics Institute of India	PG Diploma inLaw school with IP courses
Banglore University Law College	Law school with IP courses
Balaji Law College	Law school with IP courses
Cochin University of Science and Technology	Law school with IP courses
University of Delhi	Law school with IP courses
Gujarat National Law University	Law school with IP courses
Hemchandracharya North Gujarat University	Law school with IP courses
ICFAI Law School	Law school with IP courses
IGNOU New Delhi	PG Diploma in Intellectual Property Rights
Indian Institute of Management	Law school with IP courses
Indian Law Society (ILS) Pune	Law school with IP courses
National Academy of Legal Studies and Research	Law school with IP courses

Name of University/Institute	*Type of Course*
National Law School of India University	Law school with IP courses
National Law University Jodhpur (Rajasthan)	Law school with IP courses
National University of Judicial Sciences, W.B. National Law Institute University, Bhopal	Training programme on Patents and other Intellectual Property Rights (IPRs)
Patent Office of India	Law school with IP courses
Punjabi University	Law school with IP courses Diploma in Intellectual Property Law
V.M. Salgaocar, College of Law	Law school with IP courses
VMOU, Kota (Raj)	PG Diploma in Intellectual Property Rights
Symbiosis Law College Pune	Diploma in Intellectual Property Rights
Tamil Nadu Dr. Ambedkar Law University	Law school with IP courses
Lucknow University	PG Diploma in Intellectual Property Laws
Andhra University, Waltair	P.G. Diploma in Patent Litigation
Bangalore University	Diploma in Intellectual Property Rights
Calcutta University	Law Degree with IPR Knowledge
South Gujarat University, Surat	Law Degree with IPR Knowledge
Osmania University, Hyderabad	Law Degree with IPR Knowledge
Sri Venkateswara University, Tirupati	Law Degree with IPR Knowledge
Mangalore University	Law Degree with IPR Knowledge
Madras University	Law Degree with IPR Knowledge
University of Calicut	Law Degree with IPR Knowledge
Nagpur University	Law Degree with IPR Knowledge
Symbiosis Society's Law College	Law Degree with IPR Knowledge
I L S Law College, Pune	Law Degree with IPR Knowledge
Pondicherry University	Law Degree with IPR Knowledge
University of Kerala, Thiruvananthapuram	Law Degree with IPR Knowledge
Guru Gobind Singh Indraprastha University, Delhi	Law Degree with IPR Knowledge
Shivaji University, Kolhapur	Law Degree with IPR Knowledge
University of Mumbai	Law Degree with IPR Knowledge
National Law Institute University	Law Degree with IPR Knowledge
	Law Degree with IPR Knowledge

The various organization/institute promoting or providing such studies include:

- ✰ World Intellectual Property Organisation (WIPO)
- ✰ Industrial Trademark Association,
- ✰ IIPS
- ✰ AIPS

References

Agitha, T G(2013): Impact of IP on Public Health: The Developed Country Scenario. JIPR 18(4): 382- 389

Ganguli,P.,Intellectul Property Rights, tata MnGraw Hill.

Gupta,V.K., chem. Indian news,1995.

http://www.usto.gov/web/offices/com/seehes

http://ipindia,nicin/ipr/patent

http://www.bits-pilani.ac.in/uploads/Patent_Manual

http://www.wipo.int/

http://www.wto.org/english/tratop_e/trips_e/intel1_e.htm

Kannan (2010) Importance of Intellectual Property Rights. International Journal of Intellectual Property Rights 1(1): 1-5

Reddy, G B and Kadri, Harunrashid A (2013): Local Working of Patents - Law and Implementation in India. JIPR 18(1): 15-27

Chapter 11

Patent Claims: A Tool for Defining the Patent Protection

Payal Thaorey

Post Graduate Teaching, Department of Law, RTM Nagpur University, Nagpur 440001
e-mail: payal.mundafale@gmail.com

"Name of the game is the claims"

— *Justice Giles S. Rich*

ABSTRACT

A patent is a document, issued, upon application, by a government office (or a regional office acting for several countries), which describes an invention and creates a legal situation in which the patented invention can normally only be exploited (manufactured, used, sold, imported) with the authorization of the owner of the patent. This patent application is made in the form of patent claim. The patent claim is the heart and soul of a patent. The claims demarcate in words the boundary of invention, just like a picket-fence defines the extent of land covered by a deed for a piece of land. The purpose of patent claim is to establish the scope of a useful economic right that reflects the patentee's business needs and goals.

The claims may be broad or narrow in their scope or breadth. Normally, broad claims include fewer elements or limitations than narrow claims do, and can be very valuable because they can cover a range of valuable products or situations, but can be more difficult to obtain and to enforce because there may be a broader range of prior art that may block or invalidate them. Narrow claims are generally very specific to one particular element or product. In general, a narrow claim specifies more details than a broader claim.

These claims are of paramount importance in both patent prosecution in the Patent Office and patent litigation in the courts. Therefore, during claim drafting the choice of words used in the patent claims should be dealt in a great understanding and thought so as to define the nature and scope of the patent. Anything which is described but not properly and carefully claimed becomes freely available for public use. Claim drafting is a highly specialized skill, and it is not recommended that inventors try to draft their own claims. Casual claims drafting makes the patent more vulnerable for infringement. Utmost precautions needs to be taken while drafting the patent claim, as anything which remained unclaimed may hamper the claimed protection.

Hence in the light of above discussion, the researcher in present research paper has focus on the significance of patent claims and its role in extending the scope for patent protection. The emphasis is made on understanding the crafting of patent claims then merely focusing on the drafting of patent claims.

Keywords: *Patents, Claims, Protection, Infringement, drafting.*

Introduction

Claims are at the heart of almost every critical question in patent law. Most notably claims determine a patent's rights of exclusion. Yet, despite their importance, there is no reliable way to determine the ultimate boundaries of a patent. During litigation, these claim-based boundaries can be pushed and pulled dramatically. The result is a system that is hard to predict and appears judge-dependent. Some judges favour narrower patents, some favour broader. In other words, the fight over how broadly a patent should exclude drives uncertainty. What has not been recognized is that there is also confusion over the fundamental meaning of claims. There is a question over how we should interpret patent claims. Patent law has not clarified exactly what the patent applicant is communicating via claims.

This chapter will be classified into three sections wherein the First section will deal with the concept of patent, its theoretical approach and patent claim format. The second section will discuss the most vital part of patent claim *i.e.* the patent claim construction as well as the intrinsic and extrinsic evidence used for deriving its meaning for defining the scope of patent protection. The third section will emphasise on the various claim sets as well as several types of patent claims in brief. These sections will together help in understanding the crafting of patent claims instead of merely focusing on the drafting of patent claims.

Section-1

Concept of Patent Claim

WIPO defines the Patent Claims as, "the legally-operative part of a patent application; and everything else revolves around it"[1]. According to Article 6 of the Patent Cooperation Treaty the patent claim is "The claim or claims shall define the matter for which protection is sought. Claims shall be clear and concise. They shall be fully supported by the description"[2]. The claims mark the boundaries of the protection provided by a patent, just as a physical boundary such as a fence, marks the limits of a parcel of real property. Thus, the claims are a written approximation of the abstract inventive concept created by the inventor. The claims define the scope of protection provided by a patent. While jurisdictions around the world may apply differing legal doctrines for claim interpretation, in the most prevalent theory the claims set forth the outer limits of patent protection.

---

1 WIPO Patent Drafting Manual, IP Assets Management Series, http://www.wipo.int/edocs/pubdocs/en/patents/867/wipo_pub_867.pdf accessed on 12 March 2018.

2 Refer Article 6 of Patent Cooperation Treaty 1970 for details.

The section 10[3] of Patent Act, 1970 mandates that complete specification ends with one or more claims defining the scope of the invention. The patent protection and the process of defining claims or terms used in claims to resolve this 'scope of invention' is termed as claim construction or interpretation. Claims identify the metes and bounds of an inventor's monopoly. The process of adjudicating any infringement action in the patent law deals with the verification of the claim scope covering the infringing technology. In other words, claims maintain their significance throughout the life of a patent and serve to protect the rights of the patent owner[4]. It is important to note here that, The Patent Act 1970 did not define the term Claims. In India, like USA the whole concept of Patent Claims depends upon the Courts to define its scope and meaning.

Theoretically, the patent system gives inventors exclusive rights in exchange for inventions. The process for receiving these exclusive rights starts with the patent application, the core of which is the patent specification[5]. The applicant is first instructed to provide "a written description of the invention" as well as "[how] to make and use [that invention][6]. This written description is the quid pro quo of the patent system. The inventor discloses the invention in detail to prove that they did in fact invent something and so that others can later reproduce and use it. In return, the inventor gets (for a limited time) valuable exclusive rights. After providing this description, the patent document turns to the inventor's quo the exclusive rights. Patent applicants are instructed to "conclude" the specification with "one or more claims particularly pointing out and distinctly claiming the subject matter which the inventor regards as the invention."[7]

Claims are the most important part of the patent document. The claims demarcate in words the boundary of invention, just like a picket-fence defines the extent of land covered by a deed for a piece of land. The purpose of patent claim is to establish the scope of a useful economic right that reflects the patentee's business needs and goals. As held by the Supreme Court of United tates of America in Aro Mfg., Co. v. Convertible Top Replacement Co[8], the claims are used to define the extent of the exclusive rights. Claims "are the sole measure of the grant."

---

3 Refer section 10 of Patent Act, 1970 for details.

4 Adarsh Ramanujan (2009), Methodology of Claim Construction after Philips V. AWH Corp: The Need for Alternative Approach. Vol 14, January, Journal of Intellectual Property Rights, pp 28-45. http://www.niscair.res.in/ScienceCommunication/ResearchJournals/rejour/jipr/jipr2k9/jipr_jan09.asp#28 accessed on 13 March 2018.

5 Oskar Liivak (2016). The Unresolved Interpretive Ambiguity of Patent. Vol. 49, Claims University of California, Davis, https://lawreview.law.ucdavis.edu/issues/49/5/Articles/49-5_Liivak.pdf accessed on 16 March 2018.

6 *Ibid.*

7 *Ibid.*

8 365 U.S. 336, 339-40 (1961)

Usually, the claims are directed to the competitors of the patent holder and their function is to define the scope of the invention claimed, during the term of a patent and tell patent the competitor as to what exactly should be refrained from doing as that act could lead to an infringement of the patent[9].

The remarkable thing to note here is that the meaning to a patent claim is given during the patent lawsuit. When a patent claim's validity is at issue, the patent owner may want the claim to be construed narrowly, so it does not include a certain piece of prior art that would render the claim invalid as claiming something that is not "new". When infringement of the claim is at stake, the patent owner may want the claim to be construed broadly so as to encompass the defence of its product or method.[10] Since, the Acts are silent about the concept of claim, it is at the liberty and discretion of the court to define its scope. The courts dig into the claim construction for deciding the scope of patent protection. The construction of the patent claim becomes integral and vital at the time of disputes, it is important to discuss its aspects in detail in this chapter.

Patent Claim: Traditional Theoretical Approach

For a long time, the patent claims have been analogized both to statues and contracts. The two main categories of traditional interpretive theories in the fields of statutory interpretation and contract interpretation are textualism and intentionalism, which were used to define the patent claim. Textualism (Text-Oriented Interpretation) is the view that language conveys meaning "only because a linguistic community attaches common understandings to words and phrases, and relies on shared conventions for deciphering those words and phrases in particular contexts."[11] Whereas Intentionalism (Author-Oriented Interpretation) is a theory of legal interpretation which holds that the legal texts such as contracts and statutes must be interpreted according to authorial intention. It asserts "that the meaning of a text is identical to the meaning that its author intended it to/.communicate."[12] The two theories may achieve the same result in many cases, however, they "will yield different verdicts when the hypothetical interpreter has access to evidence that trumps or supplements the linguistic evidence." Let us understand the approaches of these two interpretation:

A. Text-Oriented Interpretation: Under the "ordinary meaning first" approach, claim terms are given their "ordinary and accustomed"

9 Ruchi Tiwari (2000). Interpreting Claims in a Patent Specification. Vol 5, January, Journal of Intellectual Property Rights, pp 132-136, http://nopr.niscair.res.in/bitstream/123456789/19495/1/JIPR per cent 205 per cent 283 per cent 29 per cent 20132-136.pdf accessed on 13 March 2018.

10 Donald M. Cameron (2015). Claim Construction, In. Patent and Trade Secrets Law, http://www.jurisdiction.com/patweb04.pdf accessed on 16 March 2018.

11 Huang Yan (2013). A Dynamic Framework for Patent Claim Construction: Insights From A Philosophical Hermeneutic Study. 21 Tex. Intell. Prop. L.J. 1, Texas Intellectual Property Law Journal, http://www.tiplj.org/wp-content/uploads/Volumes/v21/v21p1.pdf accessed on 15 March 2018

12 *Ibid.*

meaning—"Accordingly, a technical term used in a patent claim is interpreted as having the meaning a person of ordinary skill in the field of the invention would understand it to mean."[13]

B. Author-Oriented Interpretation: The purposive approach requires the court to reconstruct the patentee's hypothetical objective intent to describe and demarcate the scope of protection. "The task for the court is to determine what the person skilled in the art would have understood the patentee to have been using the language of the claim to mean."

Although the traditional theories specify some goals to be pursued and identify their preferred sources of evidence, there still remain a number of unresolved issues:

1. The text-oriented theory presumes that there is a conventional usage of a word among the scientific and technological community. But in some cases, the ordinary meaning fails to capture the distinctiveness of the invention and would yield no conclusions about the scope of protection[14].
2. The intent-oriented theory presumes that meaning is the patentee's objective intent. However, it is not only hard to find and identify the objective intent, but also unsatisfactory to regard the scope of protection as merely what the patentee communicated.

In the beginning of Nineteenth century the patents did not have claims and the scope of the patented invention was determined in court proceedings during patent infringement litigation by reviewing the specification filed by the inventor. Not surprisingly, this process eventually became unworkable and the process of patent claiming was born as a means for providing greater notice of the boundaries of the patent. Additionally, in a substantive examination patent system the claims are reviewed by a patent examiner, which provides the courts and the public with some assurance that a typical patent claim does not exceed the maximum scope of protection the inventor should receive. Thus, the claims were originally based on the concept that they were to serve as a guideline to explain what the inventor perceived as his invention at the time he made his invention and filed his patent application. Today, the claims define the protection given by a patent and lie at the heart of any invention. In fact, claims are typically the first portion of the patent application examined and scrutinized by a patent examiner or anyone studying the patent.

Patent Claim Format

A patent claim has three parts: the preamble, the transitional phrase and the body.

---

13 *ibid*

14 *Ibid.*

A) The Preamble

A preamble is an introductory phrase that identifies the category of the invention protected by that claim[15]. The preamble typically introduces the subject matter of the claim, and may also describe the intended purpose of the invention. Ordinarily, the preamble is viewed merely as a statement of purpose, in which case it does not have a limiting effect on the claim, and plays essentially no role in an infringement analysis[16]. However, in rare cases, the preamble may be viewed as a claim limitation.

The preamble may not necessarily be accorded the same weight during patent litigation as the body of the claim and the weight given to preambles can vary from jurisdiction to jurisdiction. In some jurisdictions the courts will look at whether the preamble "breathes life" into the claim as a whole and, if so, the preamble will be accorded patentable weight[17]. In deciding whether a preamble term is "necessary to give life, meaning, and vitality to the claim," a court may consider a number of factors, including 1) the overall claim structure, 2) whether the claim would be understandable in the absence of the preamble term at issue, 3) the use of the term as antecedent basis for subsequent limitations in the claims, and 4) the prevalence of the term in describing the invention throughout the application.

B) Transitional Phrase

There are two types of transitional phrases: open-ended and closed phrases. Open-ended phrases do not exclude any additional, unrecited elements or method steps[18]. In other words, open-ended phrases are inclusive, not exclusive. In the US for example, open-ended phrases include the terms "comprising," "including," "containing," and "characterized by." These terms have been construed or interpreted to mean "including the following elements but not excluding others."[19]

Closed phrases are the opposite of open-ended phrases. Closed phrases, such as "consisting of," limit the claim to nothing more than the specifically-recited elements. The claim covers only the elements named and nothing more[20]. In regular practice the closed claims are rarely used because infringers can easily avoid infringement by simply adding another element to the existing claims.

---

15 WIPO Patent Drafting Manual, IP Assets Management Series, http://www.wipo.int/edocs/pubdocs/en/patents/867/wipo_pub_867.pdf accessed on 12 March 2018.

16 Shawn Kolitch (2015). Patent Claim Construction: The Neglected Preamble, Vol. 8, No. 1, Intellectual Property Newsletter, http://www.khpatent.com/wp-content/uploads/2015/12/9492SJK_Patent_Claim_Construction.pdf accessed on 21 March 2018.

17 *Ibid.*

18 WIPO Patent Drafting Manual, IP Assets Management Series, http://www.wipo.int/edocs/pubdocs/en/patents/867/wipo_pub_867.pdf accessed on 12 March 2018.

19 *Ibid.*

20 *Ibid.*

C) The Body of the Claim

The body of a claim is the portion that follows the transitional phrase. The body of the claim recites the elements and limitations of the claim. The body also explains how the different elements exist in relationship to one another. Basically, the body of the claim recites and inter-relates all the elements of the claim. A patent claim cannot be merely a list of parts. They must be connected in some manner to each other. The Controller of Patents will not allow patent claims that are merely listed in parts.

Section-2

Patent Claim Construction

There is no straight jacket formula for construction of a patent claim. Construction of patent claims depends on each invention. It depends on what protection the Applicant seeks to claim on that invention. Depending on the protection sought by the applicant the claim may be constructed in a broad or narrow manner in reference to existing prior art. However, care must be taken to ensure that the patent claims are neither too broad (it cannot include what the applicant has not invented) nor too narrow (where the applicant may lose out on a necessary protection). In the *Delhi Network of Positive People* v. *Respondent Union of India and Ors*[21] the High Court of Delhi held that patent claim application must contain the inventive concept.

According to Huang Yan, "The Patent claim construction has its unique features unlike the other legal texts, such as defining invention and providing public notice about the exact patent scope of exclusivity."[22] Claims are always constructed in a single sentence that can include commas, colons, and semi-colons. Each of these "sentences" is preceded by a number that becomes the claim's identifier, *e.g.* "Claim 1." The patent claim language can be an amalgam of multiple vocabularies and perspectives. However, a claim can only have one period at the end (except for abbreviations).

To comply with this requirement the claim must be:

- Precise
- Clear
- Correct, and
- Unambiguous

The claims are written at the end of the patent and are introduced with language such as:

- What is claimed is:

---

21 W.P.(C) No.2867/2014

22 Huang Yan (2013). A Dynamic Framework for Patent Claim Construction: Insights From A Philosophical Hermeneutic Study. 21 Tex. Intell. Prop. L.J. 1, Texas Intellectual Property Law Journal, http://www.tiplj.org/wp-content/uploads/Volumes/v21/v21p1.pdf accessed on 15 March 2018.

- ✰ I claim:
- ✰ We claim:
- ✰ Claims:

The claims of a patent can be directed to:

- ✰ A machine,
- ✰ An article of manufacture,
- ✰ A process, or
- ✰ A composition of matter

Since the claims are the principal determinant of the scope of the monopoly, how they are to be interpreted is frequently the nub of a dispute. In *CTR Manufacturing Industries Limited* Vs. *Defendants Sergi Transformer Explosion Prevention Technologies Pvt. Ltd. and Ors.* the Bombay High Court held that "the claim construction should not be done in such a manner that it will restrain the future improvements"[23]

The construction of a claim cannot be done in isolation from the rest of the specification. Claims are intended to be pithy delineations of the scope of monopoly, and they are drafted in the light of much more detailed text of description. The patent specification must always be read as a whole[24]. All the terms which have a special meaning in the art, or are given a special definition, must be read in their particular sense. For this, there are categories of evidence which help them in interpreting the claims. In *TVS Motor Company Limited* Vs. *Bajaj Auto Limited*[25] it was held that the patent claim construction must emphasized on the 'Purposive Construction' of patent claim instead of ordinary construction as the later may narrow down the scope of patent protection.

Claim Interpretation vis-à-vis Claim Construction

In every patent claim drafting, the drafter has to take due cognizance about its clarity of interpretation as well as totality of construction. At times, there exists an ambiguity in our understanding of patent claims. Importantly, this interpretive ambiguity is separate from the construction of claim which defines the ultimate patent scope. Asking whether a claim drafter is making a request for exclusion with their claim or instead stating what they claim to have invented is a matter of interpretation. The aim of interpretation is to understand the message the author intends to convey to the reader via the text. It provides the "set of ideas and concepts that are communicated by the language to a member of the intended audience".[26]

---

23 Motion No. 497 Of 2014 in Suit No. 448 of 2012.

24 *Ibid.*

25 CIVIL APPEAL No. 6309 of 2009.

26 Oskar Liivak (2016). The Unresolved Interpretive Ambiguity of Patent. Vol. 49, Claims University of California, Davis, https://lawreview.law.ucdavis.edu/issues/49/5/Articles/49-5_Liivak.pdf accessed on 16 March 2018.

Having interpreted the text, the next step is construction. This entails determining the legal effect of the text. And although interpretation and its linguistic meaning often provide a good start toward legal effect, linguistic meaning may not answer all relevant questions. It is said that, "Construction is the activity of determining the legal meaning and effect of a text".[27] Claim construction is the "thickly normative" process of moving from the linguistic meaning of a text to rendering a legal decision with actual impact on legal actors.

The interpretation-construction distinction does not tell us how to resolve these disputes over legal effect. Rather, the payoff of drawing the distinction is antecedent: it tells us which issues are problems of linguistic meaning, and which issues are problems of legal effect. This is important because the two types of problems call for different solutions.

Sources for Deriving Meaning of Claims

The Patent Claim Jurisprudence in India is still at a very infant stage. Whereas the European and American Laws are far more developed in this regard and therefore we rely on them for deriving the meaning of patent claim to a great extent. After the landmark judgement of *Philips* v *AWH Corp*[28], a drastic change has been witnessed in the interpretation of Patent Claims by the US courts. They started interpreting the Claim construction on the basis of categories of evidence *i.e.* Intrinsic and Extrinsic. Earlier the consideration of extrinsic evidence was limited to educating the court in case of doubt about the technology. In 2002, the United States Federal Circuit Court appeared to elevate dictionaries, a special category of extrinsic evidence, to a central role in claim construction. The court emphasized, however, that extrinsic evidence must be considered "in the context of the intrinsic evidence [,]" but is "less reliable than the patent and its prosecution history in determining how to read claim terms."[29] The law is clear that intrinsic evidence serves as the principal source for claim construction and the extrinsic evidence will be served as secondary source for claim construction which will complement the intrinsic evidence.

a) Intrinsic Evidence

"Intrinsic" evidence refers to the patent and its file history, including any re-examinations and reissues. Intrinsic evidence also includes related patents and their prosecution histories. The Courts treats the prior art that is cited or incorporated by reference in the patent-in-suit and prosecution history as intrinsic evidence.

---

27 *Ibid.*

28 363 F. 3d1207, 1209, (Fed. Cir. 2004).

29 Huang Yan (2013). A Dynamic Framework for Patent Claim Construction: Insights From A Philosophical Hermeneutic Study. 21 Tex. Intell. Prop. L.J. 1, Texas Intellectual Property Law Journal, http://www.tiplj.org/wp-content/uploads/Volumes/v21/v21p1.pdf accessed on 15 March 2018.

i) Specification

The patent specification provides a written description of the invention and the manner and process of making and using it. It includes the field and background of the invention, the drawings, detailed description of the invention, preferred embodiments, best mode of practicing the invention and the patent claims[30].

ii) Prosecution History

Beyond the specification and other claims, an important source of evidence in claim construction is a patent's prosecution history. A "prosecution history" consists of "the complete record of the proceedings before the Patent Office and includes the prior art cited during the examination of the patent.

iii) Related and Foreign Applications

Some patents issue from single applications, with a single prosecution history. Other patents are members of large families of related patents, with a web of underlying patent applications, along with counterparts filed in foreign countries. In such instances, when one patent is in suit, parties may find statements in its related patents and patent applications, and in its foreign counterparts, that bear on claim construction[31].

b) Extrinsic Evidence

"Extrinsic evidence" refers to all other types of evidence, including inventor testimony, expert testimony, and documentary evidence of how the patentee and alleged infringer have used the claim terms. Dictionaries are considered to be "extrinsic" evidence[32]. There are five ways[33] in which the extrinsic evidence can be explored in patent claim construction. They are:

1. First, extrinsic evidence by definition is not part of the patent and does not have the specification's virtue of being created at the time of patent prosecution for the purpose of explaining the patent's scope and meaning.
2. Second, while claims are construed as they would be understood by a hypothetical person of skill in the art, extrinsic publications may not be written by or for skilled artisans and therefore may not reflect the understanding of a skilled artisan in the field of the patent.

---

30 *Ibid.*

31 Peter S. Menell, Matthew D. Powers, and Steven C. Carlson (2010). Patent Claim Construction: A Modern Synthesis And Structured Framework, Berkeley Technology Law Journal [Vol. 25:2, https://poseidon01.ssrn.com/delivery.php?ID=24803102406408308 10881221120791231010100400720 5801703406606411 4120083095112083071066063000002000122001112002065109100081070088052047036085068088127097125093092070081086006029089008111126097007084099027117031100065027018092106085087080000029118081 and EXT=pdf accessed on 02 April 2018.

32 Southwall Techs., Inc. v. Cardinal IG Co., 54 F.3d 1570, 1578 (Fed. Cir. 1995).

33 *Ibid.*

3. Third, extrinsic evidence consisting of expert reports and testimony is generated at the time of and for the purpose of litigation and thus can suffer from bias that is not present in intrinsic evidence.
4. Fourth, there is a virtually unbounded universe of potential extrinsic evidence of some marginal relevance that could be brought to bear on any claim construction question.
5. Finally, undue reliance on extrinsic evidence poses the risk that it will be used to change the meaning of claims in derogation of the "indisputable public records consisting of the claims, the specification and the prosecution history," thereby undermining the public notice function of patents.

Where the specification supports two interpretations of a disputed claim, extrinsic evidence can be used to confirm which interpretation is more consistent with what a person having ordinary skill in the art would have understood at the time of invention. Also the Expert Opinions can be taken into consideration only when they are in tune with the intrinsic evidence.

Section-3

Types of Claim Sets

A set of claims in a patent specification will normally include one or more independent (or main) claims and a number of dependent or subsidiary claims (or sub claims) which depend on one or more preceding independent claim(s). According to WIPO, "All patent applications must contain at least one "independent" claim directed to the essential features of the invention, *i.e.* those features necessary to satisfy the legal requirements of novelty and inventive step"[34]. Each independent claim may be followed by one or more dependent claims concerning more specific embodiments of the invention recited in the independent claim. The following are the various types of claims:

A) Independent Claims

The independent claims in a patent represent the broadest claims. Some independent claims are broader than other independent claims but a given independent claim is always broader than any claim that depends on it. An independent claim is a claim that stands alone and does not need a limitation from another claim in order to be complete. Each claim set begins with an independent claim.

A patent application may have more than one independent claim. For instance, sometimes a single invention might encompass several different inventive concepts, in which case it may not be possible to have one broad claim that covers all the

---

34 WIPO Patent Drafting Manual, IP Assets Management Series, http://www.wipo.int/edocs/pubdocs/en/patents/867/wipo_pub_867.pdf accessed on 12 March 2018.

different inventive concepts. In general, it is wise to have several independent claims, each of which separately covers a different inventive concept[35].

An independent claim should typically specify the essential features needed to define the invention except insofar as such features are implied by the generic terms used, *e.g.* a claim to a bicycle does not typically need to mention the presence of wheels. Where patentability depends on a technical effect the claims should typically be drafted so as to include all the technical features of the invention which are essential for the technical effect[36]. In other words, claims must be clear and be directed to the heart of the invention.

B) Dependent Claims

A dependent claim is one that depends from another claim – either an independent claim or another dependent claim. Such dependencies are signalled by the identification of parent claim. By reciting another claim, the dependent claim is saying that it includes everything from the parent claim plus whatever is newly-recited in the dependent claim itself. Dependent claims tend to be considerably shorter than independent claims[37].

Dependent claims should be grouped together in the most appropriate way possible. The arrangement must, therefore, be one which enables the association of related claims to be readily determined and their meaning in association to be readily construed. In no way can a dependent claim extend the scope of protection of the invention defined in the corresponding independent claim. While drafting the dependent claim, the "amended" word indicates a change to the claim, the brackets () show deleted words and the underlining shows newly-added words.

Dependent claims are always narrower than the claim from which they depend. A dependent claim can only add elements or limitations to the claim to which it refers. It cannot subtract any elements or limitations from the same. This claim would be incorrect because it subtracts an element from the independent claim, namely the light. Again, dependent claims may not subtract any elements or limitations from the claim on which it depends. It is important to remember that if the independent claims are considered allowable over prior art by a patent examiner, the dependent claims will also be allowable over prior art. Dependent claims can be used to make independent claims more clearly broader.

C) Multiple Dependent Claims

Multiple dependent claims provide another format for dependent claims. The preamble of a multiple dependent claim refers to more than one claim in the alternative. For example, a preamble of a multiple dependent claim might read "the apparatus of Claim 1 or Claim 2" or "the apparatus of one of Claims 1 and 2."

---

35 WIPO Patent Drafting Manual, IP Assets Management Series, http://www.wipo.int/edocs/pubdocs/en/patents/867/wipo_pub_867.pdf accessed on 12 March 2018.

36 *Ibid.*

37 *Ibid.*

Here, Claims 1 and 2 are referred to in the alternative – meaning the claim depends on Claim 1 or Claim 2 but not both. Like dependent claims, the body of a multiple dependent claim narrow's the claim from which it depends[38]. In Novartis Ag and Anr Vs. Defendant Cipla Ltd[39] the High Court of Delhi held that an injunction may be granted in respect of a single claim even though other claims in the specification are not prima facie valid.

In some jurisdictions one multiple dependent claims may not depend on another multiple dependent claim. Like many aspects of patent practice, different jurisdictions may have different formatting requirements for multiple dependent claims and the patent agent must make his claims conform to the precise requirements for the jurisdictions of interest to his client.

Apart from these claim sets, there are various other types of claims which are recognised in different jurisdictions. They are discussed briefly below:

Specific Types of Claims

For many inventions, claims in more than one category are needed for full protection. The WIPO's Patent Drafting Manual[40] provides some of the various types or categories of claims that offers the inventor a complete scope for defining the Paten Claim protection extensively. They are given as follows:

1. *Apparatus or Device Claims:* An apparatus or device claim protects embodiments of an invention in the form of a physical apparatus, system or device. For instance, a claim that covers a tripod for a camera or a window crank is an apparatus claim.
2. *Method Claims or Process Claims:* Method claims are claims that recite a sequence of steps which together complete a task such as making an article of some sort. However, note that in many jurisdictions the steps performed in a method claim are presumed to occur in any order, unless otherwise stated, for both prior art and infringement purposes.
3. *Product-By-Process Claims*: Claims for products defined in terms of a process of manufacture are allowable in some jurisdictions provided that the products as such fulfil the requirements for patentability, *i.e.* they are new and inventive. A product is not typically rendered novel merely by the fact that it is produced by means of a new process. A claim defining a product in terms of a process will be construed as a claim to the product as such in many jurisdictions. The claim may for instance take the form "Product X obtainable by process Y." Irrespective of whether the term "obtainable," "obtained," "directly obtained" or an equivalent wording

38 WIPO Patent Drafting Manual, IP Assets Management Series, http://www.wipo.int/edocs/pubdocs/en/patents/867/wipo_pub_867.pdf accessed on 12 March 2018.

39 I.A. No.24863/2014 IN CS(OS) 3812/2014.

40 WIPO Patent Drafting Manual, IP Assets Management Series, http://www.wipo.int/edocs/pubdocs/en/patents/867/wipo_pub_867.pdf accessed on 12 March 2018.

is used in the product-by-process claim, it is still directed to the product per se and confers absolute protection upon the product.

4. *Design Claims*: In those jurisdictions that allow design patents, generally only one claim is permissible. The drawings are usually the critical element for a design patent since the protection provided pertains to ornamental design.
5. *Plant Patent Claims*: As noted earlier, some jurisdictions allow patenting of new varieties of plants. Not all jurisdictions permit such patents. Some jurisdictions allow for protection of new plants using essentially the same type of claims that one would use for a biotechnology invention, *e.g.* a deposit made according to the Budapest Treaty. Other jurisdictions allow for the patenting of plants under certain conditions such as by asexual propagation.
6. *Composition Claims:* Claims related to compositions are used where the invention to be claimed has to do with the chemical nature of the materials or components used.
7. *Biotechnology Claims*: Biotechnology inventions may include cDNA, recombinant DNA, DNA fragments, protein, monoclonal antibodies, anti-sense DNA and RNA, recombinant vectors and expression vectors. Many jurisdictions have special requirements for inventions related to biotechnology inventions and for sequence listings and deposit rules. Where an invention involves a biological material and words alone cannot sufficiently describe how to make and use the invention in a reproducible manner, access to the biological material may be necessary for the satisfaction of the statutory requirements for patentability. The Budapest Treaty[41] on the International Recognition of the Deposit of Microorganisms for the Purposes of Patent Procedure was established in 1977 to facilitate the recognition of deposited biological material in patent applications throughout the world. The Treaty requires signatory countries to recognize a deposit with any depository which has been approved by WIPO.

8. *Use Claims*: Some jurisdictions permit claims to new uses of known substances, particularly second or subsequent medical uses or indications of known substances and compositions. These use claims are also known as Swiss-type claims since Switzerland was the first country to allow them. Use claims are not permitted in all jurisdictions. Such claims are permitted in the EPO, even though the EPO generally does not allow claims directly to a method of treating the human body. Such claims, however, are not permitted in the US or India.

---

41 The Budapest Treaty on the International Recognition of the Deposit of Microorganisms for the Purposes of Patent Procedure, or Budapest Treaty, is an international treaty signed in Budapest, Hungary, on April 28, 1977. It entered into force on August 9, 1980, and was later amended on September 26, 1980. The treaty is administered by the World Intellectual Property Organization (WIPO).

9. *Software Claims*: Patent applications related to computer software and/or hardware devices that execute specialized algorithms typically include apparatus and method claims. Such applications also often contain some specialized claim formats for software inventions. The acceptable claim formats for computer software inventions may vary from country to country. Some acceptable formats may include computer-readable medium claims, data structure claims and propagated signal claims.
10. *Omnibus Claims*: "Omnibus" claims include a reference to the description or the drawings without providing any specific limitations.
11. *Means-Plus-Function Claim*: It is a claim including a technical feature expressed in functional terms of the type "means for converting a digital electric signal into an analog electric signal". A variant known as a "step-plus-function" claim style may be used to describe the steps of a method invention ("step for converting. step for storing.")

    Means-plus-function claims are governed by the various statutes and laws of the country or countries in which a patent application is filed.
12. *Markush claim*: Markush claim or structure is a claim with multiple "functionally equivalent" chemical entities allowed in one or more parts of the compound, mainly but not exclusively used in chemistry. If a compound being patented includes several Markush groups, the number of possible compounds it covers could be vast. Markush claims were named after Eugene Markush, the first inventor to use them successfully in a U.S. patent. In Bristol-Myers Squibb Company and Ors v. BDR Lifesciences Pvt. Ltd. and Anr[42] the High Court of Delhi discussed the Markush claim exclusively.

Conclusion

From the above discussion it is clear that the Patent claims does hold a significant place in defining the scope of patent protection. Across jurisdictions there are many approaches which contributes in defining the scope for patent protection. Traditional interpretive theories that attach a fixed and static meaning to the claim terms do not fit well with the dynamic nature of claim construction. In India, the meaning and scope of patent claim is usually based on the construction of patent claims document as well as the interpretation given by the judiciary. There is no defined laws available in the Indian law which provides the framework for drafting the claims. What is to understand here is that, the claim being the primary document, utmost care has to be taken while drafting it by considering all the peripheral perspectives impacting on its scope. It is suggested that the claims should not be made unduly complex. The claim must be given a desired meaning which will help in its best possible interpretation.

---

42 I.A. No.15720/2009 in CS(OS) No.2303/2009, I.A. No.5910/2013 in CS(OS) No.679/2013.

Chapter 12

IPR Necessitate in Agriculture

R.K. Kalaria

Aspee Shakilam Biotechnology Institute,
Navsari Agricultural University, Surat (Gujarat) 395 007
e-mail: risheekal@nau.in

ABSTRACT

Agriculture plays a vital role in India's economy as backbone of GDP. Agriculture employs nearly 60-70 per cent of the population and it is a principal provider to India's economic output. In 2016, agriculture contributed around 17.35 per cent to the India GDP[2,3]. A current economic survey expressed anxiety on the decline in the share of the agricultural sector's as capital formation in GDP[10].

Increasing and accelerating economic growth require enhancing strengthening of new agricultural practices to convene the increasing needs for food. Recent literature reported that some of the existing practices have led to stress on natural bio resources including water and soil [13]. Inconvenience leading to decline of soil health and declining water resources are some of the crucial areas needing more innovations approaches to make agriculture more sustainable in current scenarios [12,15]. The required demands would be in terms of the quantity and quantity of food produced using conventional and non conventional crop improvement programmes [13].

Keyword: IPR, Agriculture, PVPFR, CBD and GM crops.

Introduction of IPR in Agriculture Prospect

In nineteenth century, several countries started patent legislations. From few decades, genetic engineering became a vital part of breeding activities for patents on plants and animals or their parts, such as genes or gene sequences, have gained an increasingly significant role. This improvement has attracted criticism, from different society groups worldwide. Intellectual property rights (IPR) in agriculture have existed for almost many years. In the present era of liberalization, globalization and fast paced information technology, IPR have appeared as a new worldwide phenomenon during the process of crop improvements[9].

In India, patents are obtainable for new processes in respect of agriculture ie agrochemicals, growth promoters and regulators *etc.* but not to all products under Section of the Patents Act, 1970 with some restrictions[5]. The main concern in the agricultural sector is innovations are incorrectly appropriable. In recent years, IPRs are obtained by scientists and corporate sector on traditionally used biological resources such as Neem, Turmeric, Tulsi *etc.* A competent and efficient IPR management could balances individual inducement and benefits with the wider needs of the society. Several forms of IPRs including patents, plant varieties protection, trademarks, trade secrecy rights and plant breeders' rights employed in the sector of agriculture challenge to address this concern.

Increasing crop productivity has long been the objective of agricultural research. Few current trends in agricultural research are essential to understand the ongoing debates concerning the range of plant variety protection. The first is the biotechnology revolution leds to advances in GM (Genetically Modified) crops due to genetic engineering. This new technology makes potential development of novel plant varieties with higher productivity and disease-resistance characteristics that might helpful in sustainable agriculture.

The environmental protection concerns derived from GM products is also a subject of consideration. GM organisms pose recent threats to the conservation of biodiversity. The likelihood of genetic contamination is a recent type of pollution that consequence altered living organisms into the open ecosystem. The Cartagena Protocol on Biosafety to the Convention on Biological Diversity (CBD) is the main international legal instrument addressing concern related to the introduction of GM organisms. In India, the thought of commercialization of technology from resarch is relatively new in agriculture sector[13].The Government of India has recently declared the "National Intellectual Property Rights (IPR) policy[1].

India is among the initial countries in the world to have passed legislation granting farmers' rights in the form of the Plant Varieties Protection and Farmers' Rights Act, 2001 (PVPFR). Law is exclusive aims to protect both farmers' and breeders' rights [9]. The Plant Varieties Protection and Farmers' Rights Act, 2001, establishes a exclusive system by extending the idea of Plant Breeders Rights (PBRs), which is at present applied to novel varieties of plants, held by farmers, NGOs and other public sector institutions[8].

IPR Laws in India Agriculture

Several form of the IPRs mainly patents, plant breeders' rights, trademarks, geographical indications and trade secrets *etc.* are applicable to the agricultural sector in that they can be used to defend goods or services produced in the agricultural sector. India being an affiliated to the various international conventions and agreements is bound to enact/amend relevant domestic laws to gear up and face the challenges of globalization. The IPRs related laws in India are undergoing transformation in order to authenticate the conditions in the TRIPS Agreement.

Patent Act of 1970 is one of the significant landmarks in the history of IPR laws in India. The government brought amendments to the Patent Act in 1999, 2002 and 2005. The main alter brought through the amendments do not substantially affect traditional knowledge, farmers' rights and biodiversity. The food sector in India is also facing new challenges in implementing new patent rule [16].

The Biological Diversity Act, 2002 was implemented following India's endorsement of the Biodiversity Convention (CBD). It aims to preserve biodiversity, sustainable use of biological resources and justifying sharing of benefits that occur from their use or traditional information. It mandates the setting up of institutions at national, state and local levels, for the reason of regulation of biological diversity. For entrance and transport of biodiversity records, foreigners and industrial establishments have to take authorization from the national authorities. The Act attempts to control access to biodiversity for industrial purposes, to fight biopiracy and distinguish community human rights over conventional knowledge and biodiversity.IPRs on biological resources are the solitary annoyed subject in the overall IPR. [5]

Plant Varieties Protection and Farmers Rights (PVPFR) Act, 2001 was enacted under the obligations set out in Article 27.3(b) of the Agreement on Trade Related Intellectual Property Rights (TRIPS) which provide authorization the protection of plant varieties either by patents or by an effective sui generis system or a combination of both. The Indian legislation on Plant Varieties Protection (PVP) is being perceived as a progressive legislation. In India, the PVPFR Act in addition to offering protection to plant rights, also protects the rights of the farmers to save, use, sow, re-sow, exchange, share or sell farm produce including the seeds of any unprotected variety, with an exemption to prevent the sale of branded seeds.[6]

The Geographical Indications of Goods (Registration and Protection) Act, 1999 was enacted as a sui generis system, post Basmati rice case (1997) in which India challenged the patent granted by the American Rice Company, on its claim of producing basmati rice grains. The Act was brought in to defend the prohibited use of geographical indications with respect to agricultural goods.

The Seeds Bill, 2004 was proposed as a substitute for the existing Seeds Act, 1966. The stated purpose of the proposed law is to control the seed market and certified seeds of "quality". With the proposed changes, the seed law would be harmonized with other seed laws around the world. The rationale for a new Act can be traced back to the relatively quick changes that are taking place in the seed sector in the past couple of decades. These include in particular the growing role of private seed companies and the progressive introduction of transgenic.[14]

International Conventions and Treaties on Agricultural Produce and Patent Rights

The NICE Agreement concerning the International Classification of Goods and Services for the Purposes of the Registration of Marks was a multilateral international treaty, came into force on April 8, 1961, and it was revised at Stockholm on July 14, 1967, and at Geneva on May 13, 1977 ("The Geneva Act"). It contains information

regarding registration of pesticides used in agriculture and allied fields were mentioned. As a result, the farmers need to register their innovation, trade name under the Trademarks Act by following the Rules of 2002.[4]

TRIPS Agreement

Trade Related Aspects of Intellectual Property Rights (TRIPS) Agreement, 1994 is an annex 1C of the Marrakesh Agreement establishing the World Trade Organization is concerned with the overall intellectual property branches which provide a new phenomenon for the international registration of product and innovations. Regarding agricultural aspect, it is a welcome relief for India, as the government was struggling to protect basmati rice, turmeric, neem, tea and various agricultural produces under IPR regime.

The World Conference held in Havana in 1947 had established the General Agreement on Trade and Tariffs (GATT) as a temporary body for Multilateral Trade Negotiations (MTNs). The 1986 GATT Round, popularly known as the Uruguay Round (UR) provided for a opportunity for formation of diverse coalitions to advance their interests, bringing new elements into trade discussion, especially relating to agriculture. One of the most important agreements of UR relates to the granting of IPR on biological materials embodied in the TRIPS. It specifically requires member nations to grant patents on micro-organisms, non-biological and micro-biological processes as well as an effective IPR protection for plant varieties. The TRIPS agreement recognizes the creation of IPR as vital regime for the development of mankind[5,6].

TRIPS agreement consist of different part as discuss below in brief. **Part I** of TRIPS agreement contains the basic principles on accord for National Treatment and granted Most-Favored Nation Treatment. **Part II** then goes through each type of intellectual property individual at a time, describing the principles and privileges in each case. These include: Copyrights of books, paintings, computer programs *etc.* **Part III** goes on to explain how member countries must afford efficient means for implementing these IPR and capable to penalties to frighten on further violations. **Part IV** deals with the achievement and preservation of IPRs, **Part V** provides for argument on prevention and settlement. To concern these, the **Part VI** identifies numerous transitional arrangements for member countries. Developing countries like India were given the option to fulfil till 2005 under transitional arrangements.

Plant Variety Protection

The International Convention for the Protection of New Varieties of Plants of December 2, 1961 is also called as UPOV Convention 1961. The Convention provides grant for plant breeder's rights to the adhering states under their domestic laws. UPOV is closely associated with the WIPO (World Intellectual Property Organisation).The issue of Plant Varieties Protection (PVP) is important and can be understood in two ways. Firstly, where protection of plant variety is vital to offer incentive to commercial breeders for developing new plant varieties. Secondly, where Plant Varieties Protection (PVP) has direct connection with the rights of the farmers who have traditionally improving plant varieties as per their local environmental conditions. Researcher in 2015 enlisted some crop species notified for registration in india (Table 12.1)[6]. Thus, with respect to the protection of plant varieties, TRIPS agreement understandable that plants and animals may be excluded from patentability. India is bound by all the provisions of TRIPS Agreement, which force the country to enact/amend relevant domestic laws.

Table 12.1: Crop Species Notified for Registration

Sl.No.	*Group*	*No.*	*Crop Species*	*Gazette Notification No.*
1	Cereals	9	Bread wheat, Rice, Pearl millet, Sorghum, Maize	S.O.1884(E), 1 November 2006
			Durum wheat, Dicoccum wheat, *Triticum species* (other than *Triticum aestivum* L., *Triticum durum* Desf and *Triticum dicoccum* L.)	S.O.1913(E), 18 August 2011
2	Legumes	7	Chickpea, Green Gram (Mungbean), Black Gram (Urad bean), Field pea, Kidney Bean (Rajmash), Lentil, Pigeon pea	S.O.1884(E), 1 November 2006
3	Fibre Crops	6	Diploid cotton (two species), Tetraploid cotton (two species), Jute (two species)	S.O.2229(E), 31 December 2007
4	Oilseeds	11	Indian mustard, Karan rai, Rapeseed, Gobhi sarson, Groundnut, Soybean, Sunflower, Safflower, Castor, Sesame, Linseed	S.O.993(E), 30 April 2010
5	Sugar Crops	1	Sugarcane	S.O.1874(E), 3 August 2009
6	Vegetables	14	Ginger, Turmeric	S.O.1874(E), 3 August 2009
			Tomato, Brinjal, Okra (Lady's finger), Cauliflower, Cabbage, Potato, Onion, Garlic	S.O.2883(E), 2 December 2010
			Bitter Gourd, Bottle Gourd, Cucumber, Pumpkin	S.O.1093(E), 15 April 2014
7	Spices	4	Black pepper, Small cardamom	S.O.993(E), 30 April 2010
			Coriander, Fenugreek	S.O.1093(E), 15 April 2014
8	Fruits	14	Mango, Almond, Apple, Pear, Apricot, Cherry, Walnut	S.O.2883(E), 2 December 2010
			Grapes, Pomegranate, Indian jujube (Ber)	S.O.1093(E), 15 April 2014
			Acid Lime, Mandarin, Sweet Orange, Banana	S.O. 2664 (E), 16 October 2014
9	Plantation crop	8	Coconut	S.O.1913(E), 18 August 2011
			Eucalyptus (2 crop species), Casuarina (2 crop species)	S.O.1093(E), 15 April 2014
			Tea (3 crop species)	S.O. 2664 (E), 16 October 2014

Plant Varieties Protection and Farmers' Rights Act, 2001:

In compliance with the requirement under TRIPS, India developed its own sui generis system of law to protect plant variety. It has been considered essential to identified and protect the right of the farmers in respect of their contribution made maintain and improving plant genetic resources for the development of new plant varieties. In current scenarios, to accelerate agricultural productivity, it was felt essential to protect plant breeders' rights to promote investment for research and development of new plant varieties. The law introduced as Protection of Plant Varieties and Farmers' Rights Act, 2001 (PVPFR Act). The PVPFR Act 2001 came into existence to provide for the establishment of an effective system for the protection of plant varieties, the rights of farmers and plant breeders and to encourage the development of new varieties of plants[8].The Act makes provisions for such farmer's varieties to be registered with the help of NGO's so that they are protected against being scavenged [11].

The Acts and Offices to implement and deal with IPR components in India:

- The Patents Act, 1970 (amended in 1999, 2002 and 2005) through the Patent Offices at Kolkata (HQ), Mumbai, Chennai and Delhi.
- The Designs Act, 2000 through the Patent Offices at Kolkata (HQ), Mumbai, Chennai, and Delhi.
- The Trade Marks Act, 1999 through the Trade Marks Registry at Mumbai (HQ), Chennai, Delhi, Kolkata and Ahmedabad.
- The Geographical Indications of Goods (Registration and Protection) Act, 1999 through the Geographical Indications Registry at Chennai.

In 2007, Modernization of IP administration in india started as E-filing facility for patent and trademark applications has been introduced.

Role of IPR in Agriculture

In 2002, the UK company patented a procedure for the identification of broccoli plants that have an increased glucosinolate per cent through the European Patent Office. That patent, however, include not only the use of special marker genes to breed broccoli, but also the vegetable plants and the broccoli seed obtained by means of this process. Farmers' groups and NGO in contrast, stand in opposition to such undermining of the patent law. In 2009 and 2010, applied for patents on pig and fish processed product in which feed supplied contains a certain proportion of omega-3 fatty acids derived from genetically modified soya, sunflower, oilseed rape or maize.

IPRs provide an inducement for private research and development for crop improvement techniques, thereby reducing the necessitate for government funding to subsidize these activities. Before the advent of modern technologies in the agricultural sector, inventions based on living organisms were considered as natural and obvious discoveries that could rarely be copied and did not required any protection. Developments in biotechnology have led to change the circumstances dramatically. Biotechnological inventions require extensive investments, and their processes and products can easily be copied. The develpment definitely look for returns on their investments to support and provide incentives for their future innovations. IPR provides a way for ensuring financial revenues, and also protects novel innovations and crop material from illegal commercial duplication [7].

Conclusion

IPR protection in agriculture should continue improving enforcement, access to resources and technology; benefit sharing, equity and justice in order to give consequence to the national agricultural policy and the intrinsic basic principles of the Indian laws. It is important that the government should make such amendments in the Acts which efficiently and adequately preserve and keep the attention of individuals and do not exclude domestic industries, farmers, scientists and market and at the same time are in the interest of the larger section of society. Patent rights must be seen as an inducement system, in which encourages the innovator to expand new technologies and publicly disclose his resulting innovations[5]. Farmers should be given their well deserved rights and incentives as well as protection of their developed variety. It is also important to note that developed economies benefit greatly from an organized IPR system due to their intrinsic capabilities to capitalize on such opportunities. The target for various agricultural goods having export prospects should be more enhanced competitiveness together with increased production particularly for high value commercial crops, spices, medicinal and aromatic plants.

References

1. Anonymous, (2016a) https://www.statista.com/statistics/271329/distribution-of-gross-domestic- product-gdp-across-economic-sectors-in-india/accessed on 26.03.2018.
2. Anonymous, (2016b) National Intellectual Property Rights Policy. Department of Industrial Policy and Promotion. Ministry of Commerce and Industry, Government of India. accessed on 26.03.2018
3. Anonymous, (2018) Food and Agriculture Organization in India, http://www.fao.org accessed on 26.03.2018.
4. Cullet, P (1999) Revision of the TRIPS Agreement concerning the Protection of Plant Varieties, 2 Journal of World Intellectual Property, p. 617.
5. Dewan, M (2011) IPR Protection in Agriculture: An Overview.Journal of Intellectual Property Rights, 16:131-138
6. Hanchinal, RR (2015) Providing Intellectual Property Protection to Farmers' Varieties in India under the Protection of Plant Varieties and Farmers' Rights Act, 2001 Journal of Intellectual Property Rights,20:7-18
7. Meyer, H (2009) The role of intellectual property rights in agriculture. Previously unpublished study on behalf of The Federal Ministry for Economic Cooperation and Development (BMZ), Paper 314. Sector project 'Welternährung und Agrobiodiversität' [Global food security and agrobiodiversity] of GTZ. Eschborn.

8. Ramanna, A (2003). India's Plant Varieties and Farmers' Rights Legislation: Potential impact on stakeholder's access to Genetic Resources, EPTD Discussion pg. 39, Washington, USA.(http://www.ifpri.org/publication/india per cent E2 per cent 80 per cent 99s-plant-variety-and farmers per cent E2 per cent 80 per cent 99-rights-legislation)

9. Ramanna, A (2006). *Farmers' Rights in India - A case study*, FNI Report, Norway, p.1-89 (https://www.fni.no/getfile.php/131801/Filer/Publikasjoner/FNI-R0606.pdf)

10. Rajput, A (2018). Economic Dev. and Policy in India, published online in School of open learning, University of Delhi, New Delhi accessed on 26.03.2018.

11. Sophy, KJ (2015) Farmers' Rights under Plant Variety Protection Legislation in India: A Critical Study, Rostrum's Law Review 2(2):1-5.

12. Sastry, RK, Rashmi, HB and Rao, NH (2010). Nanotechnology for enhancing food security in India. Food Policy 36(3): 391-400.

13. Sastry, RK (2017). Intellectual Property Rights In Indian Agriculture. 105th FoCARS, ICAR-National Academy of Agricultural Management. Hyderabad. accessed on 26.03.2018

14. Vandna, S (2014), Sacred Seed, Global Peace Initiative of Women, Deradhun. accessed on 26.03.2018.

15. Verma, S and Bodh, PC (2016) Agricultural Situation in India, Directorate of Economics and Statistics Department of Agriculture, Cooperation and Farmers Welfare ministry of Agriculture and Farmers welfare, government of India. New Delhi pp:1-6.

16. Overwalle, GV (1999) Patent protection for plants: A comparison of American and European approaches, IDEA-Journal of Law and Technology, 39 (2):143-194.

Chapter 13

Comparative Analysis on Changing Scenario in Geographical Indications: An Indian Perspective

Rahil Mathakia and Viralkumar B. Mandaliya

Gujarat National Law University, Gandhinagar-382426 (Gujarat) INDIA
e-mail: viral_mandaliya@yahoo.com

ABSTRACT

In India, the registration of Geographical indication (GI) was enforced after the GI Act, 1999. Since its enforcement, out of 617 application, 320 products/goods were registered in five distinct group *i.e.* Handicraft (including Textiles) products, Agricultural products, Manufactured products, Foodstuff products and Natural products. In this study, the registration of GI is analyzed for various modes like year-wise, category-wise and state-wise. It is pertinent that there is the highest registration of GI from the State of Karnataka. The present analysis has summarized the wealth of original products/goods from various states/UTs of India.

Keywords: *Geographical indication, GI Act, 1999, Geographical indication registry.*

Introduction

A geographical indication (GI) is a sign used on products that have a specific geographical origin and possess qualities or a reputation that are due to that origin. In order to function as a GI, a sign must identify a product as originating in a given place. In addition, the qualities, characteristics or reputation of the product should be essentially due to the place of origin. Since the qualities depend on the geographical place of production, there is a clear link between the product and its original place of production[1].

---

1 http://www.wipo.int/geo_indications/en, accessed on 4 July 2018.

As per the (Indian) Geographical Indications of Goods (Registration and Protection) Act, 1999[2] "Geographical Indication", in relation to goods, means an indication which identifies such goods as agricultural goods, natural goods or manufactured goods as originating, or manufactured in the territory of a country, or a region or locality in that territory, where a given quality, reputation or other characteristic of such goods is essentially attributable to its geographical origin and in case where such goods are manufactured goods one of the activities of either the production or of processing or preparation of the goods concerned takes place in such territory, region or locality, as the case may be[3].

Geographical Indications of Goods (Registration and Protection) Rules, 2002[4] was notified by Ministry of Commerce and Industry, GoI on 8th March 2002 while. Geographical Indications of Goods (Registration and Protection) Act, 1999, which came into effect on September 15, 2003.

This chapter summarizes the goods registered since the Act is enforced in the country. The information for registered goods were taken from Geographical Indication Registry of India[5]. This registry was searched on 19th July 2018 to analyze the current status of GIs in India from year 2003-18. The state-wise registration details of GIs applications[6] were analyzed for various parameters in this study. This state-wise registration details were comprised of details of GIs registration up to 31st March 2018.

Analysis of Total Number of GI Application from year 2003-18

The total number of GI application received by registry was 617 on 19th July 2018 (Table 13.1). The number of registered GI was 320 out of total application of 617. It is observed that the number of pending application *i.e.* 273 which is as half of total application (Figure 13.1). This 320 registered GIs were taken in the subsequent analysis.

Table 13.1: The Status of Total Number of GI Application from Year 2003-18

Status of GI Applications	
Refused	6
Registered	320
Withdrawn	5
Abandon	13
Pending	273
All	**617**

2 https://indiacode.nic.in/bitstream/123456789/1981/1/199948.pdf, accessed on 6 July 2018.

3 http://www.ipindia.nic.in/writereaddata/Portal/IPOAct/1_49_1_gi-act-1999.pdf, accessed on 8 July 2018.

4 http://www.ipindia.nic.in/writereaddata/Portal/IPORule/1_27_1_gi-rules.pdf, accessed on 10 July 2018.

5 http://www.ipindia.nic.in/registered-gls.htm, accessed on 14 July 2018.

6 http://www.ipindia.nic.in/writereaddata/Portal/Images/pdf/Registered_GI_March_2018.pdf, accessed on 19 July 2018.

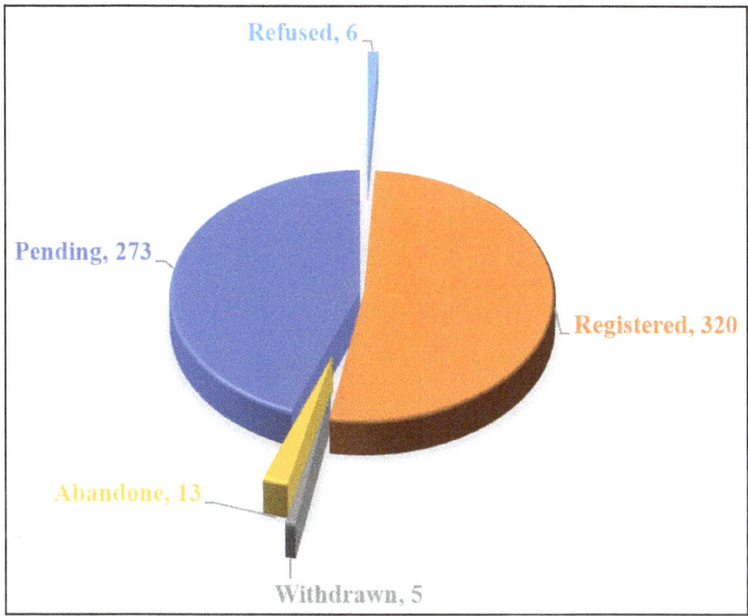

Figure 13.1: Analysis of Total Number of GI Application from Year 2003-18.

Analysis of Year-wise Number of Registration of GIs from 2003-18

A total 320 Geographical Indications (GIs) have been registered since 2003. It is observed that lowest number of GIs were registered in 2004-05 (n=3) and 2006-07 (n=3), while highest number of GIs were registered in 2008-09 (n=45) and 2016-17 (n=43) (Table 13.2). The linear trend line in this timeline graph indicate that there is a steady development of registration process from 2010-11 (Figure 13.2).

Table 13.2: Status of Year-wise Number of Registration of GIs from 2003-18

Year	*Registered Geographical Indications*
2004-05	3
2005-06	24
2006-07	3
2007-08	31
2008-09	45
2009-10	14
2010-11	29
2011-12	23
2012-13	21
2013-14	22
2014-15	20
2015-16	26

Year	Registered Geographical Indications
2016-17	33
2017-18	26
Total	**320**

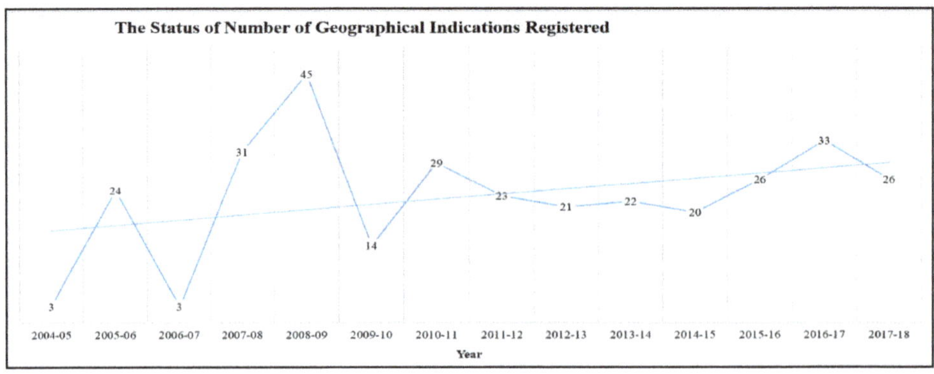

Figure 13.2: Year-wise Registration Status of GIs from 2003-18.

Analysis of Year-wise Registered Type of Goods as GIs from 2003-18

A product/goods which is registered as GIs were categories in 5 distinct group *i.e.* Handicraft (including Textiles) products, Agricultural products, Manufactured products, Foodstuff products and Natural products (Table 13.3). The categorical distribution has shown that 62 per cent was from Handicraft (including Textiles) products, 28 per cent was from Agricultural products, and 10 per cent was comprised of remaining three categories *i.e.* Manufactured, Foodstuff and Natural products (Figure 13.3). Furthermore, year-wise products were enlisted and graphically presented in Figure 13.4. From this it is elucidated that top most registration of Handicraft (including Textiles) products was in year 2008-09 and top most registration of Agricultural products was in year 2016-17.

Table 13.3: Year-wise Registration of Kind of Goods as GIs from 2003-18

Year	Registration Details of Geographical Indications					Total
	Handicraft (including Textiles)	Agricultural	Manu-factured	Foodstuff	Natural	
2004-05	2	1				3
2005-06	18	2	4			**24**
2006-07	1	2				**3**
2007-08	19	11	1			**31**
2008-09	33	10	1	1		**45**
2009-10	7	5	1	1		**14**
2010-11	15	7	4	3		**29**

Year	Registration Details of Geographical Indications					Total
	Handicraft (including Textiles)	*Agricultural*	*Manu-factured*	*Foodstuff*	*Natural*	
2011-12	15	4	4			**23**
2012-13	18	2	1			**21**
2013-14	17	4	1			**22**
2014-15	5	11	1	2	1	**20**
2015-16	17	9				**26**
2016-17	13	14	1	5		**33**
2017-18	17	7	1	1		**26**
Total	197	89	20	13	1	**320**

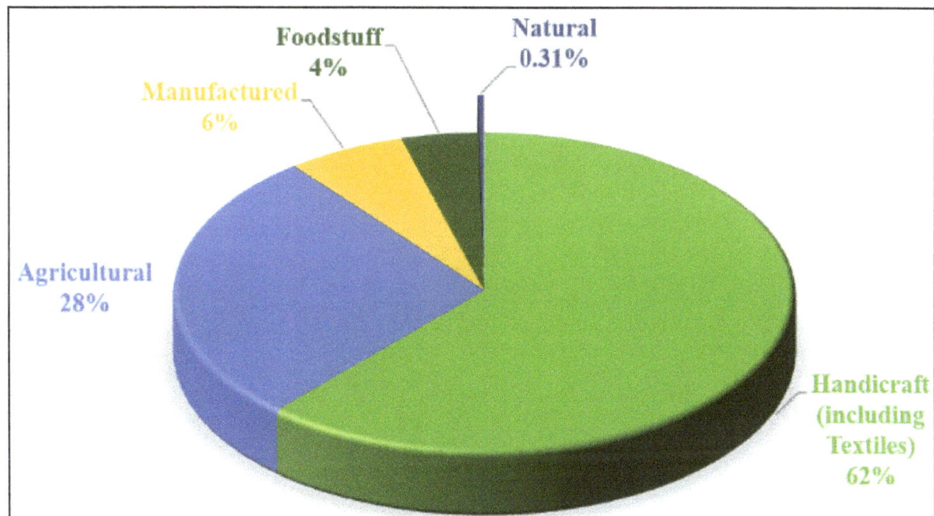

Figure 13.3: The Kind of Goods Registered as GIs (2003-18).

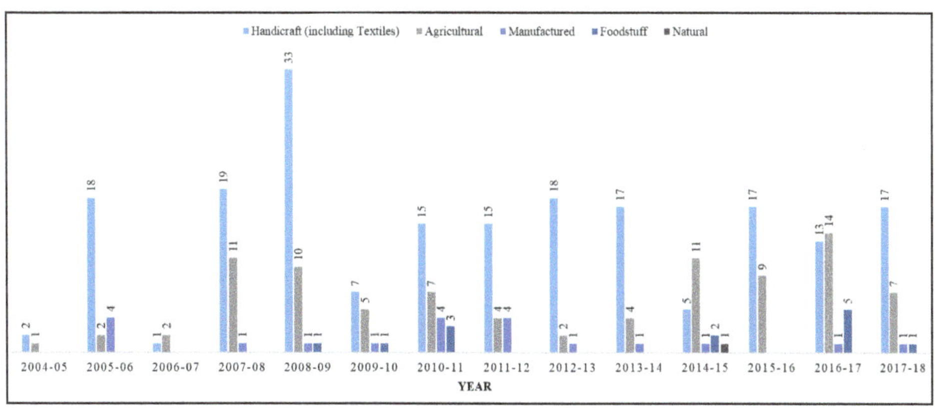

Figure 13.4: Year-wise Distribution of Goods that Registered as GIs (2003-18).

Analysis of Year-wise Registered GIs in different Regions

A total 320 Geographical Indications (GIs) have been registered which comprised of contribution from nations *i.e.* States and Union Territories of India as well as across the nations *i.e.* from foreign countries. According to this study 307 products is registered by India (Figure 13.5), and 13 products is registered by foreign states. The number of registered GI was lower *i.e.* n= 1 from Tripura, Sikkim, Mizoram, Goa and Arunachal Pradesh, while higher number *i.e.* n>30 was from Karnataka and Maharashtra (Table 13.4; Figure 13.6). Further analysis on Karnataka and Maharashtra has shown that number of registered products were higher in year 2006-08 (n=13) and 2016-18 (n-13), respectively (Figure 13.7).

Jammu and Kashmir 7
Himachal Pradesh 6
Chandigarh
1 Punjab
Haryana
Uttarakhand 1
National Capital Territory of Delhi
Sikkim 1
Arunachal Pradesh 1
Rajasthan 14
Uttar Pradesh 25
Assam 6
3 Nagaland
2 Meghalaya
Bihar 11
4 Manipur
Jharkhand
Gujarat 13
9 Madhya Pradesh
West Bengal 21
1 Tripura
Mizoram 1
Chhattisgarh 5
Odisha 15
Daman and Diu
Dadra and Nagar Haveli
Maharashtra 30
Telangana 13
Goa 1
Karnataka 39
Andhra Pradesh 19
2 Puducherry
Kerala 27
Tamil Nadu 28
Lakshadweep
Andaman and Nicobar Islands

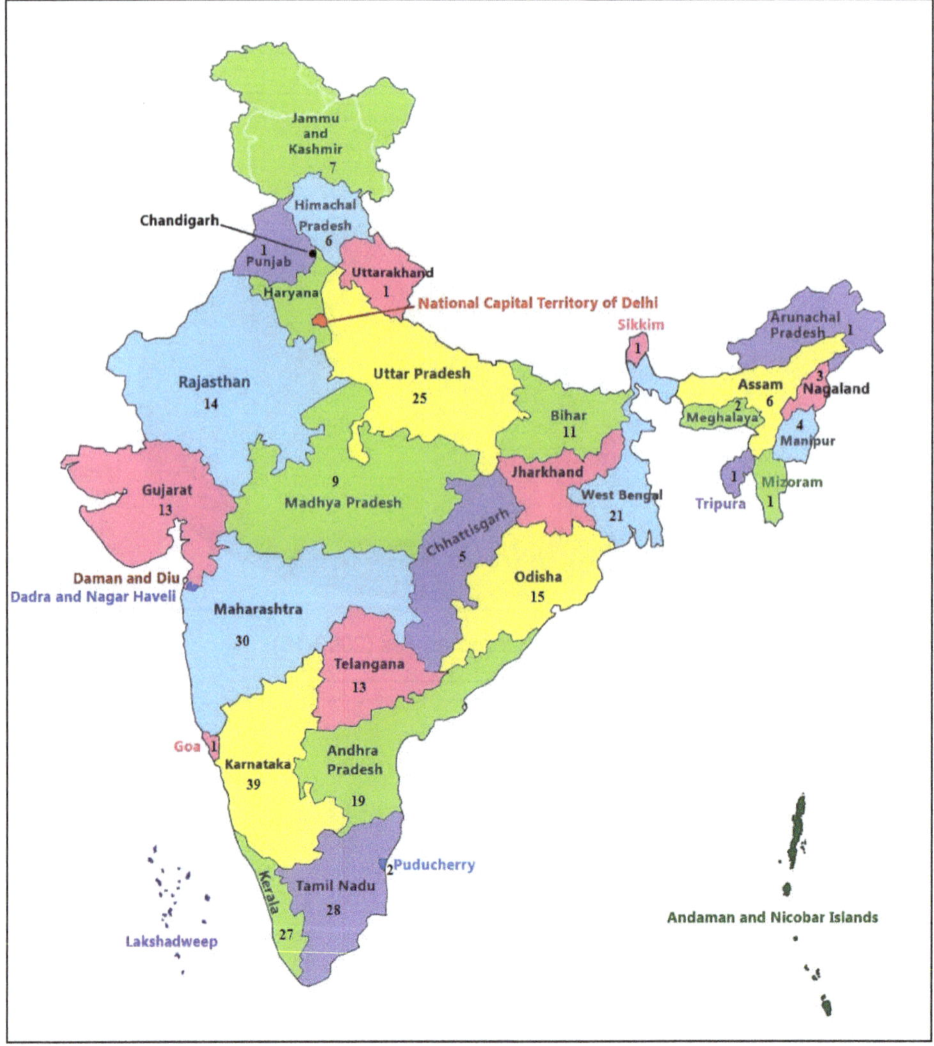

Figure 13.5: Map of India indicating the Number of GIs registered from 2003-18 (Data was taken from GI registry and prepared by the authors).

Table 13.4: Regions and Year-wise details of GIs from 2003-18

State	*2004-06*	*2006-08*	*2008-10*	*2010-12*	*2012-14*	*2014-16*	*2016-18*	*Total*
Andhra Pradesh	2	1	5	3	2		6	19
Arunachal Pradesh						1		1
Assam		1	1		1	2	1	6
Bihar		4			1		6	11
Chhattisgarh			3	1	1			5
Goa			1					1
Gujarat			4	4	1	3	1	13
Himachal Pradesh	2		1	1	2			6
India (Basmati)						1		1
Jammu and Kashmir			3	3			1	7
Karnataka	10	**13**	4	4	1	6	1	39
Kerala	1	5	7	7	1	5	1	27
Madhya Pradesh	1		3		2	3		9
Maharashtra	2		1	4	3	7	**13**	30
Manipur					3	1		4
Meghalaya						2		2
Mizoram						1		1
Nagaland			1			1	1	3
Odisha	2		3	4	6			15
Pondicherry				2				2
Punjab				1				1
Rajasthan	1		4	3	1	1	4	14
Sikkim						1		1
Tamil Nadu	5	7	6		6	3	1	28
Telangana		1	3	5	1		3	13
Tripura						1		1
Uttar Pradesh		1	3	1	10	6	4	25
Uttarakhand							1	1
West Bengal	1	1	5	2		1	11	21
Foreign			1	7	1		4	13
Total	27	34	59	52	43	46	59	320

Analysis of Kind of Goods as GIs from different Regions (2003-18)

In this analysis, the type of goods that registered as a GIs were classified region-wise and tabulated in Table 13.5. The goods wise registration of GI was highest from Tamil Nadu, Maharashtra and Foreign regions in Handicraft (including Textiles), Agricultural and Manufactured products, respectively (Figure 13.8). It is very

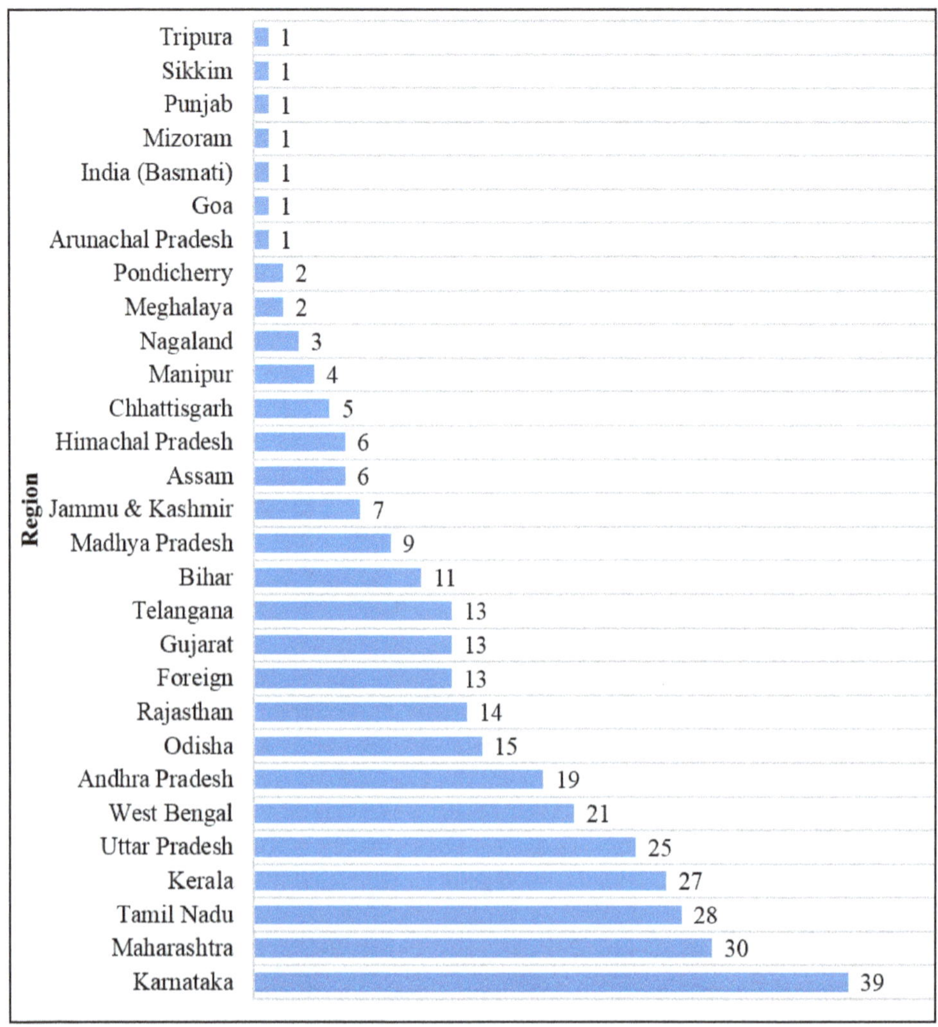

Figure 13.6: Region-wise Number of Registered GIs in India and Abroad (2003-18).

astonishing that only one GI is from Natural goods category and it is "MAKRANA MARBLE" that registered by Rajasthan[7] (Figure 13.9).

Conclusion

Geographical indication (GI) increases the visibility of the goods/product of the origin. The GI registration were facilitated by Geographical Indication Registry, GoI after enactment of GI Act, 1999. Since then 320 products/goods were registered by various states/UTs of India and abroad. The highest number of GIs (n=45) were

7 http://ipindiaservices.gov.in/GirPublic/Application/Details/405, accessed on 25 July, 2018.

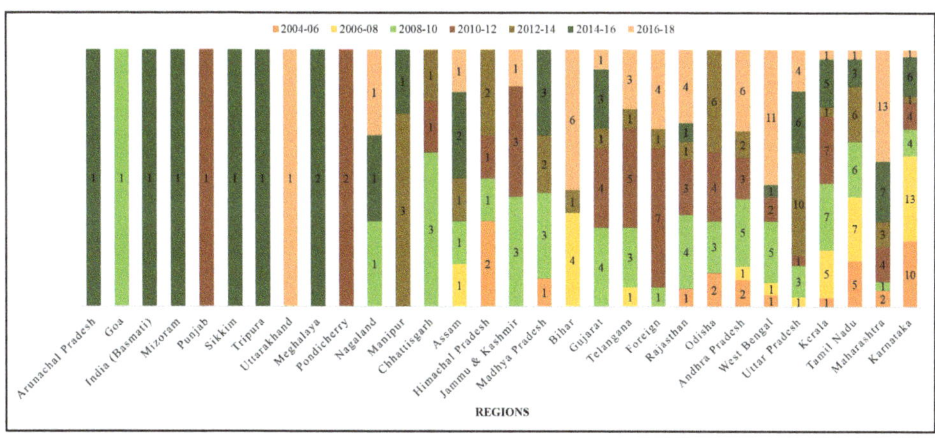

Figure 13.7: Year-wise Growth of Registered GIs in different Regions (2003-18).

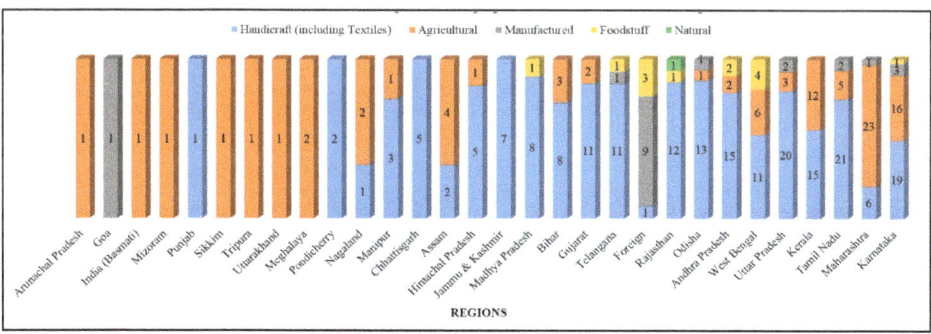

Figure 13.8: Goods-wise Distribution of Registered GIs in different Regions (2003-18).

Table 13.5: Kind of Goods/Products as GI from Various Regions (2003-18)

Regions	*Registration Details of Geographical Indications*					
	Handicraft (including Textiles)	*Agricultural*	*Manu-factured*	*Food Stuff*	*Natural*	*Total*
Andhra Pradesh	15	2		2		19
Arunachal Pradesh		1				1
Assam	2	4				6
Bihar	8	3				11
Chhattisgarh	5					5
Goa			1			1
Gujarat	11	2				13
Himachal Pradesh	5	1				6
India (Basmati)		1				1
Jammu and Kashmir	7					7

Regions	*Registration Details of Geographical Indications*					
	Handicraft (including Textiles)	*Agricultural*	*Manu-factured*	*Food Stuff*	*Natural*	*Total*
Karnataka	19	16	3	1		39
Kerala	15	12				27
Madhya Pradesh	8			1		9
Maharashtra	6	**23**	1			30
Manipur	3	1				4
Meghalaya		2				2
Mizoram		1				1
Nagaland	1	2				3
Odisha	13	1	1			15
Pondicherry	2					2
Punjab	1					1
Rajasthan	12			1	1	14
Sikkim		1				1
Tamil Nadu	**21**	5	2			28
Telangana	11		1	1		13
Tripura		1				1
Uttar Pradesh	20	3	2			25
Uttarakhand		1				1
West Bengal	11	6		4		21
Foreign	1		**9**	3		13
Total	197	89	20	13	1	320

registered in 2008-09. The top most registration was shown by the State of Karnataka and the number was 39. The registered GIs were categories in five distinct group *i.e.* Handicraft (including Textiles) products, Agricultural products, Manufactured products, Foodstuff products and Natural products. There was only one GI is registered in Natural goods category and it was "MAKRANA MARBLE" registered by the State of Rajasthan.

Acknowledgment

The authors are thankful to Geographical Indication Registry, Government of India for keeping the records in public access. The authors are also thankful to Prof. Dr. Bimal N. Patel (Director) and Prof. Dr. Ranita Nagar (Dean, Research), Gujarat National Law University for their continuous support and encouragement towards the research. Last, authors would like to thank Information and Communication Technology (ICT) Division, Gujarat National Law University, Gandhinagar for providing uninterrupted internet facility during the course of entire study.

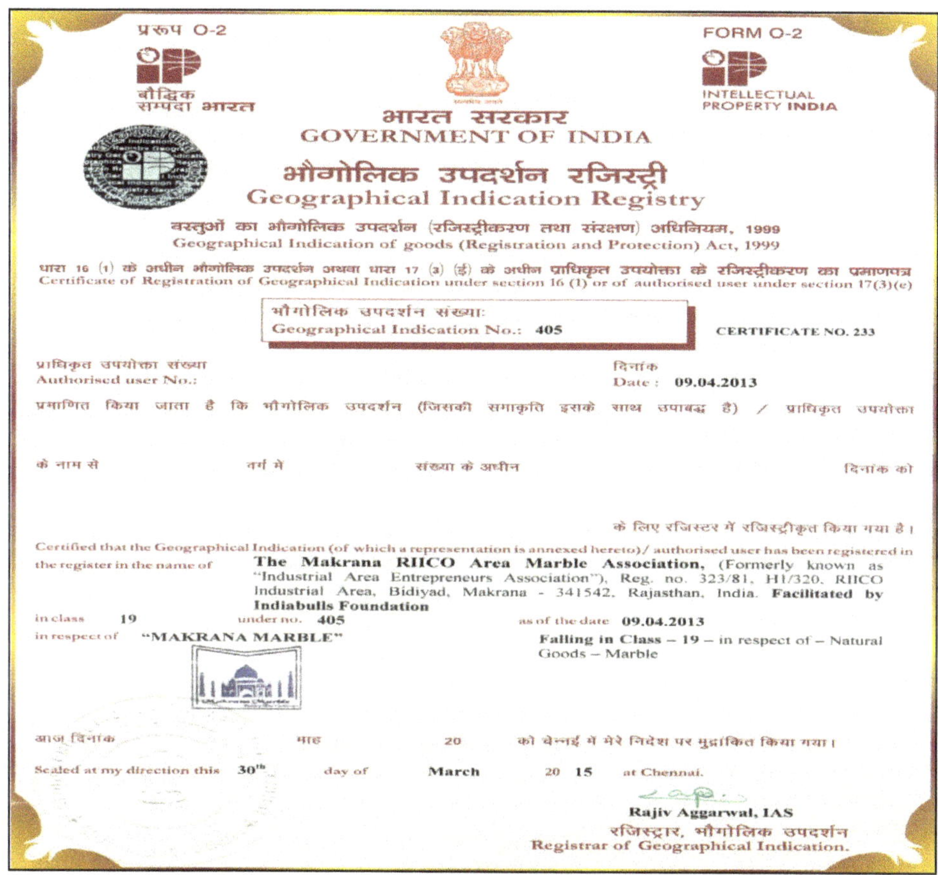

प्ररूप O-2

FORM O-2

बौद्धिक सम्पदा भारत

INTELLECTUAL PROPERTY INDIA

भारत सरकार

GOVERNMENT OF INDIA

भौगोलिक उपदर्शन रजिस्ट्री

Geographical Indication Registry

वस्तुओं का भौगोलिक उपदर्शन (रजिस्ट्रीकरण तथा संरक्षण) अधिनियम, 1999

Geographical Indication of goods (Registration and Protection) Act, 1999

धारा 16 (1) के अधीन भौगोलिक उपदर्शन अथवा धारा 17 (3) (ई) के अधीन प्राधिकृत उपयोक्ता के रजिस्ट्रीकरण का प्रमाणपत्र

Certificate of Registration of Geographical Indication under section 16 (1) or of authorised user under section 17(3)(e)

भौगोलिक उपदर्शन संख्या:

Geographical Indication No.: **405**

CERTIFICATE NO. 233

प्राधिकृत उपयोक्ता संख्या

Authorised user No.:

दिनांक

Date : **09.04.2013**

प्रमाणित किया जाता है कि भौगोलिक उपदर्शन (जिसकी समाकृति इसके साथ उपाबद्ध है) / प्राधिकृत उपयोक्ता

के नाम से वर्ग में संख्या के अधीन दिनांक को

के लिए रजिस्टर में रजिस्ट्रीकृत किया गया है।

Certified that the Geographical Indication (of which a representation is annexed hereto)/ authorised user has been registered in the register in the name of **The Makrana RIICO Area Marble Association,** (Formerly known as "Industrial Area Entrepreneurs Association"), Reg. no. 323/81, H1/320, RIICO Industrial Area, Bidiyad, Makrana - 341542, Rajasthan, India. **Facilitated by Indiabulls Foundation**

in class **19** under no. **405** as of the date **09.04.2013**

in respect of **"MAKRANA MARBLE"** **Falling in Class – 19** – in respect of – Natural Goods – Marble

आज दिनांक माह 20 को चेन्नई में मेरे निदेश पर मुद्रांकित किया गया।

Sealed at my direction this **30th** day of **March** 20 **15** at Chennai.

Rajiv Aggarwal, IAS

रजिस्ट्रार, भौगोलिक उपदर्शन

Registrar of Geographical Indication.

Figure 13.9: The GI Registration Certificate of "MAKRANA MARBLE" under Natural Goods Category from the State of Rajasthan.

Chapter 14

Agricultural Biotechnology in Indian Food Sector: Possible Risks and Benefits

Saumya Verma

Advocate at Madhya Pradesh High Court, Jabalpur, India - 482001
e-mail: saumya.verma91@gmail.com

ABSTRACT

It is interesting to analyse the relation between the approach of Norman Borlaug and M.S. Swaminathan for agricultural biotechnology. Where, Borlaug has considered biotechnology as "inevitable", Swaminathan elaborates it as "natural and necessary". During 1980s, country was able to attain self sufficiency in food sector; a trend growth rate of 2.6 per cent per year in 1980s reveals this fact. At the juncture, when world is facing food crisis, the biotechnological innovations are a ray of hope in dealing with the existing constraints. It has been more than 29 years when green revolution happened with the advent of high yield variety Mexican seeds which aided Indian economy to achieve optimum agricultural growth and thereby, food security. For materialising the policies to achieve food security within country, government is continuously trying to come up with various legislations, guidelines, schemes with a considerable amount of investment incapacity building and catalysing research and development process for the same. But they lack a single view on the application of GM technology in agriculture. The country needs a robust road map to leverage biotechnology. Regulatory approvals are not given on time, and multiple regulatory bodies cause inordinate delays. Currently, 91 applications for field trials are pending for approval, 44 of which are for GM food crops. To overcome such delays, the government proposed to set up Biotechnology Regulatory Authority of India (BRAI), an independent regulator under the Ministry of Science and amp; Technology, but the proposal is still waiting for Cabinet approval. Going ahead, the challenge for the government will be to establish an effective regulatory system and a communication mechanism on GM foods, which can help allay fears about the safety of such crops, while ensuring higher productivity and remuneration to farmers. Because farmers constitutes as a nucleus of the application of biotechnology in agriculture. They are the real consumers of any technology which is going to be applied on agriculture. The purpose of the present genesis is to recognise the potential of biotechnology in addressing food production which is one of the formidable economic challenges before

India till date. The article has been divided into three important parts which has several sub-parts. The first part of article explains as how the food sufficiency can be achieved through agri-biotechnology.The challenges of the expanding market of the agri-biotechnology like food safety issues have been dealt under second part and the last part analyses the role of biotechnology in eradication of hunger and malnutrition. It concludes that the risks associated with the use of biotechnology in agriculture and food sector are needed to be experimented continuously to reap out the complete benefits of this new technology.

Keywords: *Agriculture biotechnology, Genetically modified food, Food sufficiency, Food safety, Biotechnology laws.*

"Without food, man can live at most but a few weeks; without it, all other components of social justice are meaningless."

— Norman Borlaug

1. Introduction

During 1980s, country was able to attain self sufficiency in food sector; a trend growth rate of 2.6 per cent per year in 1980s reveals this fact. Overall increase in agricultural GDP during 1980s remained 4 per cent led by tremendous progress in agricultural productivity of certain crops like oil seeds, sugarcane, cotton, horticultural products including fruits, livestock products including poultry, fisheries *etc.*[1]

Apart from share of agriculture GDP in economic growth, there are other associated sacrosanct goals to which Indian agricultural has made major contribution *i.e.* food sector. It has been tested that agricultural biotechnology possess immense potential in bringing revolutionary changes in food sector in regards to ensuring food security. One of the veterans molecular genetics at Tuskegee considers biotechnology as not only the gift of future but nostalgia.[2] It is interesting to analyse the relation between the approach of Norman Borlaug and M.S. Swaminathan for agricultural biotechnology. Where, Borlaug has considered biotechnology as "inevitable", Swaminathan elaborates it as "natural and necessary".[3] It has been currently said that necessity is the mother of invention. At the juncture, when world is facing food crisis, the biotechnological innovations are a ray of hope in dealing with the existing constraints. It has been more than 29 years when green revolution happened with the advent of high yield variety Mexican seeds aided Indian economy to achieve optimum agricultural growth and thereby, food security.

1 Swaminathan, M.S. (2010). Achieving food security in times of crisis. New Biotechnology. Available at: https://pdfs.semanticscholar.org/5201/fca40e31a7104a35a895235897a5fcb35dd0.pdf [Accessed March 20, 2017].

2 Swaminathan, M.S. (2010). Achieving food security in times of crisis. New Biotechnology. Available at: https://pdfs.semanticscholar.org/5201/fca40e31a7104a35a895235897a5fcb35dd0.pdf [Accessed March 20, 2017].

3 Swaminathan, M.S. (2010). Achieving food security in times of crisis. New Biotechnology. Available at: https://pdfs.semanticscholar.org/5201/fca40e31a7104a35a895235897a5fcb35dd0.pdf [Accessed March 20, 2017].

In order to face the current challenges in food sector, Indian government has placed strong reliance on agricultural biotechnology which is estimated to bring desired leaps in food production once was seen during 1960s green revolution. For materializing the policies to achieve food security within country, government is continuously trying to come up with various legislations, guidelines, schemes with a considerable amount of investment incapacity building and catalyzing research and development process for the same.But one important thing to note down here is that farmers constitutes as a nucleus of the application of biotechnology in agriculture. Since they are the real consumers of any technology which is going to be applied on agriculture, the significance of pre sent technology in fulfilling the needs of farmers in overcoming agrarian crisis is to be assessed.

Agricultural Biotechnology and Food Sufficiency in India

Indian Agricultural Profile

India with its 1.21 billion population growing at 1.4 per cent as reported constitutes world's largest democracy.[4] Rich diversity and federal set up with its 28 states and 7 union territories possess exceptional terrain comprising of different agricultural conditions. The classification of different geographic zones can be put as –The Great Himalayas of North, The Indo-Gangetic Plain or Northern Plains, Fertile plain of Eastern India, peninsular Plateau called Deccan Plateau called Deccan plateau, Central highlands, the Great Indian Desert and the Coastal Plains which includes Eastern and Western Ghats.

Agriculture is the backbone of Indian economy. Since 58 per cent of the rural household sustenance, agricultural GDP forms the core of the economic growth. Even after the liberalisation era too, the contribution of agricultural sector in economic growth is quite significant. Along with other crucial sectors like fish culture, poultry, horticulture and forestry, agriculture is one of the largest contributor, to national gross domestic product. According to economic survey 2016-17, the overall growth rate for the agriculture and allied sectors has been estimated as 4.1 per cent.[5] According to central statistical organisation of India, the total food grains production during tariff season of 2016-17 has been estimated as 8.9 per cent which was on expected lines.[6] India is the largest producer and exporter of spices and the second largest producer of fruits in the world.10 per cent of country's export is shared by agricultural sector.[7] It is department of agriculture is the central body to take initiatives for ensuring development in agricultural sector in bodies like National Dairy Development Board.

---

4 BBC (2017), 'India country profile' BBC News.

5 IBEF [2017], 'Economic survey of India 2016-17' <https://www.ibef.org/economy/economic-survey-2015-16> accessed 25 March, 2017.

6 IBEF [2017], 'Economic survey of India 2016-17' <https://www.ibef.org/economy/economic-survey-2015-16> accessed 25 March, 2017.

7 IBEF [2017], 'Economic survey of India 2016-17' <https://www.ibef.org/economy/economic-survey-2015-16> accessed 25 March, 2017.

Biotechnology Revolution: The Next Green Revolution

It has been rightly pointed out by veteran economist, Amartya Sen that the famine in India was not because of the food but because of the inability of the poor to acquire food.[8] Rigid social structure proved to be inefficient in preventing the localisation of money to the rich farmers. It had direct implications on small farmers who without money were unable to improve their socio-economic status.

Green revolution and commercialization of agriculture led to a drastic change which farmers had a difficult time with. Revolutionising agricultural practices and techniques with modern technology needs adequate training and knowledge which India was deficient at that point of time. Professor A R Vasavi states about incapability of public agencies in India to equip the significant portion of people with training and education.[9] Witnessing the negative implications of green revolution taught us that technology is necessary but not sufficient. Biotechnology in agriculture is at the hinge and knocks for the next green revolution. To be truly attaining success in eliminating poverty, starvation and malnutrition, policymakers need work with land so as to increase overall agricultural production and addressing food concerns. World is developing at a faster pace where we cannot manage with old technology.

Biotechnology in agriculture has come up as a boon for the developing countries like India. With the application of modern biotechnology, many transgenic plants have been genetically improved, reduced dependence of farmers on pesticides and fertilisers led to higher crop production to achieve food security. Modern biotechnology techniques like cell culture and protoplast fusion have given rise to hybrid/cybrid plant breeds. Present technology has proved to be quiet effective in devising bio fertilisers like green manuring, algalisation, seed bacterization *etc.* which has reduced the dependency of farmers on synthetic pesticides and insecticides. Three most important practical processes which are being applied under agricultural biotechnology are:[10]

Tissue Culture

The process of regeneration of plants from diseased free plant parts or one which allows for reproduction of disease free planting material is called tissue culture.It involves utilizing of explants *i.e.* small pieces of plant tissues cultured in nutrient medium under sterile conditions contains pineapples, bananas, coffee, papaya *etc.* are a few examples which are produced using tissue culture technique.

---

8 Sebby, K. (2010).The Green Revolution of the 1960's and Its Impact on Small Farmers in India. University of Nebraska at Lincoln.

9 Sebby, K. (2010).The Green Revolution of the 1960's and Its Impact on Small Farmers in India. University of Nebraska at Lincoln.

10 ISAAA.Tissue Culture Technology, <http://www.isaaa.org/resources/publications/pocketk/14/default.asp> accessed 23 March, 2017 and Clark, D.P. and Pazdernik,N. Biotechnology: Applying the Genetic Revolution. (2edn, ISBN: 978- 0-12-385015-7).

Marker Aided Selection

Marker aided selection technique includes the application of traditional genetics and molecular biology. On the basis of morphological or DNA/RNA variations, a trait of interest here. Such method is applied in agricultural biotechnology to get desired traits in plants for example disease resistance *etc.*

Genetic Engineering

Genetic Engineering, conjointly called biotechnology or recombinant DNA technology was first applied within the seventies. This technique under biotechnology permits designated individual genes to be transferred from on e organism into another and conjointly between non-related species. It is one among those ways which aids in introducing novel characteristics or traits into microorganisms, plants and animals. The product obtained from this technology area unit normally referred to as genetically modified organisms (GMOs).

In the year 1986, the department of biotechnology was established by the ministry of science and technology for the event of biotechnology in India.DBT is responsible for the development of such centres within country which could harness the potential of new skilled persons and enhance research and development in private sector. Indian government's initiatives to sponsoring the areas like recombinant DNA technology, tissue culture, bio-fertilizers, agricultural and medical sciences, genetics, environment, bioprocess engineering and many more will have a long lasting impact in the wholesome development of biotechnology industry. 2005 amendments to Indian patent law signifies major changes in Indian approach towards introduction of new initiatives like biotechnology.

Plant biotechnology is that technique which is employed to manipulate the genetic makeup of plants to get desired characteristics within it. In basic agricultural practices we tend to typically watch for natural production of offspring which will have fundamental quality. However, in plant biotechnology we tend to choose the required quality of an attribute to clump with different quality to supply multiple qualitative traits in one offspring. For the given purpose, the plant biotechnology encompasses a fine number of techniques that includes genetic engineering, tissue-culture, cell-culture, protoplast technique, somatic hybridization, marker assisted selection *etc. e.g.* Tissue culture technique, plants are grown under a nutrient medium and sterile conditions. Biotechnology is a highly emerging field which is proving advantageous in diverse areas like forestry, environment clean-up, food processing, household products, forensics *etc.*

Future Global Demands and Unleashed Potential of Biotechnology

The demand for the cereals is estimated to grow by about 560 million metric tons over 23 years period 1997-2020 for developing countries.[11] Whereas, the developed

---

11 Rosegrant, M.W., Paisner, M.S., Meijer, S. and Witcover,J. 2020 Global Food Outlook Trends, Alternatives, and Choices. International Food Policy Research Institute Washington, D.C., <http://ageconsearch.umn.edu/record/15916/files/mi01ro01.pdf> accessed 22 March, 2017.1

countries are anticipated to have an increase by 100 million metric tons in their food demands as its obvious with the current demographics which is showing an increase of 1.2 billion.[12] With rapid urbanization and increased household incomes and the increased per capita consumption of food is on increase which most importantly include dairy products, poultry products and meat, cereals like wheat, rice, soybean and maize *etc.* To keep pace with such growing demands of food especially cereals, the domestic yield within developing nations like India will have to be addressed in such a manner so as to attain self-sufficiency in food sector rather than depending on imports from OECD region. Now the issue arises as how to meet such augmenting demands in regards to agricultural products and other livestock products. Devising measures of assessing agricultural benefits in terms of additional intensive in its inputs and introducing basic reforms to agricultural and food systems are a few arguments to address the food sufficiency issues in India.

It has been expressly said by some GM protagonists that agri-biotechnology is a success at the hinge of the door to food security and better economic growth. They consider "agro-biotechnology" as a next green revolution in regards to crop productivity and attainment of food security. It has been observed that the yield of maize, rice and other staple grains enhanced in the duration of 1970- 1990.[13]However, it declined within late nineties which showcased a symptom of poor agricultural growth, food crisis and hence the declined economic growth rate. In opposition to it, GM antagonists plead that the traditional varieties are still a success and GM technology is not needed to redress the seed crisis.[14] Thus, it is needless to mention that farmers in developing countries like India are confronting to several issues that technology is not enough to redress *e.g.* political and socio-economic constraints on equity, animal- husbandry and its management, degradation of environment and natural wealth, poor infrastructure *etc.*

To achieve a sustainable agricultural growth is a huge challenge for policymakers as well as farmers. It is valid here to say that conventional plant breeding carves out its own niche in regards to its quality, suitability and accessibility. However, increasing population and its growing demands are outweighing such conventional techniques and compel us to look for some better alternative *i.e.* agricultural biotechnology which can be an important and successful tool in improving plant breeding programmes.

Food Safety and Human Health: Issues and Challenges

General technique of the production of biotechnologically derived foods involve transfer of the desired genes or genes in combination with a promoter and a gene

---

12 Rosegrant, M.W., Paisner, M.S., Meijer, S. and Witcover, J. 2020 Global Food Outlook Trends, Alternatives, and Choices. International Food Policy Research Institute Washington, D.C., <http://ageconsearch.umn.edu/record/15916/files/mi01ro01.pdf> accessed 22 March, 2017.

13 Ministry of Agriculture (2015). Government of India, 'Agricultural statistics at a Glance 2014.(Oxford University Press) <http://eands.dacnet.nic.in/PDF/Agricultural-Statistics-At-Glance2014.pdf> accessed 25 March 2017.

14 Kruft, D. (2001). Impacts of Genetically-Modified Crops and Seeds on Farmers. <https://pennstatelaw.psu.edu/_file/aglaw/Impacts_of_Genetically_Modified.pdf> accessed 25 March, 2017.

for a selectable marker trait to the host whose cells are to be transformed. For this, the cells which are needed to be transformed isolated from those other cells in the host organism. There are several key issues which are arising due to insertion of foreign genetic material into the host genome, where it has been derived that transgene are inherently toxic and results into unintended mutagenic effects. There could be many factors which leads the transgene to cause unintended implications over host genome which is as follows:

- ✰ Over-expression of host towards pharmacologically active substances.
- ✰ Silencing of host genes.
- ✰ Alterations in host metabolic pathways.

However, it isn't new to the agricultural sector to come across such hazards as these are not only appearing in agricultural biotechnology but are also inherent in conventional breeding methods."Bio safety" has been defined as such policies and procedures which are applied to confirm the environmentally sound application of biotechnology. In India, department of biotechnology has employed National Biotechnology Development Strategy".[15]

As started from 2007 it acts as a guiding document for the programmes to be undertaken to address an umpteen number of issues relating to research and development, technology transfer, IPRs, regulation standards, public standard of biotechnology *etc.*[16] Release of biotechnologically derived foods possess potential risks to human health and environment. It is necessary to be assured to the people at large that biotechnologically derived foods are completely safe before it could come to the actual use. A responsible government body should be constituted which could give clearances to such international institutions and companies to carry out further development of agriculture biotechnology. Controversies have made its space with respect to the following points:

- ✰ Safety of GM foods and environment.
- ✰ Business interests behind GM crops
- ✰ Human health and biotechnologically derived foods.
- ✰ GM foods and Intellectual Property Rights.

Controversies and Moratoriums Associated with GM Crops in India – Timeline

GM crops were first introduced in India in the year 2002 in the form of BT Cotton. It was in 2006 when GM crops faced the public interest litigation filed by the activists against commercialisation of GM crops in the apex court of India. Later on

---

15 Department of Biotechnology. (2015). Government of India, 'National Biotechnology Development Strategy 2015-2020', <http://www.dbtindia.nic.in/wp-content/uploads/DBT_Book-_29-december_2015.pdf> accessed 22 March, 2017.

16 Department of Biotechnology. (2015). Government of India, 'National Biotechnology Development Strategy 2015-2020', <http://www.dbtindia.nic.in/wp-content/uploads/DBT_Book-_29-december_2015.pdf> accessed 22 March, 2017.

issues arose with respect to the commercialisation and consumption of BT Brinjal also which faced stay in its release due to lack of consensus among scientists and farmers of brinjal growing states.[17]As a result, the then environment minister Shri. Jairam Ramesh blocked its release. It was ministry of environment and forests which was responsible for the mass commercialisation and issuance of clearances for the release of genetically modified crops earlier. Now it is carried out by department of science and technology.

New crop trials in relation to genetically modified crops began in 2013 after which a supreme court appoint a panel recommended suspension of trials for 10 years for fortifying regulator and monitoring systems. Following the recommendations, the environment minister Jayanthi Natarajan put on hold to such new crop field trials.[18]Her successor, Veerappa Moily took an opposite stand and approved one acre field trials. In March, 2014, the UPA government with under GEAC approved trials for eleven crops that included mainly sorghum, cotton, wheat, rice, maize *etc.*In the same year, 21 new GM crop varieties got approval under NDA government for field trials.GM mustard controversy came into picture in 2016 when GEAC approved its field trial. However, SC stayed the order and sought for public opinion.[19]

Genetically Modified Crops in India

BT Cotton is the only genetically modified cash crop under commercial cultivation till now. Other crops under trial like wheat, maize, sorghum *etc.* have not been approved and considered fit for public consumption.

(a) BT Cotton

BT Cotton was the first ever GM crop released for public consumption in 2002 and is the only GM crop under cultivation in country. It is an insect pest resistant GM variety developed by Monsanto, USA. It is formed as result of isolation of gene from Bacillus Thuringiensis and its development into fully grown plant. [20]It is 355 promoter from cauliflower mosaic virus that the plasmid construct comprising Cry1AC is extracted. It imparts the characteristics into plant so as it could lead producing BT Protein. The npt II gene is used to select the transformed cells in plant containing antibiotic kanamycin. AAD gene encodes the selectable mark enzyme 3″ (9) - Oaminoglycoside Adenyltransferase and facilitates the selection

---

17 ClearIAS, Science and Technology Notes. (2016). 'Genetically Modified Crops and Regulations in India', <http://www.clearias.com/genetically-modified-crops-and-regulations-in-india/> Accessed 15 March, 2017.

18 ClearIAS, Science and Technology Notes. (2016). 'Genetically Modified Crops and Regulations in India', <http://www.clearias.com/genetically-modified-crops-and-regulations-in-india/> Accessed 15 March, 2017.

19 ClearIAS, Science and Technology Notes. (2016). 'Genetically Modified Crops and Regulations in India', <http://www.clearias.com/genetically-modified-crops-and-regulations-in-india/> Accessed 15 March, 2017.

20 Qaim, M. Bt Cotton in India: Development of Benefits and the Role of Government Seed Price Intervention.12 (2). AgBioForum, <http://www.agbioforum.org/v12n2/v12n2a03- sadashivappa.htm > accessed 22 March, 2017.

of bacteria containing the above given plasmid. It is done over a certain medium which contains streptomycin.[21]

(b) BT Brinjal

It is only in 2007 when GEAC gave the green signal for the commercial release of BT Brinjal. It was produced by Mahyco (Maharashtra Hybrid Seeds Company) as a team with the Dharwad University of Agricultural University.[22]However, the process was halted in 2010.The then minister for environment and forests restrained the commercialisation of BT Brinjal which broke out into a controversy and Indian government construct data extracted out of field tests of BT Brinjal to an RTI application and Delhi High Court orders. It was contended that without maintaining strict testing standards and GEAC approval was being considered as a 'shame' by some activists. Consequently giving rise to a huge legal mess.

(c) GM-mustard

Dhara Mustard Hybrid-11 or DMH-11 is a genetically modified variety of mustard developed by Delhi University's centre for genetic manipulation of crop plants.[23] GM mustard has been in news recently due to huge uproar against its commercialisation by many environmentalist and health experts on the belief that it is likely to have negative effect on health and environment. Geneticists have been suggesting that it is likely to increase yield and many varieties are pest resistant. Hence, a good proposition for farmers as it is likely to improve productivity. And reduce input cost thereby maximising profit. As a result, farmers are committing suicide due to failure of BT Cotton crops. The similar thing may get repeated here to. Government intends to use GM foods to solve problems of sustainable agriculture, food security and malnutrition. However, there is leading to disillusionment among young scientists researchers from entering this field.

Arguments in Favour of GM Foods

First and foremost positive aspect of introduction of GM crops is control over the occurrence of certain diseases. By the Process of modifying DNA of these foods, the allergens could be eliminated successfully. Biotechnologically derived foods have been reported to have faster growth than traditional varieties of foods. This property of biotechnologically derived foods is being seen as a ray of hope of coping up with the food security issues. These foods are boon for those drought prone regions, areas with less fertile soil and with extreme climatic conditions. Though seeds are expensive but reduce the dependency of farmers on harmful pesticides and insecticides which is counted as an environment friendly agricultural practice. It has also been reported that GM foods have high nutritive value with higher

---

21 Qaim, M. Bt Cotton in India: Development of Benefits and the Role of Government Seed Price Intervention.12 (2). AgBioForum, <http://www.agbioforum.org/v12n2/v12n2a03- sadashivappa.htm > accessed 22 March, 2017.

22 Centre for Environment Education, MoEF, [2010].National Consultations on BT Brinjal: A Report. Government of India

23 Mohani, V., 2017. Mustard set to be India's first GM food, gets regulator nod. The Times of India.

content of vitamins and minerals. These are some of the case studies showcasing the benefits derived from GM crops:

i. Improved Traits in Staple Crops

Food crops which are relevant to both subsistence and commercial farming. For *e.g.* sorghum, maize, soyabean *etc.* are showing significantly lower yield than in the developed countries, reasons behind of include poor seed quality, recalcitrant soil, environmental degradation, pests and diseases, lack of fertilisers, inadequate water control and so on. Substantial improvements can definitely be achieved by adopting better irrigation techniques, integrated pest management or agricultural extension services. But still non-GM approaches have limitations as compared to their GM counterparts which are potentially contributing in raising crop yield.[24]

ii. Improved Micronutrients in Rice

Professor Ingo Potrykus and Dr.Peter Beyer of Swiss federal Institute of Technology developed a distinct variety of rice enriched with Beta- Carotene called Golden Rice by transferring one bacterial gene and two daffodil genes into a variety of rice.[25]Beta- Carotene is an important micronutrient which is converted into Vitamin-A in body. So, the purpose of developing such variety of rice was to help prevent the deficiency of Vitamin-A which causes Xerophthalmia. It has been estimated that more than 14 million children under 5 years were suffering from this disease.

iii. Herbicide Tolerance

Herbicide tolerant plants could be witnessed being grown in Argentina during 2002.It was soyabean plant which was genetically modified which was tolerant to a specific weed killer. Thus, GM Soyabean has ascertained the possibility of depending upon use of the environmentally damaging herbicides.[26]

iv. Improved Resistance to Viruses in Sweet Potato

A GM variety of sweet potato developed by Kenya Agricultural Research Institute (KARI) in collaboration with Monsanto and other universities of USA which is resistant to the feathery mottle virus. This crop is still being tested under several field trials which are being conducted in some African countries. [27]

---

24 Lok Sabha Secretariat. (2012), New Delhi, 'Cultivation of Genetically Modified Food Crops: Prospects and Effects, <http://164.100.47.134/lsscommittee/Agriculture/GM_Report.pdf> accessed 21 Mar, 2017.

25 The Golden Rice Project. (2016), 'Golden Rice is part of the solution', <http://www.goldenrice.org/> accessed 25 March, 2017.

26 Lok Sabha Secretariat. (2016), Cultivation of Genetically Modified Food Crops: Prospects and Effects, New Delhi, <http://164.100.47.134/lsscommittee/Agriculture/GM_Report.pdf> accessed 21 Mar, 2017.

27 Mohani, V. (2014), Scientists bring a 15-point resolution in favour of GM crop technology. The Times of India. New Delhi.

v. Improved Nutritional Value

A rice variety developed which contains enhanced levels of beta -carotene called Golden rice is proving to be a boon in treating the deficiency of Vitamin-A causing Xerophthalmia especially among children.[28]

vi. Improved Resistance to Diseases in Bananas

In case of bananas also, the commercial plant breeding has been found to be ineffective to produce crops that are resistant to bacterial or viral infections. It is the GM technology which has offered possibilities of increasing resistance to pests and diseases.GM technology for bananas is effective in increasing its varieties so as to slow down the impact of pests.[29]

The father of green revolution, Norman Borlaug has strongly supported genetically modified food to control hunger and starvation. As it is clear from his statement - **"It is better to die eating GM food instead of dying of hunger."**[30]Recognising the very thought of Norman Borlaug, former prime minister, Manmohan Singh saw biotechnology as a key to achieve food security. President Pranab Mukherjee has emphasized for the proper testing of biotechnologically derived foods before releasing them for consumption among public which is quite obvious from what he stated as-

"The concerns over their (GM crops) perceived risks should be addressed by following internationally accepted procedures for addressing safety parameters. ICAR, which is involved in developing useful products and technologies in this field, must contribute to the public discourse and provide clarity on this sensitive issue."[31]

There are also a few groups like Greenpeace India and gene campaign which strive against GM foods and focussing towards environmental concerns.[32]Institutions like IARI and ICAR have also demanded the field trials for GM crops as it ensures the safe consumption and better environmental concerns as a priority.[33]A 15-point resolution in favour of GM crops by some of the scientists of National Academy

---

28 The Golden Rice Project. (2016), Golden Rice is part of the solution,<http://www.goldenrice.org/> accessed 25 March, 2017.

29 Qaim, M. (2010), The Benefits of Genetically Modified Crops—and the Costs of Inefficient Regulation. Resources for the Future, <http://www.rff.org/blog/2010/benefits-genetically-modified-crops-and-costs- inefficient-regulation> accessed 18 March, 2017.

30 Modi, A., 2014. Seed of Doubt. Business Today. Available at: https://www.businesstoday.in/magazine/features/genetically-modified-crops-controversial-challenges-ahead/story/204944.html [Accessed March 20, 2017].

31 Address by the Hon'ble President on the Occasion of the 85th Foundation Day of Indian Council of Agricultural Research (ICAR). Press Information Bureau, Government of India, http://pib.nic.in/newsite/mbErel.aspx?relid=97242 accessed 25 March, 2017.

32 Greenpeace. Stopping genetic junk, <http://www.greenpeace.org/india/en/What- We-Do/Sustainable-Agriculture/GE-campaign/> accessed 20 March, 2017.

33 Lok Sabha Secretariat. (2012), Cultivation of Genetically Modified Food Crops: Prospects and Effects. New Delhi, <http://164.100.47.134/lsscommittee/Agriculture/GM_Report.pdf> accessed 21 March, 2017.

of Agricultural Sciences (NASA) is a progressive step towards safe introduction of GM crops in public.[34]

Arguments in against of GM Crops

It has been reported that GM foods may cause harm to human health by developing such diseases which are immune to antibiotics. Issue arises because of unknown long term effects of these foods on human health, since these are newly invented. Manufacturers tend to derived and may affect their business as it is not recognised in public much because of ethical and legal issues attached with it. It involves ethics and morals when one talks about a notion of transferring animal genes into plants and vice versa.

Cross pollination method is regarded as harmful to other organisms which thrive in this biosphere. Emergence of superbugs, super weeds as a result of recombinant technology is a matter of concern. It all depends on selective pressure when it is strong enough; the resistance shows for example due to prolonged use of herbicides, the surrounding weeds could develop a resistance to the herbicide tolerant by the plants.[35]

Health risks which are associated with GM foods are toxicity, allergic reactions, antibiotic resistance, immune-suppression, cancer and loss of nutrients. Genetic engineering is different from natural breeding as it uses genes from bacteria and viruses to be inserted into plants to develop into GM plants like soyabean, corn, cottonseed, canola *etc.*[36] It has been claimed that BT-Toxin is harmless to human health and other mammals as it employs natural bacteria to be inserted in the process. However, on the contrary to it, scientists have proved that BT has powerful immune responses which causes allergic reactions and leaves intestines damaged. BT Cotton is one of its examples whose allergic properties have been witnessed in India only.BT Corn triggers immune responses while implemented over mice and rats. In regards to this, the world health organisation has called for a screening protocol for GM soybean, corn and papaya.[37] In the year 1980s, more than 100 Americans were reported to have developed sickness and disability because of a contaminated brand of GM food supplement called L- tryptophan.[38] This is just a beginning of the challenges associated with GM food crops and toxicologists need to go way ahead to assess whether foods derived through genetic engineering qualify human health standards or not.

34 Mohani, V. (2014), Scientists bring a 15-point resolution in favour of GM crop technology. The Times of India. New Delhi.

35 Odum, M. (2015), Arguments Against GMOs, <http://www.resilience.org/stories/2015-05-22/arguments-against-gmos/> accessed 20 March, 2017.

36 Odum, M. (2015), Arguments Against GMOs, <http://www.resilience.org/stories/2015-05-22/arguments-against-gmos/> accessed 20 March, 2017.

37 ClearIAS, Science and Technology Notes. (2016), Genetically Modified Crops and Regulations in India, <http://www.clearias.com/genetically-modified-crops-and-regulations-in-india/> accessed 15 March, 2017.

38 Institute of Responsible Technology. Health Risks, <http://responsibletechnology.org/gmo-education/health-risks/> accessed 20 March, 2017

Regulatory Mechanism for GM Crops in India

GEAC (Genetic Engineering Approval Committee) is the chief biotechnology regulator in India functioning as a statutory body under environment protection Act, 1986 of Ministry of environment and forests. It is responsible for granting clearances to field trials and commercial release of GM crops. Other competent authorities provided under rules of 1989 are given below:[39]

- ☆ Institutional safety Committees (IBSE)
- ☆ Review Committee of genetic Manipulation (RCGM)
- ☆ Genetic Engineering Approval Committee (GEAC)
- ☆ District Level Committee (DLC)

Genetic Engineering Appraisal Committee (GEAC)

1. It works as a statutory body under the Ministry of Environment and Forests for giving clearances to the activities which are susceptible to harm the environment due to the use of large scale of hazardous biological material and recombinants in research and industrial production. Such clearance is issued by assessing the commercialization of biological matter and recombinants from environmental point of view.[40]
2. It is also concerned with the approval of release of genetically modified organisms into environment under the provisions of Rules of 1989.
3. Rules of 1989 are also applicable on the release and utilization of such living modified organisms which falls under risk category III to which the functions of GEAC extends. It deals with the manufacture and use of recombinant pharma products and also where the end product of any pharmaceutical product is a living modified organism.
4. The Committee has an option to co-opt the other experts of GEAC as per Section 4, para 3 of Rules of 1989 as it is deemed fit.[41]
5. Subgroups or subcommittees or such other expert committees may also be appointed by it as needed to ensure bio safety of the LMOs and GMOs.
6. A quorum of GEAC comprises of a third of its members which are entrusted with a task to initiate meeting
7. A "Statement of Confidentiality" is required to duly signed by GEAC as per Rules of 1989 to carry out its functions in a proper manner.

---

39 ClearIAS, Science and Technology Notes. (2016), Genetically Modified Crops and Regulations in India, <http://www.clearias.com/genetically-modified-crops-and-regulations-in-india/> accessed 15 March, 2017.

40 MoEF, Government of India. (2016), Genetic Engineering Approval Committee (GEAC), <http://www.moef.nic.in/division/genetic-engineering-approval-committee-geac> accessed 18 March, 2017.

41 MoEF, Government of India. (2016), Genetic Engineering Approval Committee (GEAC), <http://www.moef.nic.in/division/genetic-engineering-approval-committee-geac> accessed 18 March, 2017.

8. Tenure of the Committee remains of three years from the date of issue of notification
9. Representatives of other Ministries experts might be invited as 'Special Invitees' on the call of GEAC to participate in the meeting sessions of the GEAC. It depends on the issue which is going to be discussed.

Eradicating Hunger and Malnutrition: Role of Food Biotechnology

World is continuing to be suffered from food crisis and malnutrition. It has been reported that at least 800 million people are suffering from malnutrition. Because of insufficient income among people as estimated to be 1.3 billion, they are unable to afford adequate diet.[42]

Global food crisis is the prominent cause behind the recurring problems of malnutrition especially in the Sub-Saharan parts of Africa where infant mortality rate has been reported to be 9.2 per cent. About three million children in such African nations have gone blind due to the deficiency of vitamin A.[43] Following such crisis, it has been tested out that genetically modified crops possess potential to relieve the world of hunger and malnutrition. But issues and challenges regarding the benefits of genetically modified crops are still there.

In hospitability for the efficiently producing agricultural products in their respective regions is one among the important factors behind so many countries suffering from hunger and starvation. Most of the nations which are suffering from the hunger and malnutrition are located in tropical and desert regions where agricultural activities are very less due to lack of growing conditions. Other endemic problems constitutes of costly pesticides and fertilisers, soil erosion, inadequate storage *etc.* which are difficult to cope up with by small and marginal farmers who are generally involved in agricultural practices in developing nations. Plant virus contributes to one of such factors which make the region vulnerable to poor crop productivity. It has been reported that in the year 1999, the mosaic plant virus destroyed 60 per cent of Africa's cassava crop by inducing infection in it.[44] By keeping these situations in mind, it was devised by the scientists that agriculture biotechnology may play a vital role not only in conquering the pest and virus attacks but also enhancing the yield of the crop. Through the process of genetic engineering it has become possible to manipulate the genetic makeup of the staple crops of developing nations like rice, maize, potatoes, cassava *etc.* to make them more resistant to the pests, viruses and diseases induced by them, making them more nutritive and increasing the crop yield.

---

42 Centrone, M.J. Biotechnology: Putting an End to World Hunger. AgBioWorld <http://www.agbioworld.org/biotech-info/articles/interviews/freerepublic.html> accessed 20 March, 2017.

43 Centrone, M.J. Biotechnology: Putting an End to World Hunger. AgBioWorld <http://www.agbioworld.org/biotech-info/articles/interviews/freerepublic.html> accessed 20 March, 2017.

44 Thresh, J.M. and Cooter, R.J. (2005), Strategies for controlling cassava mosaic virus disease in Africa Authors. 54 (5). Plant Pathology <http://onlinelibrary.wiley.com/doi/10.1111/j.1365-3059.2005.01282.x/full> accessed 20 March, 2017.

Bioengineered crops can be elaborated as possessing their own inbuilt pesticides and herbicides which helps farmers to secure crops from the infliction of diseases for example bacterial blight and in enhancing the crop produce. Genetically modified crops are advantageous to be grown in the water scarce areas too which help the farmers to use the fallow and drought prone lands. Such crops don't need the till farming and any other heavy equipments to be used to make up the field ready for the cultivation. It simply works on the normal soil content where its vaccinated seeds possess herbicide to kill weeds and pesticides to manage pests. Earlier, traditional breeding practices led to a vast number of plant varieties and hybrids which contributed to have a greater crop yield, crop stability and lucrative income. Even having such efficient conventional methods of plant breeding and green revolution along with it, food crisis has remained unresolved. Visualising the competency of biotechnology in agrarian sector, Indian government is proactive in taking initiatives in encouraging biotechnological research in agricultural sector so as to carefully address the battle of food security aiming to feed hundreds of millions miserably poor people.The environmental impacts of introduced GMOs can be either ecological or genetic and may include:[45]

Environmental and ecological concerns relating to genetically modified crops are also needed to be analysed here. Because genetically modified crops may potentially harm the biodiversity and ecological balance by killing the organisms other than the pests and plants which are beneficial as has been recently studied. It is also apprehended that genetically modified crops may lead to the reduction of soil fertility. It may transfer the insecticidal qualities to its wild relatives too which pose danger to the biological diversity. Following could be the adversities on the environment because of genetically modified crops:[46]

- ✰ Unintended impact on the population dynamics as a result of lack of exclusivity in the insecticidal actions of GM crops which may occur because of the changes in land use and agricultural practices.
- ✰ Effects on biogeochemistry because of the adverse action of genetically modified crops on the soil texture and content leaving it either more acidic or alkaline which is unfit to grow any crop. Interference with the soil microbial populations is also included under this concern which is associated with the changes in nitrogen, phosphorous and potassium content in the soil.
- ✰ Gene flow through cross pollination has been questioned since long which may lead to the transfer of genetic material to other domesticated or native populations.

---

45 Office of Director-General, FAO. GMOs and the environment.FAO Corporate Document Repository, <http://www.fao.org/docrep/003/X9602E/x9602e07.htm > accessed 18 March, 2017.

46 National Research Council (US) Committee on Environmental Impacts Associated with Commercialization of Transgenic Plants. Environmental Effects of Transgenic Plants: The Scope and Adequacy of Regulation. (National Academies Press (US), Washington (DC)).

Keeping the above implications in mind it is essential to have an efficient regulatory framework to regulate the release and consumption of genetically modified organisms. Nevertheless, the biotechnology is advantageous in various areas *e.g.* livestock management, reduction of use of herbicides and pesticides, enhancing crop yield and many others. But developing countries like India have to be competent enough to properly harness the worth of biotechnology in agriculture which is possible only with a strong regulatory framework.[47]

One recent report of the Food and Agriculture Organization states that 854 million people which are 12.6 per cent of the total population of the world are malnourished. Out of such figure, children are among the most vulnerable. Incidences of malnutrition magnify the impact of every disease, including epidemics like measles and malaria.[48] One example which tells us how biotechnology can contribute to combating global hunger and malnutrition is of Golden Rice explained in detail below:

Golden Rice

It has been estimated to be 140 million children belonging to 118 countries with lowest per capita income who are suffering from the deficiency of vitamin –A. Such low- income group countries are mostly African and South-East Asian countries. According to a report of World Health organisation, there are about 2.5 lakh to 5 lakh children are losing their eye sight every year and it poses a huge challenge to the countries to combat the deficiency of Vitamin A and associated ailments.[49] A transgenic variety of rice called Golden Rice has been created by the researchers of Germany and Switzerland developed by the combination of three genes- two from the daffodil and one from a bacterium which helps in producing vitamin A. Transgenic rice is available for the mass distribution by waiving the patent rights of biotechnology companies by keeping in view the need of food and nutrition especially in those countries which are famine prone. Golden rice is counted to be one among the biotechnology products which has a potential to contribute to the society at large.

According to Peter Rosset, director of Food First, "People do not have Vitamin A deficiency because rice contains too little Vitamin A, but because their diet has been reduced to rice and almost nothing else."It can derive from the statement which takes into account of the present situation of food insecurity that it is abject poverty which is the root cause of global hunger. From sources of wealth to technological landscape everything has been monopolised by the private sector which leave little or no room for the people to afford even two times meals in worst cases.

---

47 Ania Wieczorek, 'Use of Biotechnology in Agriculture—Benefits and Risks' [2003] 3 () College of Tropical Agriculture and Human Resources (CTAHR).

48 FAO, IFAD, WFP. (2015), The State of Food Insecurity in the World, <http://www.fao.org/3/a-i4646e.pdf> accessed 18 March, 2017.

49 Qaim, M. and Kouser, S. (2013), Genetically Modified Crops and Food Security. 8 (6), <https://www.ncbi.nlm.nih.gov/pmc/articles/PMC3674000/> accessed 19 March, 2017.

Continuing incidences of monopolisation of genetic material by biotechnology firms and companies is landing all the developing countries at a worrisome stage. If farmers will have to purchase the seeds everytime before the season of sowing the same, it will drastically affect their economic condition and thereby standard of living. Seed patents and regimes like UPOV which protects the rights of breeders have put the agricultural research and development at a disadvantage. This is ultimately endangering the livelihoods of marginal farmers belonging to the regions like Africa, Latin America and Asia where they rely upon saving the seeds from the harvested crop to use it again for the next season. However, after an umpteen number of cases of protest against the commercialisation of terminator seeds which are also known as "Suicide Seeds", top biotech companies like Monsanto and AstraZeneca have taken back the commercialization of such seeds which "switch off" a plant's ability to germinate a second time.[50] It is to be noted that the biotechnology industry collectively owns at least 38 patents that features controlling seed or plant germination processes.

In developing countries, there may be a potential negative impact from Intellectual Property Rights (IPR) over biotechnological products or the processes used in producing them. IPRs have been held not only by private companies, but also by some public organizations making it impossible to use any aspect of biotechnology for improving major crop species without infringing a patent somewhere in the process.

Because of IPRs, it has not always been possible to separate the biotechnology prospects from the business interests involved. A major consequence of IPR in agricultural biotechnology is that many developing countries which have not yet invested in biotechnology may never be able to catch up in the future.It is not possible to separate the biotechnology industry prospects from the business interests because of the involvement of the intellectual property assets. Increasing privatisation in agricultural research and monopolisation of seeds is a matter of concerns for the developing countries which would put them at disadvantage as far as food security is concerned.

Conclusion

To achieve a sustainable agricultural development, a robust management strategy is a prerequisite. In addition to a responsible management of biotechnology industry, a strong regulatory framework for the purposes like environment clearance and release covering the food safety concerns is needed to be established. Witnessing the past experiences relating to the commercialization of the BT crops, it is a high time to lay down a strong legal regime for the better regulation of food safety and standardization of GMOs and LMOs. Apart from setting up of individual national regulatory frameworks, international cooperation to provide scientific and financial support to the developing and least developed nations

---

50 Warwick,H.(2000), Syngenta Switching off farmers' rights? Genetics Forum. Genewatch, UK <http://stopogm.net/sites/stopogm.net/files/SyngentaSwitching.pdf> accessed 19 March, 2017.

is important so that such nations could grow up in capacity building terms and develop indigenous technology. Biotechnology in agriculture has been relied upon by the Indian government as a sunrise sector. Recognising its capability to reduce the hunger and malnutrition, the Indian government has taken initiatives to devise a number of schemes to deal with the food safety concerned with GMOs and their commercialization. In between all, the public debate on the risks associated with the consumption of the GMOs cannot be neglected. It is often advised to tolerate certain residual risks because a completely risk free technology is not possible at all. It must not be forgotten that the utilization of the benefits of the biotechnology in agriculture can have lots of positive implications as far as human health and environment are associated for example, reduction of the use of chemicals like pesticides and insecticides. Countries like USA, China and South Africa have already started demonstrating the benefits of GM crops.

Technology acquisition and seed monopolization are some of the important concerns to determine the feasibility of the agriculture biotechnology to address the food needs and treating the serious issues like poverty, hunger and malnutrition. Developed countries are obliged to transfer the technology in biotechnology so as the developing and least developed nations could utilise their genetic resources well. Biotechnology holds tremendous potential to combat with increasing hunger and famine worldwide especially for India it will prove to be a boon to achieve the food security feeding 121 crore people together. However, ill effects of biotechnology have to be experimented and researched continuously to avoid any of the incidences of the failure of the objective of food safety and security.

Chapter 15

The Relation Between Pharmaceutical Companies and IP Laws – Patent Laws in Relation to Ayurvedic Products: Need or Greed

Shikhar Bhardwaj[1], *Prateek Sharma*[2], *Vikram Nagpal*[3] *and Yogeshwar Purohit*[4]

Himachal Pradesh National Law University, Shimla, Himachal Pradesh 171011
e-mail: [1]*bhardwajshikhar420@gmail.com*, [2]*pratik.messi222@gmail.com*, [3]*vikramnagpal4@gmail.com*, [4]*yogeshwarpurohit280@gmail.com*

ABSTRACT

Patent rights and their influence on the global market have increased with the globalisation of the world. The concept was introduced to acclaim the inventor for his great innovation but, it has become a puppet in the hands of corporate big shots to gain profits. We see that now foreign companies are claiming patents on use of cloves, turmeric and other ayurvedic ingredients, which we Indians are using since generations. If the patents are awarded to them then the usage of these ingredients will not be seen in the local ayurvedic market. Today granting patent does not acclaim the inventor but just makes the invention a commodity hence, a tool for generating profits rather than social welfare. The need of patent is a question itself. By claiming patents, you just want to create a monopoly in the market. The inventor gets his royalty and the firm to which it has been sold earns the profit. Instead, by deleting the clause of patents the commodity will become more accessible for the customers.

Specifically, the ayurvedic market is the worst hit of this patent-monopolising policy. The American companies seek monetary benefits by patenting these centuries old methods which in consequence deprives the native who are using these techniques over the years. This is a sensitive issue which demands amendment in the prevalent laws and intervention from international organisations. This paper focuses on the ayurvedic market and the impact of patent law over it under the ambit of role of various international organisations governing it.

Keywords: *patent laws, ayurvedic market, social welfare*

Introduction

Patent rights and their influence on the global market have increased with the globalisation of the world. It was initially introduced to acclaim the inventor for his creation, provided invention should be made in public welfare but, in todays time it is more of a puppet in the hands of corporate big shots which they exercise to expand their business and to increase their revenue the initial concept of public welfare is out of the whole discussion. Thus, we want to bring that concept of public welfare back not on papers neither in provisions because they are already present there, we are urging to get this thing settled in the minds of corporate companies, who are exploiting the provisions for patents to gain their financial benefits.

When we talk about patents in medicinal use and in particular to ayurvedic products the basic question raises in our mind is do we really need patents for such natural products? Or for say any other IPR law. For example- there is hardly any place in this world where we cannot grow neem or tulsi from the fertile lands of North America to lands of South Africa. Providing patents or covering such topics under IPR hampers the basic concept behind these laws. We don't see any sort of new invention or creative work behind using neem or tulsi for their medicinal use, because we have been doing those things since ages and asking or granting patents over such ayurvedic medicines is completely unacceptable and highly criticisable.

The role of international organisations also becomes really important while discussing patent or IPR laws. The regulations on which international patent laws and IPR functions are determined by WTO (World Trade Organisations) and further regulated by TRIPS (Trade -Related aspect of Intellectual Property Rights). These organisations have a shallow scope for protecting ayurvedic products from the web of IPR laws. The basic contention for which we seek international organisations to pay heed is to the cause that there should be no provisions for granting patents to natural resources and in particular to ayurvedic products. Cases in the history have shown that the regulations of these organisations have been misused by the developed countries and the companies belonging to developed countries for their own benefit and riches.

Intellectual Property Rights: A Necessary "Evil"

An invention must be new and useful to be patentable. Notably, laws of nature, natural phenomena, and abstract ideas are excluded from patent-eligible protection[1], because these naturally-occurring matters are discovered rather than invented. Natural products would not be awarded a patent merely for their discovery. Patent eligibility is essentially different from patent eligibility. Patent eligibility means that the invention is an item that can seek a protection under patent law. In contrast, an invention becomes patentable when it meets the necessary requirements, such as novelty, inventiveness, and industrial applicability, and a patent can eventually be granted as well. Hence, a non-natural compound is patent-eligible, but becomes unpatentable if it is known.

---

1 Wong, A. Y.-T., and Chan, A. W.-K. (2014). Retrieved May 10, 2018, from https://www.ncbi.nlm.nih.gov/pmc/articles/PMC4086272/

The patent eligibility of natural products isolated or purified from natural materials is less affirmatively defined. The US patent law protects new, useful, and non-obvious chemical compounds and compositions[2], encompassing isolated and purified products from natural materials. It has been intensively discussed in the Courts whether a product isolated from natural materials is patent-eligible or represents another kind of substance that should be exempted from the "product of nature" doctrine. However, the Courts adopt inconstant grounds and standards for determining the patent eligibility of isolated natural products, which leaves doubt about exactly how different an isolated natural product needs to be from its natural counterpart to be sufficient for exemption[3].

The "product of nature" doctrine was seen in Association for Molecular Pathology v. Myriad Genetics[4], which invalidated a patent on an isolated DNA molecule from the human cancer-susceptibility gene BRCA. The Supreme Court affirmed that an isolated DNA molecule with an identical sequence to a natural gene is a naturally-occurring product and not patentable. On March 4th of this year, the USPTO issued lengthy guidelines ("the Guidance") to their patent examiners, instructing them to reject any patent claim to a purified natural product[5].

What Was the Status Quo Ante?

Prior to the Myriad decision, purified natural substances could be patented. The Myriad decision held that isolated DNA that has exactly the same sequence as is found in nature cannot be patented. This created doubt as to whether other purified natural substances had lost their patent-eligible status.

An early example of a patent for a purified natural substance is U.S. Patent 141,072 issued to Louis Pasteur in 1873, which claimed beer yeast "free from organic germs of disease." Likewise, Jokichi Takamine was the first to purify adrenaline, for which he was granted U.S. Patent No. 730,176. Felix Hoffman received U.S. Patent 644,077 in 1898 for purified acetyl salicylic acid, the active ingredient in aspirin[6]. Perhaps the best example of a patent for a purified natural substance is Selman Waksman's U.S. Patent 2,449,866 for the landmark antibiotic streptomycin. Waksman's claim 13 reads, in its entirety, "Streptomycin."[7]

---

2 Migrator. (2018, March 27). Advantages and disadvantages of getting a patent. Retrieved May 10, 2018, from https://www.nibusinessinfo.co.uk/content/advantages-and-disadvantages-getting-patent

3 Watson, E. (2012, January 9). What can be patented in the world of natural ingredients? Retrieved May 10, 2018, from https://www.nutraingredients-usa.com/Article/2012/01/09/What-can-be-patented-in-the-world-of-natural-ingredients.

4 Association for Molecular Pathology v. Myriad Genetics 569 U.S. 12 (2013).

5 Wong, A. Y.-T., and Chan, A. W.-K. (2014). Retrieved May 10, 2018, from https://www.ncbi.nlm.nih.gov/pmc/articles/PMC4086272/

6 Product Patent for the Indian Pharmaceutical Sector under the TRIPS regime. Retrieved May 10, 2018, from http://www.legalserviceindia.com/articles/ppch.htm

7 Landau, N. J. The New Patent Policy on Natural Products Is a Game Changer for Universities and Life Sciences Companies. Retrieved May 10, 2018, from https://www.bradley.com/insights/publications/2014/09/the-new-patent-policy-on-natural-products-is-a-g__

Countless additional examples exist. These are some of the most valuable products of the revolution in biology sparked by the discovery in the 19th Century that organisms are composed of chemicals. They include a large fraction of modern drugs and other useful materials.

What Inventions Are Affected?

The Guidance states that it applies to all "natural products" or combinations of natural products. That categorization by itself is unhelpful, as all possible inventions must contain one or more natural products (for example, an aluminum can contain aluminum, a naturally occurring element). The Guidance provides some clarification by providing the following non-exclusive list of materials that fall under the new rules:[8]

1. Chemicals derived from natural sources (including antibiotics, fats, oils, petroleum derivatives, resins, toxins, *etc.*)
2. Foods
3. Metals and metallic compounds that exist in nature
4. Minerals
5. Natural materials (rocks and soil)
6. Nucleic acids
7. Organisms (including bacteria, plants, and multicellular animals)
8. Proteins and peptides
9. Other substances found in or derived from nature

It should be noted that some categories of materials are limited to those "found in nature" or that "exist in nature," and others are limited to those "derived" from nature. However, others, such as minerals, organisms, nucleic acids, peptides, and proteins, contain no such limitations, and are apparently subject to the new rules regardless of whether they are found in nature or derived from natural sources.

The widespread perception that TRIPS flipped the patent switch from 'off' to 'on' in developing countries obscures the fact that like many international agreements, TRIPS includes room for interpretation and flexibilities. For instance, patent reform involved regulatory measures such as compulsory licensing (*i.e.* the ability to force patent holders to grant a license to domestic firms under certain conditions), formal price controls, and the right for domestic firms producing newly patented molecules to pay a royalty and continue their commercial activities. Given the threat of onerous regulations, innovating firms also sometimes preemptively modify their behavior. The mere existence of the additional regulatory tools constrains excessive price increases even without their explicit use. Perhaps as

8 Landau, N. J. The New Patent Policy on Natural Products Is a Game Changer for Universities and Life Sciences Companies. Retrieved May 10, 2018, from https://www.bradley.com/insights/publications/2014/09/the-new-patent-policy-on-natural-products-is-a-g__ 9 Product Patent for the Indian Pharmaceutical Sector under the TRIPS regime. Retrieved May 10, 2018, from http://www.legalserviceindia.com/articles/ppch.htm.

evidence of a fear of compulsory licensing, the maker of Sovaldi recently announced that it would partner with generic drug manufacturers and sell its hepatitis C cure for $900 across 90 developing countries. At that time, the US list price for Sovaldi was $84,000. In addition to the regulatory flexibilities in TRIPS, there may simply be differences between the de jure and de facto operation of product patents for pharmaceuticals in developing economies. Given the lack of a clear theoretical prediction, the net effect of the combination of regulatory features of this reform process is ultimately an open empirical question.

The consequences of having strong intellectual property laws in place were that the foreign companies or the MNCs enjoyed a complete monopoly and charged exorbitant prices, and thus dominated the Indian drug market. They were engaged mainly in the import of drugs from their country of origin. During that time the MNCs who were controlling 80 per cent of the market did not come forward with financial investment and technological help to establish drug production centers in India[9]. An American Senate Committee headed by Senator Kefauver stated in 1959 in its report that in drugs, generally, India ranks amongst the highest priced nations of the world.

Discussing Patent Laws in Purview of Medicinal Usage: IPR and Public Welfare

Patents laws and regulations have been covering lot of medicinal inventions over the years from Alexander Fleming's penicillin to Yoshinori Ohsumi, all have been granted patent over their medical invention for public welfare. But, delivering patents over ayurvedic products or medicines is unfair. Covering such elements under IPR laws which could be easily found and can be easily grown is basically hampering the whole idea of IPR laws, the inventor here is a money minded person who is using IPR laws for filling his own pocket rather, than caring more about public welfare. The applicability of laws of IPR on ayurvedic products makes the commodity very expensive for the locals to use, insignificant of the fact that they have been using it since ages. Patents gives the patent holder the exclusive right to his invention covering the making, rising, exercising, selling or distribution of the patented article or substance, as well as using and exercising the patented method or process of manufacturing an article or substance. In the case of patent of life, this implies that a patent holder can prevent others from making or using patented seeds and plants.[10]

Case Study: Patent of *Neem*

Here it become essential to talk about patent of *neem* as a bio pesticide by American pharmaceutical company named W.R. Grace and co. The properties of *neem* as biopesticide is not hidden from Indian farmers and agriculturalist. Use of neem as a natural pesticide has been observed and practiced over the centuries, providing patent to an American company who have not even invented it is in fact, intellectual "piracy" rights than intellectual property rights. Later, the patent was

---

10 VANDANA SHIVA, Patents: Myths and Reality, penguin books, India, 2001.

revoked but, this is not the only American patent covering *neem*. The first US patent was obtained by Terumo Corporation in 1983 for its therapeutic preparation from neem bark. In 1985 Robert Larson from (USDA) obtained a patent for his preparation of neem seed extract and the Environmental Protection Agency approved this product for use in US market.

The above case study of *neem* clearly embarks the arrogance of western companies and corporate giants to exploit the resources of developing countries and break the international regulations in such a manner that they gain advantage over other countries. Not only *neem*, other ayurvedic products like turmeric, cloves and *tulsi* have also faced such wrath of IPR laws. The fundamental concept behind IPR's is being challenged through such actions and grants of patents.

Medicinal Monopoly-through Patents

The major reason to seek patents for medical products by the big pharmaceuticals company is just to create monopoly in the market. By patenting they become the only provider of that particular medicine and hence, exploit the market demand. Again, the point of public welfare is in question by patenting and by monopolising the medical sector patent rights do no good to common man. The continuous patents on ayurvedic products highlights that the point is not to "provide medicines" but to "how expensive the medicines should be provided." This a game of turning patented material into a commercial product to earn money from the pockets of the people who are using it over years and patented product is what they have been using since ages.

Intellectual Piracy Rights Discussing Biopiracy

There is no accepted definition of bio-piracy it refers to the process through which the rights of indigenous cultural resources and knowledge are erased and replaced by monopoly rights.

In the recent past there have been several cases of bio-piracy of Traditional Knowledge particularly from the developing world. Developing countries, especially Latin America and Asia are rich in biological diversity and the wide genetic variability in these countries in many times exploited by the developing countries. This process of transferring of biological wealth of the third world without praying for it has come to be known as bio-piracy. India boasts a wide variety of flora and fauna which are diversified in nature. The faunal and floral richness has been one of the biggest assets of India. Available data place India in the tenth position in the world and fourth in Asia in plant diversity. With this India has long been a victim of bio-piracy.

The issue of IPRs is thus getting closely related to the issue of bio-piracy and intellectual piracy of western style IPR regimes. The lack of legal protection of biological and cultural heritage has made the indigenous communities of the third world vulnerable to bio-piracy and intellectual piracy as in the cases of neem *etc.* The existing patent regimes based on western paradigms are biased in favour of large Trans National Corporations with interests cutting across pharmaceuticals and Agri-chemicals.

International Organizations Dealing with IPR-Leaking Roof Covering the Room

There are various international organizations which deal with IPR and guide the regulations of it. Some of them are TRIPS (Trade Related Aspects of Intellectual Property Rights), WIPS (World Intellectual Property Organization) *etc.*

TRIPS among them is one of the most important organization which usually covers the area of intellectual property that covers copyrights, patent, Geographical Indications, Industrial Designs.[11] TRIPS set out minimum standard of protection to be provided by each member. This agreement sets these standards from the conventions that was held before the formation of TRIPS, some of them are the Paris Convention for the Protection of Industrial Property (Paris Convention), The Berne Convention for the Protection of Literary and Artistic Works (Berne Convention) and World Intellectual Property Organization which is generally known as WIPO. The agreement lays down some general provisions on civil and administrative procedure and remedies, provisional measures, special requirements related to border measures and criminal procedures, which specify, in a certain amount of detail, the procedures and remedies that must be available so that right holders can effectively enforce their rights and through this agreement disputes of WTO members regarding the TRIPS obligations are subjected to WTO's disputes settlement procedures.[12]

But the parliaments of various developing countries are pressuring WTO to interpret various clauses in the agreement to introduce massive reforms of the existing IPR laws in order to develop a legal framework with TRIPS conformity. A biggest flaw in the implementation of proper procedure of deciding a dispute in WTO disputes settlement procedure is the little jurisdiction defined in the agreement and therefore the first step would be to define the scope and extent of existing obligations by means of the standard methods of treaty interpretation. Therefore, a great problem is being faced by the developing countries in this regard which the developing countries are trying to clear but no process is being made in this. Not only there is a jurisdiction problem but the countries are facing problems relating to the implementation of agreement, namely the continuous use of unilateral pressures and the lack of actual implementation of Article 66.2 (incentives for the transfer of technology to least developed countries) and Article 67 (technical assistance to developing countries.

Many countries are stressing on the difficulty that they have been facing due the massive legislation changes that TRIPS is making, countries have also put forward their problems with the developed countries due to the lack of support. In this context, the implementation of Article 66.2 to the benefit of least developed countries has been raised by Egypt, India and the African Group, which noted

---

11 Overview: The TRIPS Agreement, World Trade Organization, https://www.wto.org/english/tratop_e/trips_e/intel2_e.htm. 12 *Ibid.*

13 Training tools on the TRIPS agreement: The Developing Countries Perspective, UNCTAD, Geneva 2002

that there have been no concrete steps by developed countries with regard to the fulfilment of their obligations under that article. The African Group has pointed out that Article 66.2 which says that developed country members shall provide the incentives is not a hortatory clause. Egypt also pointed out the need to review the implementation of Article 67.

For some developing countries such as Cuba, Dominican Republic, Egypt the transitional period in Article 65.2 has been For some developing countries (Cuba, Dominican Republic, Egypt and Honduras) the transitional period in Article 65.2 has been insufficient for undertaking the difficult and costly tasks related to the modernization of the administrative infrastructure (intellectual property offices and institutions, the judicial and customs systems), for drafting new laws with substantive and procedural provisions for the protection of IPRs, and for strengthening institutions and creating a culture for the protection of those rights. They have therefore requested an extension of the transition period for the developing countries.[13]

Article 23.4 of the TRIPS Agreement requires Members to undertake negotiations on the establishment of a multilateral system of notification and registration of geographical indications for wines. Different proposals have been made on the subject. The European Communities proposed an international registration of geographical indications under which registered indications would be automatically protected in the participating Member countries, subject to a procedure for dealing with opposition from any Member which considers that a geographical indication is not eligible for protection in its territory. On the other hand, the United States and Japan envisage the development of an international database of geographical indications to which Members would be expected to refer in the operation of their national systems. Both approaches have support from other Members. In addition, several countries have proposed (in the framework of the preparations for the WTO Ministerial Conference and of the built-in agenda for the TRIPS Agreement) that the enhanced protection now available for wines and spirits be extended to other products, such as agricultural products, medicines and handicrafts.[14] The Indian delegation argued that "It is an anomaly that the higher level of protection is available only for wines and spirits. It is proposed that such higher level of protection should be available for goods other than wines and spirits also. This would be helpful for products of export interest like basmati rice, Darjeeling tea, alphonso mangoes, Kohlapuri slippers in the case of India. It is India's belief that there are other Members of the WTO who would be interested in higher level of protection to products of export interest to them like Bulgarian yoghurt, Czech Pilsen beer, many agricultural products of the European Union, Hungarian Szatmar plums and so on. There is a need to expedite work already initiated in the TRIPS Council in this regard, under Article 24, so that benefits arising out of the TRIPS Agreement in this area are spread out wider."[15] Proposals relating to increase of the product is supported by Cuba, Indonesia, Pakistan, Egypt *etc.*

---

14 *Ibid.*

15 *Ibid.*

The agreement is thus creating a huge problem among the developing countries and since developed countries has great power in their hands are influencing or can say suppressing the developing countries by not following the provisions of the agreement and creating their own provisions which is beneficial for themselves and thus the problems are being faced by the small countries or developing countries.

Therefore, there is a great need to amend the article of the agreement so that equality among the countries is created and no small country is left out.

Conclusion

Ayurveda is by and large a conceptual science where concepts have been evolved around principles of health, enteropathogenesis of diseases and approaches to treatment, which include not only drug but also therapeutic diets and therapies to correct disturbed balance of the body. In this system of medicine, use of plants has been the eternal source of food and medicine since antiquity. Although local herbs and plants are used traditionally in all countries of the world, but India has been the pioneers in this field where its traditional systems of medicine have been flourishing for centuries and millennia in a well-codified form. Ayurveda is based on its own original and unique fundamental principles and it has its authentic literature including material medical. Ayurveda in India has remained in unbroken practice for thousands of years and even today the main stream of official system of medicine with huge infrastructure. In fact, in India, Ayurveda is credited as most authentic traditional knowledge of medicine. Earlier World Intellectual Property Organizations Conventions, 1967 states that 'Intellectuals Property includes the rights relating to literary, artistic and scientific works, performances and performing artists, photographs and broadcasts, inventions in all fields of human endeavour –scientific discoveries, industrial designs, trademarks, service marks and commercial names and designations, protections against unfair competition and all other rights resulting from intellectuals activity in the industrial, scientific, literary or artistic fields., but in present scenario patents being granted for indigenous knowledge and natural plants this leads to the bio-piracy.

Now a day's companies to acquire large market share and seem to be in a high stakes scavenger to collect patents which can ultimately sold for billions. Patents also attracted organizations to explore possibilities of commercial benefits with Ayurvedic traditional knowledge. The universalization of patents to cover all subject matter, including life forms, increases the scope of patents and now it has invading in forests and farms to kitchen and medical plant gardens. Tradition Knowledge which India has practise for many centuries for day to day uses such as *neem, haldi, karela, jamun, kali mirch* and hundreds of other plants used not in food but as medicine also are in danger of being patented by the western companies for commercial gain. This is also factual that at present Ayurvedic practice is being accomplished day by day and evolves as individuals and communities respond to the challenges posed by their social environment and new ailments. Therefore, it is not only desirable to develop a protection policy that documents and preserves traditional knowledge created in the past, which may be on the brink of disappearance; it is also important to consider how to respect and sustain the development and dissemination of further traditional knowledge that arises from continuing use of traditional knowledge systems. Thousands of patents on African plants have been filed. These include brazzeine, a protein 500 times sweeter than sugar from a plant in Gabon; Teff, the grain used in Ethiopia's flat 'injera' bread; and thaumatin, a natural sweetener from a plant in West Africa. The African soap berry, the Kunde Zulu cowpea and genetic material from the west African cocoa plant also make the list.

Increasingly, African countries are going to court over patents on their indigenous plants. The most celebrated case to date involves the Hoodia cactus from the Kalahari Desert. For centuries, the San people of southern Africa ate pieces of the cactus to stave off hunger and thirst. Analysing the cactus, the Council for Scientific and Industrial Research (CSIR) in South Africa found the molecule that curbs appetite and sold the rights to develop an anti-obesity drug to pharmaceutical company Pfizer. It could be worth billions.

The commercial development of naturally occurring biological materials, such as plant substances or genetic cell lines, by a technologically advanced country or transnational corporation without fair compensation to the peoples or nations of the developing world is one of the most serious cases of the externalisation of resources. The appropriation and patenting of nanotechnologies by corporations has more often than not worked against the best interests of humanity, especially in the less developed world. in many countries, patents with full monopolistic restrictions are now applicable to plant varieties, micro-organisms, and genetically modified animals. In 1972, the US Supreme Court ruled that microbiologist Ananda Chakrabarty's patent claim for a genetically engineered bacterial strain, was permissible. This legitimised the view that anything made by humans and not found in nature was patentable. Genetically altered animals, such as the infamous 'onco-mouse' of Harvard University (bred for cancer research), were also soon given patents.

Finally, several patent claims have been made, and some granted, on human genetic material, including on material that has hardly been altered from its natural state. Until very recently, these trends were restricted to isolated countries, which could not impose them on others.

Chapter 16

Security and IPR in Developing Countries

Sagun Vishan and Prakhar Srivastava

Amity Institute of Biotechnology, Amity University, Noida, Uttar Pradesh -201301
e-mail: sagunvishan@gmail.com

ABSTRACT

IPRs have become increasingly important in the past two decades in numbers of fields. This includes agriculture biotechnology as well were IPR provide a basic platform to private sector for their development. As in past few years agriculture is in most of the developing country has been getting exposed to an entirely new sets of technologies. One of the major debates with regard to food security today is the contribution of agro-biotechnology can make to meeting the food needs of today's worlds populations as there is a need of foster food securities in context of free exchange of knowledge to a system seeking the same goal on the basis of private appropriation of knowledge. The agriculture and food security are directly interlinked with each other because of extensive of IPRs to agriculture. Food security is a major problem throughout the developing nations. It is not only concern of individuals but also of the states. As food is the basic individual right but also affects the economical development in a state. Food security still remains an overwhelming concern for developing countries. Even in some part of world the some portion of population remains unnourished. The food security is not only depending on the availability of food but also an effective access and appropriate distribution of existing resources. This paper will examine the issues of food securities from narrow perspective of intellectual property and will also discuss the international legal framework in developing countries for food securities and intellectual properties.

Keywords: Argo-biotechnology, Food security and Intellectual property.

Introduction

There is no easy way to identify the policy, economic and legal linkages between food security as a goal and intellectual property rights (IPRs) as an instrument to promote and enhance human creativity and overall social well-being. But connections do exist. Food security is part of the basic human right to food, broadly defined as timely access to sufficient and nutritious food[1]. It is inextricably linked to the right to health[2]. It is linked to intellectual property (IP) inasmuch as plant variety protection (PVP; also known as plant breeders' rights) and patents, as applied to genetic resources, biodiversity components and biotechnological processes, may be limiting the possibilities of cultivators to freely grow certain crops, and of people to consume resulting agricultural products. Linkages may also be found in the overall social goals of distinct, long-established legal regimes including those protecting human rights – specifically in regard to the right to food – and IPRs. While pursuing different specific objectives, these regimes should, in theory, be complementary in advancing human welfare and development (Okediji 2007). From a strict legal perspective, IPRs should in no way undermine a very basic human right on which life – literally – depends. When applied not just to whole plants and animals but also to reproductive material including seeds, and to genetic resources in general, IPRs may affect the accessibility and availability of a large number of agricultural products. This is especially the case with IPRs such as patents which allow the rights holder to prevent third parties from commercial exploitation of the exclusive rights as defined in the patent claims[3]. Food security is also inextricably linked to poverty, as it is mostly poor people who suffer from limited access to appropriate food sources. Curiously, a considerable portion of the world's poor are farmers, which again raises issues associated with seeds and their protection through IP, including the consequences of restrictions on the use of seeds for these farmers. This is one of the themes explored in this chapter. Intellectual property protection of technologies including biotechnology may also signify that countries and their communities (especially those of technologically disadvantaged nations) are unable to enhance their agricultural processes through appropriate application of these technologies. Private and public research sectors may meanwhile be affected by legal restrictions on the use of certain technologies, thus reducing options for agricultural development. This is even more serious in a context where, increasingly, the relationship between appropriate food intake and health has become apparent in both developed and developing countries.

Intellectual Property Rights in Agriculture

Intellectual property protection has been extended in the last 25 years to a wide range of information, materials and products relevant to food and agriculture. The US Supreme Court decision in Diamond v Chakrabarty influenced national legislation and case law in many jurisdictions, opening the door for the patentability of living organisms, including microbes, plants and animals and their parts and components. In addition, the TRIPS Agreement and, more recently, a growing number of free trade agreements (FTAs) promoted by the United States of America, European Free Trade Association (EFTA) and the EU have propelled the expansion of intellectual property protection to biological materials, particularly plants. Since 1995, 40 countries have adhered to the UPOV Convention for the Protection of New Varieties of Plants, which until then had had a membership essentially limited to developed countries. The extension of IPRs to agricultural inputs and products raises a number of ethical concerns.

Intellectual Property Rights and Trade Barriers

A large part of the population in developing countries depends on the production and sale of agricultural products. In accordance with the World Development Report 2008, agriculture is called to play a central role in achieving the Millennium Development Goal of halving extreme poverty and hunger by 2015. Gross domestic product originating in agriculture is deemed to be about four times more effective in reducing poverty than that originating outside the sector (World Bank, 2007). The expansion of agricultural exports may contribute, if appropriate income distribution policies are in place, to reducing poverty and global income inequalities. During the Uruguay Round of the General Agreement on Tariffs and Trade, developed countries demanded acceptance of the TRIPS Agreement by developing countries as a quid pro quo to reduce their barriers to agricultural trade. In recent FTAs signed between the United States of America, EFTA, EU and several developing countries, the offer of preferential access to agricultural markets has also been the key card used to break such countries' resistance to admit TRIPS-plus standards of IPR protection. TRIPS-plus standards are likely to have negative impacts, inter alia, on access to medicines, educational materials and technologies essential for development.

The Right to Food: A Conceptual and Legal Background

The tragedy of hunger in many parts of the world is incomprehensible alongside the affluence and overconsumption in other parts[4]. The Food and Agriculture Organization of the United Nations (FAO) estimated in June 2009 that 1.02 billion persons were hungry, an increase of more than 150 million people in just two year[5]. Increasing food prices represent a crucial part of the explanation, and the poorest, landless and female-headed households are the hardest hit (FAO 2008, pp. 1, 22–27). Poverty is still the main explanation for hunger. Significantly, 70 per cent of the world's hungry are involved in agriculture themselves, either as smallholders or as landless labourers. These simple truths show that something is clearly wrong in how agriculture and the food system are organized, both worldwide and nationally. To ensure food security and reduce poverty levels, urgent changes and responses are needed from governments, the research community including the international agricultural research centres, the private sector, the international financial community, international cooperation agencies, the retail business and society at large. In 1996, the Heads of State and Government present at the World Food Summit defined food security as a situation that 'exists when all people, at all times, have physical, social and economic access to sufficient, safe and nutritious food that meets their dietary needs and food preferences for an active and healthy life[6.]

Three elements are important in this definition: first, its emphasis on physical, social and economic access to food; second, its emphasis on the quality of the food; third, the emphasis that the intake of food must enable everyone to live an active and healthy life, not merely surviving. Even more noteworthy is the first introductory paragraph of the Rome Declaration on World Food Security, which recognizes 'the right of everyone to have access to safe and nutritious food, consistent with the right to adequate food and the fundamental right of everyone to be free from hunger'. The leaders also committed themselves to 'reducing the number of undernourished people to half their present level no later than 2015. In contrast, the term used to quantify hunger levels in the 2000 UN Millennium Declaration is 'proportion[7]. The Millennium Declaration resolves 'to halve, by the year 2015,...the proportion of [the world's] people who suffer from hunger' (ibid., emphasis added). Hence, the 1996 Summit was considerably more ambitious than the 2000 Summit, as the former is committed to a real halving from the 800 million hungry persons in 1996 to 400 million, while the latter is committed to a reduction to approximately 500 million, based on demographic trends towards 2015. While the concept of 'food security' might still be more frequently used among decision makers, it is more relevant to analyse the relationship between IPRs and food by applying the right to food. As both human rights and IPRs are widely recognized legal regimes, any comparison between them should be done from their respective objectives and means for achieving these objectives, formulated in legal terms. Compliance with the legal obligations that States assume by ratifying international treaties and adopting legislation in the realm of human rights and IPRs is sought through the implementation of both global and national strategies. States are responsible for ensuring an appropriate balancing between these rights. In this context of balancing between rights, it is relevant to quote in full a paragraph from the UK Commission on Intellectual Property Rights (CIPR): We therefore consider that an IP right is best viewed as one of the means by which nations and societies can help to promote the fulfilment of human economic and social rights. In particular, there are no circumstances in which the most fundamental human rights should be subordinated to the requirements of IP protection[8]. IP rights are granted by states for limited times (at least in the case of patents and copyrights) whereas human rights are inalienable and universal (CIPR 2002, p. 6) A similar emphasis on the relationship between IPRs and economic, social and cultural rights is expressed by the United Nations Committee on Economic, Social and Cultural Rights (CESCR) in its General Comment No. 17 (2005, para. 35)[9]. The General Comments are not legally binding, but are frequently referred to in resolutions adopted by intergovernmental bodies, and in national strategies. A more precise understanding of human rights, in particular the right to food, is, however, needed before moving towards the linkages between IPRs and food.

Agricultural Research and Intellectual Property Rights

Recognition of the links between intellectual property rights issues and food security is increasing, as evidenced by the negotiation of a new IP policy for the CGIAR in 2012 and the recognition by the G-8 New Alliance for Food Security and Nutrition to "[e]explore opportunities for applying the non-profit model licensing approach that could expand African access to food and nutritional technologies developed by national research institutions[10]. Part of the emphasis on intellectual property rights issues comes from increasing engagement of the private sector by the traditional donor community in international development efforts. Though the private sector has participated in many, often less visible, ways in past development efforts, international development donors increasingly recognize the role the private sector can play in both focusing private sector investment on agricultural research for smallholder producers in developing countries as well as facilitating the deployment of technologies developed by public sector investments to poor smallholder producers in developing countries [11].Naseem and his colleagues reviewed policy options that could cultivate private sector investment in research and development (R&D) for agriculture in developing countries, and indicated that intellectual property rights are one important incentive to stimulate private investment in agricultural research, though the impacts on pro-poor agriculture are variable depending on a number of factors[12]. Public sector research, especially that being undertaken by the CGIAR's new research programs, contributes to the development of pro-poor technologies to improve the productivity of smallholder agriculture and/or reduce the vulnerability associated with agricultural production among poor smallholder producers [13].Through strategic engagement with the private sector, the outputs of research, both in terms of technology and knowledge, (*e.g.*, greater understanding of factors to increase technology adoption among smallholders) can potentially reach greater numbers of target beneficiaries.

Further, engagment with the private sector could potentially improve the sustainability of availability of technologies, through steady demand for pro-poor technologies, when priced and available in ways accessible to poor smallholders. To harness these opportunities available through the private sector, intellectual proprety rights are an important tool. Thus, donors have taken steps to address how and in what context intellectual property rights are asserted over publicly funded international agricultural research outputs through the negotiation of the CGIAR Principles on the Management of Intellectual Assets. During the recent reform process of the CGIAR system, intellectual property issues were raised, as individual CGIAR centers had, over time, established their own policies and procedures for managing intellectual assets and engaging with the private sector. The Principles were drafted to ensure that under the new CGIAR system, all CGIAR centers were guided by the same principles to manage their intellectual assets as these assets exist largely from decades of public sector funding. These Principles commit the CGIAR to "prudent and strategic use of intellectual property rights," such as patents or plant variety protection, that are only to be pursued in situations necessary to improve the asset or "to enhance the scale or scope of impact on target beneficiaries[14].The provisions also address exclusivity agreements that the CGIAR may undertake with third parties, to ensure there is a careful review of how and under what circumstances agreements are developed. This is a living document, subject to review and revision in two years from the adoption by the Fund Council in March 2012. The review will enable donors to learn how intellectual assets management is faring under these principles, and what new or unexpected impacts this has for how the CGIAR engages with partners, and most importantly, to examine how these evolving principles can best be structured to increase the impacts of public sector funded research on smallholder producers in the developing world.

Food Secruty to Meet Dietary Needs for Active and Healthy Lives; Ethical Considerations in Connecting Elements of FAO's Mandate FAO

It is required under its Constitution of 1945 to collect, analyse, interpret and disseminate information relating to nutrition, food and agriculture. For many years, initiatives focusing on these various elements followed their own, specialized and mostly unrelated paths. In the FAO Secretariat, nutrition was left more or less isolated in a division conducting its work rather independently of what happened in the other parts of the organization. In the light of the implications for people's diet and nutrition of globalization processes as discussed below, the recent institutional reform within FAO, which has placed nutrition together with consumer protection in the Agricultural and Consumer Protection Department, should encourage stronger linkages with production issues besides emphasis on consumer protection for good nutritional health in the age of globalization. In 1996, the Heads of State and Government at the WFS agreed on a definition of food security in a way that points to an explicit connection between the various mandates of FAO according to its Constitution. ... Food security exists when all people, at all times, have physical and economic access to sufficient, safe and nutritious food to meet their dietary needs and food preferences for an active and healthy life. ... World Food Summit Plan of Action, Para. 1 (FAO, 1998) The food security concept thus defined can serve to connect the fundamental tasks of the Organization related to food production, distribution and access, encompassing the interests of both producers and consumers, and the concern with sustainable environment. The Panel recommends that FAO use the food security definition systematically and encourage Member States to do so in the formulation of their agricultural as well as their food and nutritional policies. In particular, the recognition that agricultural production should aim at providing "nutritious foods" to meet the "dietary needs" underlines the fact that a primary purpose of agriculture and food handling is to facilitate matters so that all people can eat satisfactorily in the pursuance of health and absence of disease and thereby lead an active (implying also productive) life. This should guide the production/processing/distribution chain and serve as a point of departure for checking whether developments in agricultural and food supply policies really serve the meaning and purpose expressed in the 1996

The Challenges Ahead for Developing Countries: Ensuring Better Use of Genetic Resources and more Targeted Research and Development

The enclosure of previously free resources appears to be a recurring tendency, in terms of both the increasing privatization of genetic resources and the assertion of sovereign rights over resources under international frameworks including the CBD (and restrictive access laws as a result). While the ITPGRFA perhaps represents a counter-trend in its endeavour 'to maintain a level of openness for crops listed, commentators suggest it is still too soon to say whether the protected 'commons' within the ITPGRFA will deliver the desired benefits and help to increase R&D (Roa-Rodríguez and van Dooren 2008)[15]. To reclaim 'common heritage' in the 'plant genetic resources regime complex', some commentators have meanwhile suggested exploring open source solutions to R&D in agriculture. Meanwhile, Maskus and Reichman (2005) raise very pertinent issues on international IP standard setting and implementation. Pointing to the wording of the preamble and Article 8(1) of the TRIPS Agreement, they note that: '[T]he implementation of international IP standards is necessarily limited by criteria of reasonableness. These standards, as implemented, must not become disguised barriers to the exercise of those other police and welfare powers that are normally reserved to states'. Moreover, they hold that 'states cannot be presumed to have surrendered sovereign police and welfare powers in the course of intellectual property standard setting.In relation to the present discussion; this must be understood to imply that the full obligations of a State must be taken into account when IP legislation is to be adopted or enforced. A WTO member state ought to make sure that the flexibilities provided for in the TRIPS Agreement are fully considered and appropriately reflected. Pressures to have higher IP protection standards than those required in the TRIPS Agreement – for example, in FTAs or investment treaties – should be resisted, and it should be possible to have a review of certain paragraphs in the TRIPS Agreement in order to better reconcile the Agreement to other treaties [16]. At this point, flexibilities in national IP and ABS policies may be required to:

- ✰ Facilitate research and the development of national and community-based seed banks – these may be extremely critical for biodiversity-rich countries and centers of origin and diversification of crops, as a means to support local farmers and communities in a context of growing climate change problems;
- ✰ Stimulate collective participatory breeding – this may become a good alternative to bridge TK and local farmers needs with the scientific potential of national and international institutions; collaborative research could be explored, for example, with research institutions;
- ✰ Protect and promote the TK of indigenous communities – there is a sufficient basis in different human rights provisions in favor of a position that traditional communities and indigenous peoples who nurture and improve plants should enjoy human rights protection over their production.

Intellectual Property Rights and Trade Barriers

A large part of the population in developing countries depends on the production and sale of agricultural products. In accordance with the World Development Report 2008, agriculture is called to play a central role in achieving the Millennium Development Goal of halving extreme poverty and hunger by 2015. Gross domestic product originating in agriculture is deemed to be about four times more effective in reducing poverty than that originating outside the sector (World Bank, 2007). The expansion of agricultural exports may contribute, if appropriate income distribution policies are in place, to reducing poverty and global income inequalities. During the Uruguay Round of the General Agreement on Tariffs and Trade, developed countries demanded acceptance of the TRIPS Agreement by developing countries as a quid pro quo to reduce their barriers to agricultural trade. In recent FTAs signed between the United States of America, EFTA, EU and several developing countries, the offer of preferential access to agricultural markets has also been the key card used to break such countries' resistance to admit TRIPS-plus standards of IPR protection. TRIPS-plus standards are likely to have negative impacts, inter alia, on access to medicines, educational materials and technologies essential for development.

The Panel has also observed cases in which IPRs have been exercised by their titleholders in ways that generate inequitable outcomes. Overly broad claims interpretation and abusive measures at the border may result in developing countries losing income necessary to reduce poverty and implement development programmes.

Patents on Living Forms

Many national laws have recognized the possible conflict between the granting of patents and morality. Thus, the TRIPS Agreement expressly permits WTO members to "exclude from patentability inventions, the prevention within their territory of the commercial exploitation of which is necessary to protect ordre public or morality, including to protect human, animal or plant life or health or to avoid serious prejudice to the environment, provided that such exclusion is not made merely because the exploitation is prohibited by their law." (Article 27.2). The TRIPS Agreement also allows countries to exclude plants and animals from patentability (Article 27.3(b)). The idea of appropriation of living forms through patents may be morally unacceptable, particularly when IPRs involve living forms found in nature and a private monopoly would impede access to a public good. In these cases, the very granting of a patent may be immoral, even where the commercial exploitation was morally unobjectionable.

Appropriation of Traditional Knowledge

Several cases of inequitable appropriation through patents of traditional and indigenous knowledge have been reported. The legal fiction that considers "novel" (and, hence, susceptible of being patented) unpublished traditional/indigenous knowledge generated and used in a foreign country has ethically unacceptable consequences. As elaborated by the Committee on Economic, Social and Cultural Rights in its General Comment 17 on Article 15(c) of the International Covenant on Economic, Social and Cultural Rights, the moral and material interests of peoples, communities or other groups in their collective cultural heritage constitutes a fundamental right that needs to be protected by states (UN, 2006).

Future Prospective

Intellectual property issues are increasingly relevant to the public-sector international agricultural research landscape. Given the expected significant increases in public sector funding in the coming years to address global food security issues, and the increasing role of public-private sector engagement, intellectual property rights may be an increasingly important tool to help achieve impacts from these investments. Additional research on how and in what contexts to best use intellectual property tools to achieve the intended impacts from this expansion in international agricultural research funding will be critical for the international donor community as it strives to meets its commitment to addressing global food security

Conclusion

In this paper, we addressed a number of key concerns relating to IP and food security. In. we emphasized the need for balance between IPRs and human rights in discussing the right to food. We discussed the interface between IPRs and recent agricultural trends, focusing on how the increasing reliance on the private sector for agricultural research impacts farming communities in developing countries and biodiversity more generally. We looked especially at the impacts of patents and plant variety. Along with Socio-economic concerns, we touched on the potential environmental effects. Also outlined international frameworks governing access to plant genetic resources, and how they further impact on the commons. We then explored. Potential strategies for developing countries in ensuring better use of their genetic resources and targeting R&D efforts towards priorities including food security. The crucial balancing between access and incentives. We looked there are several cases of inequitable appropriation through patents of traditional and indigenous knowledge have been reported. The legal fiction that considers "novel" (and, hence, susceptible of being patented) unpublished traditional/indigenous knowledge generated and used in a foreign country has ethically unacceptable consequences. We also discussed about that a large part of the population in developing countries depends on the production and sale of agricultural products. In accordance with the World Development Report 2008, agriculture is called to play a central role in achieving the Millennium Development Goal of halving extreme poverty and hunger by 2015. Gross domestic product originating in agriculture is deemed to be about four times more effective in reducing poverty than that originating outside the sector (World Bank, 2007). The expansion of agricultural exports may contribute, if appropriate income distribution policies are in place, to reducing poverty and global income inequalities. We also discussed about the challenges ahead for developing countries: Ensuring better use of genetic resources and more targeted research and development, the implementation of international IP standards is necessarily limited by criteria of reasonableness. We also discussed about Recognition of the links between intellectual property rights issues and food security is increasing, as evidenced by the negotiation of a new IP policy for the CGIAR in 2012 and the recognition by the G-8 New Alliance for Food Security and Nutrition to "[e]explore opportunities for applying the non-profit model licensing approach that could expand African access to food and nutritional technologies developed by national research institutions. Part of the emphasis on intellectual property rights issues comes from increasing engagement of the private sector by the traditional donor community in international development efforts. Though the private sector has participated in many, often less visible, ways in past development efforts, international development donors increasingly recognize the role the private sector can play in both focusing private sector investment on agricultural research for smallholder producers in developing countries as well as facilitating the deployment of technologies developed by public sector investments to poor smallholder producers in developing countries. We also discussed about Future Prospective, Intellectual property issues are increasingly relevant to the public-sector international agricultural research landscape. Given the expected significant increases in public sector funding in the coming years to address global food security issues, and the increasing role of public-private sector engagement, intellectual property rights may be an increasingly important tool to help achieve impacts from these investments.

REFERENCES

1. See Article 25 of the Universal Declaration of Human Rights (Paris, 10 December 1948), G.A. Res. 217A (III), (1948), UN Doc. A/810 (1948), available at: http://daccess-ddsny.un.org/doc/RESOLUTION/GEN/NR0/043/88/IMG/NR004388.pdf?OpenElement (accessed 3 February 2010).
2. The right to health is embodied in the 1946 Constitution of the World Health Organization (WHO) (New York, 22 July 1946), 14 U.N.T.S. 185, 62 Stat. 2679 (entered into force 7 April 1948). For information on human rights treaties pertaining to the right of health, see Chapter 2. See also UN Office of the High Commissioner for Human Rights (OHCHR) and WHO, Fact Sheet No. 31: The Right to Health (June 2008), available at: http://www.ohchr.org/Documents/Publications/Factsheet31.pdf (accessed 18 March 2010).
3. Tansey (2008, pp. 7–8) discusses the changing global food system and challenges for national food policies in terms of 'ensuring a sustainable, secure, safe, sufficient and nutritious (in other words healthy), equitable and culturally appropriate diet for all'.
4. Tansey (2008, p. 3) suggests that: 'What is clear is that there are serious flaws in a food system that globally leaves more than 850 million people undernourished and over 1 billion overweight (300 million of these obese)'. He adds that: 'Some 2 billion people also suffer from vitamin and micronutrient shortages. Undernutrition in pregnant women and young babies can have irreversible effects for life, while obese people's lives are threatened by diet-related non-communicable diseases such as diabetes and heart attacks'.
5. See World Food Program, '1.02 Billion People Hungry', available at: http://www.wfp.org/news/newsrelease/102-billion-people-hungry (accessed 18 March 2010). For further details on specific figures and facts regarding world food and hunger, see the International Food Policy Research Institute (IFPRI) website, available at: http://www.ifpri.org/(accessed 18 March 2010).
6. UN Food and Agriculture Organization (FAO), Rome Declaration on World Food Security and World Food Summit Plan of Action (Rome, 13 November 1996), UN Doc. WFS 96/3 (1996), para. 1, available at: http://www.fao.org/docrep/003/w3613e/w3613e00.HTM (accessed 2 April 2010).
7. United Nations Millennium Declaration (8 September 2000), G.A. Res. 55/2, UN Doc. A/RES/55/2 (2000) [hereinafter 'UN Millennium Declaration'], para. 19(1), available at: http://www.un.org/millennium/(accessed 22 June 2009).

8.The significance of this Commission being comprised of highly recognized IP law scholars and attorneys cannot be underestimated. For details of the Commission's work, see the Commission for Intellectual Property Rights website, available at: http://www.iprcommission.org (accessed 18 March 2010).

9. Committee on Economic, Social and Cultural Rights (CESCR) 2005, General Comment No. 17: The right of everyone to benefit from the protection of the moral and material interests resulting from any scientific, literary or artistic production of which he or she is the author (art. 15, para. 1 (c)), UN Doc. E/C.12/GC/17 (12 January 2006) [hereinafter 'General Comment No. 17'], available at: http://www.unhchr.ch/tbs/doc.nsf/7cec89369c43a6dfc1256a2a0027ba2a/03902145edbbe797c125711500584ea8/$FILE/ G0640060.pdf (accessed 3 February 2010)

10. WHITE HOUSE, supra note 7.

11. Reuters describes pledge announced at May 2012 G-8 discussion of global hunger and food security, http://www.reuters.com/article/2012/05/18/us-g8-foodidUSBRE84H0O920120518, (last visited Dec 11, 2012).

12. See Anwar Naseem, David J. Spielman and Steven W. Omamo, Private-Sector Investment in R&D: A Review of Policy Options to Promote its Growth in DevelopingCountry Agriculture, 26(1) AGRIBUSINESS 143 (2010), available at http://siteresources. worldbank.org/CFPEXT/Resources/NaseemetalPrivateRDAgribusiness10.pdf.

13. See CGIAR Strategic Results Framework, http://www.cgiarfund.org/strategy_results_framework.

14. See CGIAR 7th Fund Council Meeting documents Agenda Item 9, www.cgiarfund.org/7th_fund_council_meeting.

15. The SMTAs do not cover in situ collections which are still governed by national legislation (Article 12.3(h) of the ITPGRFA).

16. Article 13.2(d) of the ITPGRFA requires that 'a recipient who commercializes a product that is a plant genetic resource for food and agriculture and that incorporates material accessed from the Multilateral System, shall pay to [a financial mechanism to be established] an equitable share of the benefits arising from the commercialization of that product, except whenever such a product is available without restriction to others for further research and breeding, in which case the recipient who commercializes shall be encouraged to make such payment'.

Chapter 17

Protection of Plant Breeders' Rights vis-a-vis Exploitation of Vulnerable and Uniformed Sector of Breeders and Farmers: A Study

Tushar Arora

National Law University & Judicial Academy, Assam, Guwahati–781031, Assam (India)
e-mail: tushash8@nluassam.ac.in

ABSTRACT

The uninterrupted proliferation of the human race and the expansion of living spaces; the human encroachment of forest lands and agriculture farms has led to the entry of the field of Biotechnology in the agricultural arena; the reasons being, making judicious use of natural resources available which are being exploited at a heavy and much faster rate than before and keeping at par with the increasing number of stomachs to fill in lesser time that what it usually takes along with the duty of keeping the nutrition intact and hence, the use of various techniques along with which money, labour, hard work is involved has led to the emergence of Intellectual Property Rights in the field of agriculture, which aims to protect and give the person his fair share and frustrate any other person from making use of his property and possession for their benefit to which he is not a beneficiary. This chapter talks about how Plant Breeders' Rights which is one of the latest developments in the field of IPR is being employed to protect the rights of persons hailing from the agriculture industry (mainly Breeders and Farmers) who put in hard work to generate new varieties of plants and it also analyses the Basmati Rice Patent Controversy Case and explains how developed nations and their MNCs try to exploit the developing/underdeveloped nations and their farmers along with which it delivers possible suggestions to safeguard the vulnerable sectors of a nation such as that of agriculture from being browbeaten by the hands of such giants. The chapter also co-relates two very important fields of law, IPR and Torts.

Keywords: *IPR, Plant breeders, Agriculture.*

Introduction

"The law, under its majestic equality, forbids the rich as well the poor to sleep under bridges to beg under the streets and to steal the bread."

'Agriculture' is one of the most important aspects of today's world not only because it feeds almost 7 billion people but also because it acts as a 'living' for all those who are engaged in it. The concept of agriculture is extremely old as traced back in 9000 BC and it still accounts as one of the prominent contributors in economic, social and political fabric of the society.

Plant breeding practices have been going on for thousands of years wherein genetics is involved and a particular trait, which is desired by the breeder, is grown. It has helped in improving the food quality by letting a particular trait evolve and discontinuing the harmful/undesired one(s). With due course of time, the inclination of corporates has significantly increased in the agricultural practices, as a result of which, genetics and biotechnology together became a key factor in advancement in the field of research (in agriculture and its offshoot industry like horticulture, animal husbandry *etc.*) due to which the complexity and competition has increased many folds which has given rise to frequent disputes over the 'rights' on the new varieties developed. Therefore, to accommodate to the interests of various farmers, breeders, stakeholders of various MNCs and the public at large, various laws were passed where in everyone's interests could be taken care of and all could enjoy mutual benefits out of the same.

The chapter is divided into the following sections. The first part of the research provides a brief introduction to the laws of plant breeding and an outline on the development of the same under Intellectual Property Rights. The second part focuses on the analysis of the Protection of Plant Varieties and Farmers' Rights Act, 2001. The third section of the chapter deals with the plant breeder's rights in India and how farmers and corporate breeders perceive it. It also discusses the famous Basmati Rice Patent Controversy and a critical overview on the same. In the next part, it emphasises on the infringement of plant breeders' rights and how it could come under tort followed by a critical remark on the same.

Plant Breeders' Rights as a Part of Intellectual Property Rights

The creator of a construction site's map, the inventor of a machine, the inventor of a new software or the composer of a new *'dhun'* practically have a 'possession' over it and that must be safe-guarded from being copied or 'being used without the permission' as it takes a lot of hard-work, time may be money and brain to create a novel idea and the owner/inventor must be given full 'credit' for that. To ensure it, Intellectual Property Rights came into existence. The main legal tools of IPR are copyrights, trademarks, patents, and industrial designs. An organization, The International Union for the Protection of New Varieties of Plants (UPOV) Geneva was established in 1961 to protect new varieties of plants under Intellectual Property Rights. Its main objective is to give credit to the breeders who develop new varieties of plants by providing them immunity under IPR on the basis of a proper set of rules recommended by the members. Plant Breeders' Rights are a part of intellectual property rights that gives immunity to a breeder to protect new varieties of plants and gives him absolute control over propagating material for example seeds. These rights also include rights to alter, produce, sell, export, import and stock.[1] Strong protection is guaranteed against infringement of the rights of the breeder where strong punishment has been prescribed ranging from serving jail terms to huge fines as penalties.

The basic requirements to get the rights are:[2]

1. If the variety is new and has not been sold without the consent of the breeder for a time-period more than what permissible by the rules. For example, in Australia it is 12 months.
2. If the new variety is stable and does not change after 'multiple propagations'.
3. If the breed is uniform, *i.e.*, all plant varieties share the same traits.

Plant Breeders' Rights is a vast area of research and it further consists of:

1. Utility Patents
2. Trade Secrets
3. Contracts
4. Trademarks
5. Protection of New Breed

Just as the laws differ from country to country, so do the term for which immunity is granted. For example, in Australia, the protection remains prevalent from 20 to 25 years, in the UK; the rights last for 25 to 30 years. Every country has its own set of laws that protects the rights of the breeders like Canada, Britain, Australia, India and so on. For example, in Canada, the act was passed in 1990 and it became a member of UPOV in 1991. Similarly, in India, the same act came into force in 2001, which is explained further, in the next chapter. But the overall motive is to protect the rights of the breeder and give credibility and acknowledgement to his works.

Analysis of the Protection of Plant Varieties and Farmers' Rights Act, 2001

The sole purpose for legislating this act was that there was no protection and safeguard to the agricultural practices in the Indian Patents Act, 1970 expressly mentioned. So, to emphatically provide for a mechanism for the protection of the same was a great step by the parliament where in it enacted the Protection of Plant Varieties and Farmers' Rights Act, 2001 and then later in the year 2003, the rules were notified and the body behind drafting was 'The Protection of Plant Varieties and Farmers' Rights Authority' which encompasses the powers of administration

---

1 Plant Breeders' Rights, https://www.ipaustralia.gov.au/, Accessed on 20 April 2018, 19:20 IST.

2 Pre-requisites for PBR, https://www.gov.uk/topic/producing-distributing-food, Accessed on 22 April 2018, 13:20 IST.

under it. India was under a duty, with the regulations as expressed under the TRIPS agreement to which it is a party, where in there must be a mechanism provided expressly to safeguard the rights of the farmers, breeders and to cover all those who are protecting or generating species through their labor, both mental and physical.[3] India thus accepted and implemented the *sui generis* system and ordained the law.[4]

This act is a win-win situation for both the farmers and the breeders as it specifically provides for the protection of farmers by giving them their share of rights, which cannot be infringed by others and balances the same with the rights of the breeders by safeguarding them against any such exploitation. It does not end here; the act expressly takes into consideration the importance of researchers' rights as well as the rights, which are utilitarian in nature, which will be in welfare for a large number of people. The farmer's rights include his traditional rights to save, use, share or sell his farm produce of a variety protected under this Act provided the sale is not for the purpose of reproduction under a commercial marketing arrangement.[5]

Benefit Sharing and Compensation

According to the **Protection of Plant Varieties and Farmers' Rights Act, 2001, "benefit sharing in relation to a variety, means such proportion of the benefit accruing to a breeder of such variety or such proportion of the benefit accruing to the breeder from an agent or a licensee of such variety, as the case may be, for which a claimant shall be entitled as determined by the Authority."**[6] Once the variety is registered, it becomes the duty of the PPVFR Authority to implement the rights of the claimer with regard to his share. The discretion of the authority shall be considered as final and that will be done after hearing both the sides, *i.e.*, the claimant and the breeder.

Besides Benefit Sharing, the other right regarding monetary benefit and claim is Compensation and is specifically awarded to those who have in a certain way contributed their share of skill, expertise, knowledge, labor in invention of a new crop, specie *etc.* **Section 41(1)** explains the right to claim compensation on fulfillment of certain requisites and examination of the claim made as to weather it is falsified or true, the compensation is granted to the claimant. **Section 25 (5) (c)** also talks about the contribution of any group of people in evolution of any variety.[7]

Biologica Diversity Act, 2002: An Overview

In a generic way, Biodiversity could be understood, as the aggregate of all the living organisms on the planet Earth. The word "*Biodiversity*' could be segregated

---

3 Carl Ritzer (1998). UPOV Convention: Past, Present and Future, International Seminar on Procedural Safeguards to the Protection of Plant Varieties, London, United Kingdom, accessed on 28 April 2018.

4 Pranav Bharti (2008). Implementation and Future Prospects of *sui generis* Plant Variety Protection in India. Journal of Intellectual Property Rights, 27 (1): 273-281.

5 J P Singhla (2002). Plant Protection vis-à-vis Seed Commercialisation and Its Impact: Analysing the Future Aspects. Current Sciences, 77 (1): 399-413.

6 Section 2(b). PPFVRA, 2001.

into two parts, *'Biological'* and *'Diversity'*, which in itself is self-explanatory and thus provides for an all encompassing meaning which includes every living organism, discovered, undiscovered, of plant, animal, microorganism or any form of live present, surviving and thriving on Earth.

The Convention on Biological Diversity, 1992 also provides for a definition under **Article 2** of the same which reads as; "**biological diversity means the variability among living organisms from all sources including, inter alia, terrestrial, marine and other aquatic ecosystems and the ecological complexes of which they are part; this includes diversity within species, between species and of ecosystems.**"

India ratified the Convention on Biological Diversity in the February 1994 and after extended discourses and matters of introspection, the Government of India in 2002 came up with the Biological Diversity Act, 2002. The aims and objectives of this act is to promote, accelerate, simply, smoothen the process of openness and approachability of the resources of genetic importance and make it available to other parties involving the concept and the notion of Benefit Sharing based on mutual agreement[8], which is deliberated upon under the previous section dealing with the Analysis of the Protection of Plant Varieties and Farmers' Rights Act, 2001. The principle was promulgated in the Convention on biological Diversity, 1992 and thus was formally legislated and given express meaning the subsequent PPVFR Act of 2001. The other objectives and goals of the Act is to also check on the judicial use of such biological diversity and that it is not exploited. The act also envisages the establishment of the National Biodiversity Authority and various State Biodiversity Boards along with a Biodiversity Management Committee where in the Boards are under an obligation to refer to and discuss and respect the suggestion given by the Committee on matters relating to the use of biological resources under their jurisdiction. The aims also includes such creation various funds at all the levels for the promotion and protection of biodiversity and also safeguard the interests of the communities involved in promotion, protection of the biodiversity and blessed with the traditional knowledge of growing certain crops or species of plants which are not only of national importance but are a heritage of the nation.

The act specifically takes care of the matters vital to the use of the biodiversity, natural or manmade so that each person, natural (for *e.g.* Humans) or juridical (for *e.g.* Corporate entity) gets their share of benefits and that no one can supersede or infringe other's rights. Prior permission has to be sought before registering and claiming for any kind of intellectual Property Right over any invention in or outside India if such an invention is based on research or any source or resource found in India.[9] Another section[10] under the act deliberates upon the concept of benefit

---

7 Sunil Khetani (2010). Prominence of the Concept of Benefit Sharing and Compensation in the Seed Industry. Journal of Emerging Trends in Science and Technology, 35(9): 144-165.

8 Article 3 and Article 15. The Convention on Biological Diversity, 1992.

9 Section 6. Biological Diversity Act, 2002.

10 Section 21. Biological Diversity Act, 2002.

sharing which in itself is the aim of the act previously discussed. The whole process of benefit sharing and claims for the Intellectual property rights will be done under the authority and supervision of National Biodiversity Authority of India.

Plant Breeders' Rights in India and its Preservance by Farmers and Corporate Breeders

The Breeders' Rights in India are well established and well defined. A breeder can file a law suit even if he feels that the packaging of the product is resembling to that of his, be it the logo, shape of the logo, colour and so on. Therefore, it is prevalent even at the basic level of packaging and the defendant, if found guilty under the law could be asked to provide compensation ranging from Fifty Thousand Rupees to Ten Lac Rupees and / or a jail term ranging from three months to two years depending on the degree of severity of the case. The severity is extremely hard that even if there is a slight suspicion of infringement of the rights of the breeder, the onus of proving innocence is directly placed on the defendant as in the case of torts where a person has faced obvious damages out of lack of care of duty which the defendant was supposed to provide, the direct responsibility goes on the defendant to prove his innocence. Here, in the same way, the burden of proof lies on the defendant to prove that the consent of the breeder was sought. The compensation, if the defendant found guilty of selling, producing the variety of another breeder (plaintiff), is shoddier in which a jail term of minimum six months is mandatory and if the crime is sought again, the jail term might get doubled and the compensation might range from one lac rupees to twenty lac rupees.

Critical Remark

The author here feels that the course of proceedings should not be extremely harsh like it is presently and there must be an equal opportunity provided to the defendant side to prove his point of view to the court. Also, the Intellectual Property Right over a specie of a crop does not guarantee the quality of the product, only guarantees the rights of it to the breeder, so if the farmer buys a variety from the breeder and if it fails in the market quality wise, some provisions of compensation to the farmers must be present so that there is an equal and proportional justice done to both the parties and the burden does not only be on the farmer. Also, it is extremely important to provide protection to someone's creation but a healthy competition should also be taken care of for the markets to prosper well. Taking the same into consideration, the Government of India in 2001 passed an act called the Protection of Plant Variety and Farmers' Rights Act (PPVFR) wherein an effective pathway to protect the rights of both breeders and farmers and to protect the new varieties of plants from getting exploited and also encouraging to create more new varieties to compensate the food scarcity running in the country.

Here, the farmer or the breeder or anybody who claims to be the inventor of the variety is legible to apply for a licence if the following criteria are fulfilled:[11]

---

11 Pre-requisites for the IPR Rights, https://newdelhi.usembassy.gov/ipr.html, Accessed on 25 April 2018, 14:02 IST.

1. **Novelty**: The variety shall be legible for registration if it has not been sold for more than a period of one year in India and more than a period of six years in case of trees abroad.
2. **Distinctiveness**: The variety must be distinct and even if it has one distinguished character as compared to any other variety, it shall be liable for registration.
3. **Uniformity**: The variety is uniform if the variation in the following generations comes out to be expected, the variety shall be registered.
4. **Stability**: If the new variety is stable and does not change after 'multiple propagations'.

If all these criterions are met, the variety shall be legible for registration and would be provided license for a period of 15 years in case of trees and vines. However, the researcher enjoys the privilege of conducting studies, researches and could use it repeatedly after taking an authorization from the licensee.

Basmati Rice Patent Controversy Case: Critical Review

The US based company Rice Tec Inc. had wanted to enter the international trade markets of rice since a long and for that it had developed a few varieties one of which is *'Texmati'* but it wanted something bigger. So, in the year 1997, it got 20 patents and one of it was that it had got the name 'Basmati' patented for its rice along with the Starch Index, Photoperiodism *etc.* Basmati had been an integral part of the kitchen in India since time immemorial and had been growing in India and Pakistan for thousands of years. Basmati to India is what Champagne is to France. Not just India had lost its trade which included export of the long grain rice to the US and European markets and all over the world but it was also a shot fired at the integrity of the country as Basmati is the 'property' of India and anyone just like that cannot get a patent on it. The government here filed a case in the patent office of the US and successfully managed to get 15 out of its 20 claims revoked. One of which was the patent on the name 'Basmati' as it violated the TRIPS agreement on the Geographical Index, which says a variety that has been growing in one country for years is its property and its wealth. No one can directly or indirectly get a claim over it in any manner. Here, there was a duty towards India and its farmers by the US based company, which it did not take care of and it got breached and as a result, the farmers and the GDP of the country had to face loss as India being an agricultural based country at first and the export of Basmati brought a good foreign exchange to the country strengthening its economy. Therefore, damages did happen. Also, the damages were foreseeable as the losses would only increase in the near future also malice could be taken into account as the long term aim of the company was to enter the international rice markets and overcome the sales of India which could be brought into being if they use the same name for their brand. For that they just did a simple thing, not much labour and intelligence was required, what they did was that they had crossed the Indian variety of Basmati rice with an *ordinary* quality rice of the US and named the variety a hybrid. This clearly shows their malice too.

Infringement of Plant's Breeders' Rights: Its Application in the Law of Torts

There are extremely strict laws to protect the rights of the breeders and the onus of proving innocence lies on the defendant or the alleged violator to prove the innocence as discussed earlier. There are various forms of punishments, which include fines ranging Rs.50 thousand to 20 lac in extreme cases. The minimum jail term that a person faces is six months and it could exceed to two years. But if the offence is repeated, the jail term could be made two years and a hefty fine up-to twenty lac, as discussed in the previous chapter. Its application in the Law of Torts is explained in the critical remark.

Critical Remark

IPR could be co-related with Negligence as in case of the plant breeders' rights, a person has a duty towards the other person of not selling his varieties to anyone without the permission of the breeder. Then if he does, it becomes the breach of the so called duty and because of that, the plaintiff faces severe damages like no credibility for the hard work he had put in to generate that new variety and it is a case of strict liability. In general, we can also say that strict liability is syn. to IPR. The plaintiff just needs to prove that the tort has happened, *i.e.*, his varieties have been sold off without his consent. Also if you take intension and motive into account, there is definitely malice otherwise a man of common prudence would never intend to sell someone else's work just like that. The intention might be to earn money and not share it with the one who actually deserves it and motive could be to make him suffer the loss, which he would bear for a long time.

Conclusion

India, predominantly being an agrarian economy, calls for a need to promulgate such strict legislations for the protection of the rights of the breeders as well as farmers and also people belonging to the indigenous tribes involved in the protection/maintenance/development of particular species. Also, ours is a model which is an ideal form of legislation and is looked upon with a very high regard and places itself as a pioneer for many other countries working towards the development of such legislations. With such regard comes a responsibility to continue monitor the efficacy of such legislations and make necessary changes as and when time requires. The best way to strengthen the applicability and efficiency of the act would be ensured when the people for whom this act has been legislated and enacted have the adequate knowledge of the same, *i.e.*, the privileges, immunities and the safeguards available to them. Although, the maxim *'vigilantibus et non dormientibus jura inveniut'* holds true everywhere and there is no remedy for those who are unaware of the law of their land but to make people efficient towards their rights is not just a duty of the sate and various NGOs and many other agencies of the government and/or private unaided bodies but is also a constitutional goal and that it must be implemented through various programmes by various bodies and authorities of the state and also a task taken up by the big corporates under their Corporate Social Responsibility (CSR) scheme which would directly lead towards minimalizing of many problems and that would in itself be a great achievement for the government and the associated bodies if everyone is aware of what the law says and what are the remedies under the same.

References'

Book(s)

1. Patrick Winkler, Providing Protection for Plant Genetic Resources, Country Law, New York, 2002.
2. Nate Winston, Philosophical Foundations of the Plant Breeders' Rights and Intellectual Property Rights, Hatfield, England, 1996.
3. Diana Richardson, Local Legacy and Intellectual Property, Netherlands, 2008.

Report(s)

1. Protection of Plant Varieties and Farmers' Rights Authority, Annual Report, 2007-2008.

Article(s)

1. Torts; Cornell University Law School, https://www.law.cornell.edu/wex/tort.
2. Vishesh Kulkarni; Probing the Plant Variety Protection and Farmers Act, 2001, https://www.google.co.in/search?client=safari and rls=en and q=infringement+of+plant+breeders+rights.
3. International Union for the Protection of New Varieties of Plants, UPOV Publication No. 422 (A), 12 July 2008, available at http://www.upov.int/en/for/pdf/pub479.pdf.

Chapter 18

Intellectual Property Rights Policy Regime and Agriculture Innovation System: Issues for Governance in the Context of India

Vikas Kumar

Central University of Gujarat, Gandhinagar, Gujarat 382030
e-mail: vikaskumarcug@gmail.com

ABSTRACT

This paper deals with the IPRs in Agriculture Innovation systems. The IPR policy plays important role in the functions of innovation system, especially in terms of investment in innovation, and to encourage diffusion of information about the principles and sources of innovation throughout the economy. Therefore, ***the objectives*** of the paper is 1) to scrutinize the strong policy hurdle created by the IPR regime and faced by India, in light of Agriculture Innovation, 2) to map out the promises over the last decade, briefly presenting the broad contours of public sector constraints in agricultural research. 3) to look the trend of R&D expenditure on Agriculture Biotechnology. ***Research Methods***: The research study is based on a quantitative research method. A quantitative method is generally used in order to collect statistical data and conduct statistical analyses (Yin, 2003). Data collection for this research was carried out from various report of IPR in the context of India. ***Findings of the*** chapter that, across agriculture sectors there has been a dramatic increase in patents filed but, granted is differ during the last decades. It is also shown in chapter that the consequences of introducing IPR differ according to sectors, knowledge bases, phases in the innovation process, and political-institutional frameworks. For instance, be a real problem with the current IPR system favouring radical innovations when biotechnology develops from early-phase, hi-tech to more generally diffused multi-tech. All this provides strong arguments against a global generic patent system.

Keywords: *IPR, Agriculture innovation, Agriculture biotechnology, Research and developments, TRIPS.*

Introduction

In India, the idea of commercialization of innovation from R&D is moderately new in many divisions; particularly in farming. The Government of India has as of late reported the "National Intellectual Property Rights (IPR) strategy (GoI, 2016). The arrangement advocates advancement of an all-encompassing and favorable environment for catalyzing the licensed innovation for monetary, socio-social improvement and securing open intrigue. The arrangement report set forth seven targets to be specific I) IPR mindfulness: effort and advancement, ii) age of IPRs, iii) legitimate and authoritative system, iv) managerial administration, v) commercialization of IPR, vi) implementation and arbitration and vii) human capital improvement. The strategy goes for reinforcing the national activities, for example, "Make in India", "Skill India", "Start-Up India", "Smart Cities", "and Digital India". The leader program of the Government like Start-Up India goes for building a solid environment for supporting developments and Start-ups in the nation Under this, Atal Innovation Mission (AIM) is the activity design visualized with the emphasis on advancement of business enterprise and development in divisions, for example, producing, farming, wellbeing and instruction (GoI, 2016).

Further, the IPR play a major to diffuse innovation in India. The idea of the innovation framework (IS) – initially created by Bengt-Åke Lundvall – is a moderately new one, and was first utilized by Chris Freeman in his investigation of Japan's blossoming economy (Freeman, 1987). The idea of a local advancement framework (RIS) showed up in the mid-1990s (Cooke 2001), roughly in the meantime as the possibility of the national development framework was ending up more far reaching, because of the books by Lundvall (1992) and Nelson (1993). Normal for a frameworks way to deal with development is the affirmation that advancements are helped out through a system of different on-screen characters supported by an institutional structure. This dynamic and complex communication constitutes what is generally marked frameworks of advancement (Edquist 1997), that is, frameworks comprehended as collaboration systems (Kaufmann and Tödtling 2001). An arrangement of minor departure from this approach have been produced after some time, either taking as their purpose of takeoff either regions (national and territorial) or particular areas or innovations (Fagerberg *et al.*, 2005).

However, the chapter has been categorized into five section including introduction. The second section deals with intellectual property regime and agriculture. Third section introduces about the present IPR law related to agriculture. The fourth section discusses about the issues of IPR and agriculture and finally, the fifth section concludes argument of the chapter.

IPR Regime and Agriculture

Development in biotechnology are, in any case, joined by a more grounded licensed innovation rights (IPR) regime. In fact, with the progressions in this innovation, the instruments that are being utilized for its assurance have moved toward becoming very exclusionist in their approach. This may posture extreme difficulties for creating nations, as advances are to a great extent happening inside the private area, and these new patterns in the IPR administration appear to dispossess the passage of latecomers into the innovation race. This dispossession is happening notwithstanding the way that, since 1995, an expansive number of creating nations have consented to a generally fresher IPR administration, and now that the due date of 2005 is finished, these administrations are completely set up in all the part nations.

Further, IPR scope of the farming part is an ongoing marvel in these nations; in numerous driving economies in Asia, including India, plant assortment security is a fairly new expansion to IPR insurance. There is a pressing need to address a portion of these issues on a need premise. The IPR administration as it is currently unfurling may not be in a situation to observe this dynamic all alone, except if government approaches are changed in accordance with make space for such retention. These improvements are all the more critical with regards to creating nations, where horticultural biotechnology is being viewed as a noteworthy instrument for defeating sustenance security concerns (Cullet, 2003). Limitations on the utilization of hereditary innovations constitute a particular test as in, when implemented, privately owned businesses will have the capacity to guarantee that ranchers completely regard IPR rules (Byerlee and Fischer, 2002).

Aside from the effect of IPR on access to innovation, there is additionally the topic of development itself. A solid IPR administration in a forthcoming territory like agrarian biotechnology may smother the inventive capacity of the creating nations. This circumstance calls for better administration of the immense scene of the IPR administration. In this unique circumstance, a few issues relating to the part of government and the space for people in general area bolstered by R&D in agribusiness – beside public– private organization – have been raised (Padolina, 2000; RIS, 2003). One thought has been that open division R&D organizations ought to grow more quality and capability in the domain of this boondocks innovation. While the presence of a solid physical framework is fundamental for the advancement of a viable R&D framework, the basic components remain the institutional set-up which bolsters this framework and the attachment between the general formative goals and the R&D tries in various streams. Truth be told, these components play an undeniably noteworthy part in wilderness advances, and in biotechnology specifically, than in customary innovations.

Current Statutory IP Laws in India vis-vis Agri-based Technologies in India

The WTO-TRIPS agreement of 1995 (WTO,2016), which is official on all part nations including India, accommodated least standards and measures in regard of security of IPR in a few classifications: licenses, copyrights, trademarks, plant assortments, land signs, modern outlines, format plans of coordinated circuits, and competitive advantages. This understanding drove India to set up an arrangement of fitting and agreeable components and instruments. A portion of the lawful instruments go by the Indian Parliament as a major aspect of consistence procedure to the TRIPS incorporate The Patents Act, 1970 (39 of 1970), The Patents (Amendment) Act, 1999 (17 of 1999), The Patents (Amendment) Act 2002 (38 of 2002), The Patents (Amendment) Act 2005 (15 of 2005), The Geographical Indications of Goods (Registration and Protection) Act, 1999 (Office of Controller General of Patents

Designs and Trade Marks,2016) and The Protection of Plant Varieties and Farmers Rights Act, 2001 (PPV FR Act) (53 of 2001) (PPV and FR Authority. 2016.) Apart from these, the Government of India likewise established an umbrella enactment called the Biological Diversity Act, 2002 (No.18 of 2003). (NBA, 2008) as a component of the nation's promise to Convention of Biological Diversity (CBD). There is no particular IPR Act to give insurance to undisclosed data (competitive advantage). The Indian Contract Act of 1872 and customary law have arrangements covering this with the Ministry of Law and Justice as the nodal organization (Kochhar, 2008).

Fund Allocation for Education and Research

The agrarian segment in creating nations is going through a troublesome stage. The difficulties go from the post-Green Revolution stagnation in essential horticultural yields to expansive scale lack of healthy sustenance and declining R&D assignments. All creating nations ponder in any event a portion of these limitations. Profitability in the vast majority of the sustenance crops, be that as it may, has been stagnating since mid-1990s, in spite of the fact that the issue of whether trim yield is moving toward a level has turned out to be progressively questionable (Ruttan, 1999; Reilly and Fuglie, 1998). However, since last decade the allocation of public fund is mostly constant and in some cases it can be see decrease in allocation (Table 18.1).

The part of government in arrangement of open administrations like farming examination instruction and augmentation is of most extreme significance, and accordingly, government assumes a noteworthy part in its financing and execution. At the national level, the genuine consumption on agrarian research and training (Ag R and E) has risen minimal under four overlap over the most recent two decades from Rs. 15 billion out of 1990-91 to Rs 68 billion out of 2010-11. The all India genuine spending on Ag R and E developed by 5.8 for every penny amid the nineties and kept up its development force amid the multi decade (7.2 per cent) as well, yet significant increment came just amid the second 50 per cent of the decade (13 per cent for each) annum between 2005-06 to 2010-11. The ongoing spurt in Ag R and E ventures have prompted a great ascent in the exploration power (offer of Ag R and E speculation to AgGDP 0.63 per cent in TE 2011). Further, disaggregating total Ag R and E use into inquire about and other consumption, the aggregate research use (net of instruction and bleeding edge expansion exercises) was evaluated to Rs. 50 billion out of 2010-11, constituting just 0.36 per cent of agribusiness total national output (Sing and Pal, 2015).

The asset assignment for rural research and training crosswise over various agro-climatic areas of the nation, plainly displays an expanded R&D consideration towards negligible generation condition (Figure 18.1). This is especially valid for the slopes and northeastern area (having research force near one for every penny) which got higher asset consideration by both ICAR and state governments. The locale requires higher research asset distribution in view of troublesome landscapes and need of area particular research. The semi-bone-dry district which constitutes the most astounding offer in nation's edited region and agrarian laborers, additionally share the biggest research assets. The interest for farming exploration keeps on being sold in these areas as their agro-environmental conditions are more mind

Table 18.1: Sector-wise Plan Allocation for Agriculture Research by DARE/ICAR 2012-2017 (*Rs in Lakh)

Sectors	*2012-13*		*2013-14*		*2014-15*		*2015-16*		*2016-2017*	
	RE	*Actual*	*RE*	*Actual*	*RE*	*Actual*	*RE*	*Actual*	*RE*	*Actual*
Crop Science	41300.00	40058.59	37500.00	36898.47	38000.00	37059.60	49500.00	48168.7	43656.00	43420.94
Horticulture Science	14500.00	14355.17	14900.00	13988.03	14435.00	13758.04	18000.00	17553.76	16000.00	15880.54
Natural Resource Management	26000.00	23965.86	24500.00	23272.53	23500.00	22099.21	32100.00	27471.43	27850.00	26793.37
Agricultural Engineering	5200.00	5158.83	5500.00	5459.76	6500.00	6461.66	8200.00	8078.92	7800.00	7701.37
Animal Science	19400.00	19163.50	18998.00	19022.50	16000.00	15398.35	22600.00	20856.99	20100.00	19446.04
Fishery Science	6900.00	6881.92	7000.00	6977.68	6500.00	6373.26	7800.00	7640.00	7800.00	7765.99
Agriculture Education	43891.25	52593.02	41615.00	37102.53	38000.00	37444.71	56000.00	51437.29	65040.00	56472.96

Source: Compile by Author, 2018 through Lok Sabha Unstarred Question.

Note: RE: Revised Estimates., BE: Budget Estimates.

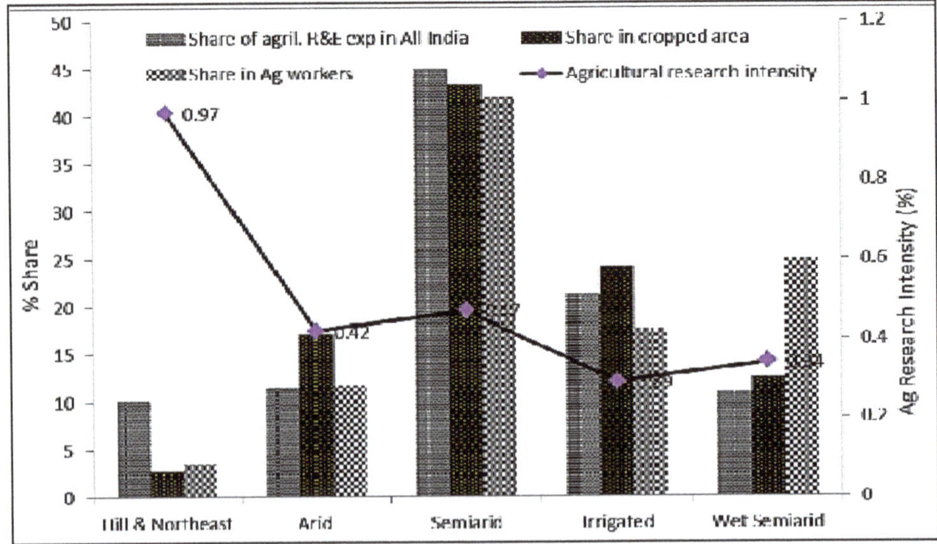

Figure 18.1: Agriculture Research and Education Investments in Different Agro Climatic Region of India (2010-2011) (*Source*: Sing, 2015).

boggling and chance inclined. New leaps forward are required in water sparing advancements in development, improvement of land profitability, normal asset administration and atmosphere flexible agribusiness.

Plant Variety Protection

IPR is important in horticulture, yet its application must be constrained in local Acts exchange. Plant assortments, for example, Hybrids can be ensured under a sui generis framework. The arrangement for Plant Variety Protection (PVP) made under the TRIPs Article 27.3(b), enables nations to give such assurance either through patent, or a powerful sui generis PVP framework or any mix of the two. Copyrights and related rights, then again, might be enrolled for databases, bioinformatics, qualities and quality groupings, amino corrosive arrangements, antibodies, and so on. Utilization of mechanical outlines and the geographies of incorporated circuits would be significant, especially in farming designing.

In India, the Patents Act, 1970, constituted the fundamental Principal Act regarding the matter. India is bound by every one of the arrangements of the TRIPs Agreement, which oblige the nation to sanction/change applicable local laws. These incorporate authorization of new enactments on Protection of Plant Varieties and Farmers' Rights Act, 2001 and Geographical Indications of Goods (Registration and Protection) Act, 1999, and revision of Patents Act, 1970 out of 1999 and 2002. The Biological Diversity Bill, 2000 is presently establishment and correction of the Seeds Act, 1966, is likewise accepting consideration (NAAS, 2003). As far as licenses in farming, the quantity of field applications is for the most part changed in all the year appeared in Table 18.2.

Table 18.2: Year-wise Distribution of Patent Applications Filed and Granted in the Areas of Agriculture

Year	*Number of Patent Applications Filed*			*Number of Patent Applications Granted*		
	Indian	*Foreign*	*Total*	*Indian*	*Foreign*	*Total*
2009-10	40	106	146	4	2	6
2010-11	20	48	126	1	5	3
2011-12	77	62	183	1	1	3
2012-13	103	87	209	3	1	5
2013-14	112	122	218	0	2	2
2014-15	120	109	226	1	1	2
2015-16	268	N.A	N.A	2	N.A	N.A
2016-17	245	N.A	N.A	4	N.A	N.A

Source: Computed by Authors, 2016 through various report of IPR.

It can be seen from Table 18.2 that, the quantity of patent application is high however patent conceded is low. So also, one can see from the table that the quantity of licenses allowed is consistent (2) in the time of 2010, 2011 and 2014 altogether. So also, Figure 18.2. demonstrates the quantity of trademarks recorded and enrolled on Agriculture, Horticulture and Forestry Products and Grains.

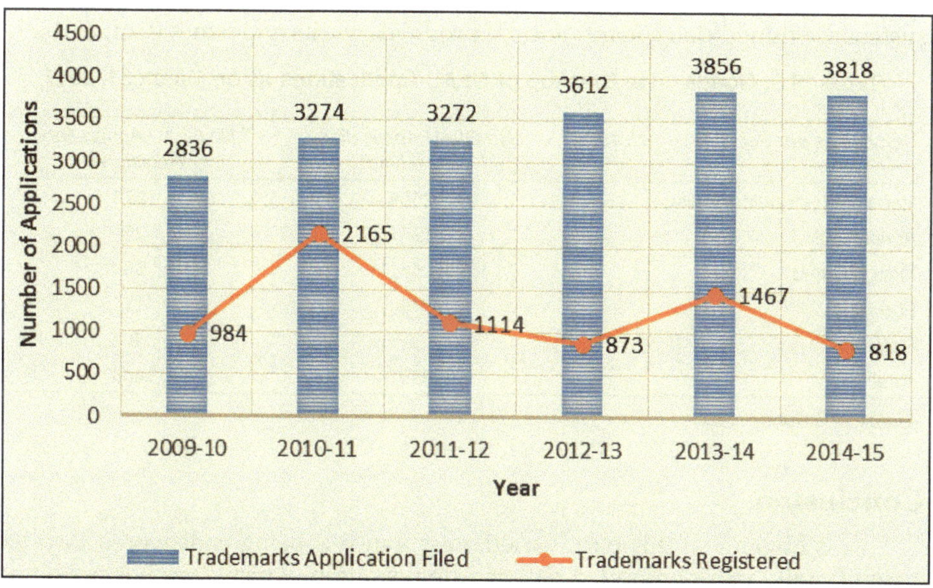

Figure 18.2: Year-wise of Trademarks Filed and Registered on Agriculture, Horticulture and Forestry Products and Grains (*Source*: Computed by Authors, 2016, through various IPR reports).

It could be said, unmistakably agrarian developments can be secured by IPRs that empowers the trend-setters to bar others from making, utilizing, or offering the new item or process. Private firms that participate in rural R&D would thus be able to be relied upon to depend on this assurance when settling on venture choices. IPR is the main apparatus to draw in private division in farming R&D (Kumar and Sinha, 2015).

Geographical Indications Registry and Agriculture

The Geographical Indications Registry is set up for organization of the Geographical Indications of Goods (Registration and Protection) Act, 1999 with the question give enrollment and better insurance of land signs identifying with merchandise. The GI Registry is arranged at Chennai. The Registry began accepting GI applications for Registration since fifteenth September 2003. It has gotten an aggregate number of 575 GI Applications as on March 31, 2017. The Registry has likewise begun getting GI Authorized User applications from May 2009 and has gotten 3897 GI Authorized User Applications as on March 31, 2017. A sum of 294 Geographical Indications (GIs) have been enrolled since fifteenth September 2003. An aggregate number of 1466 GI Authorized User testaments have been issued. From April 01, 2016 to March 31, 2017, the Office has gotten 32 Geographical Indications. Applications and 1548 Geographical Indications Authorized User Applications. 34 Geographical Indications and 282 Geographical Indications Authorized Users have been enrolled. The Registry has been sorting out Awareness programs all through India to advance Indian GIs. The parts being engaged are; tea, espresso, flavors, farming and agriculture items, handloom items, handiworks, materials, prepared sustenance things, dairy items, normal products, spirits and wines (GoI, 2016).

Table 18.3: Goods-wise Breakup of GI AU Applications as on March 31, 2017

Goods as per Sec. 2(f) GI Act, 1999	*No GI AU Applications Received*	*No GI AU Applications Registered*
Handicraft (including textiles)	2554	1374
Agricultural	1271	25
Manufactured	56	56
Foodstuff	16	11
Natural	0	0
Total	3897	1466

Source: IPR Report, 2017.

Conclusion

As is obvious in this part, varietial assurance is being endeavored through a significantly more grounded patent administration, which does not permit an agriculturists' or even research exclusion, and is much smaller in its extension than the plant licenses or plant assortment insurance. It merits reviewing that at the WTO, the verbal confrontation is as yet stuck at Article 27.3(b), which alludes to the patent administration or a successful sui generis framework for the assurance of plant assortments. In the interim, the creating nations are occupied with debating the different parts of sui generis frameworks, specifically as it has turned out to be certain that there are discussions, other than the WTO, where IPR related advancements are characterizing new forms of licensed innovation insurance that are in the long run legitimized through FTAs. The ceaseless inclination in the US toward a more grounded IPR administration – as is perceptible through a sharp development in the utility licenses – and comparable systems for the assurance of biotechnological innovations in Europe – as proposed by the Biotechnology Directive of the EU – ought to be a reason for concern. Aside from this, there is additionally a developing pattern toward protecting examination instruments. Consequently in light of the advancements in biotechnology, the profile of patent administrations is changing rapidly in created nations. Obviously, a huge piece of this exploration is exuding from the private segment.

These progressions have extreme ramifications for creating nations. Effectively battling with the usage obstacles of the TRIPs administration, there are numerous creating nations, including India, which presently can't seem to set up national enactment to position themselves opposite the worldwide arrangements at the WTO. There have been a few purposes behind this postponement, however now it is by all accounts clear that national enactment would not just unfavorably influence the entrance to innovation essentially yet the licensing of research devices would likewise avoid the latecomers in the innovation race from impersonation or item advancement in any shape. In this specific circumstance, the part of open research organizations turns out to be progressively pertinent. In creating nations profitability levels presently can't seem to draw any nearer to those accomplished in created nations. This requires the proceeded with upkeep of budgetary help for open research foundations in creating nations, and may even require an expansion to take care of the demand.

In past years, open plant reproducing programs have developed with a free trade of germplasm and agreeable logical undertakings. The post-Green Revolution rural creation situation appears to represent a few difficulties for sustenance security in creating nations. Ample opportunity has already past that horticultural R&D designs organized venture on new advances so as legitimately to adjust – or, rather, supplement – the customary methods with new innovations, for example, biotechnology. Ensure that open plant reproducers/research centers approach the best science and germplasm. Essentially, limit in broad daylight plant rearing ought to be improved. This expanded limit ought to be coordinated towards those harvests which are not prone to pull in private venture.

REFERENCES

Cooke, P. 2001, Regional Innovation Systems, Clusters, and the Knowledge Economy. *Industrial and Corporate Change*, 10(4), 945–74.

Cullet, P. 2003. *Food Security and Intellectual Property Rights in Developing Countries. IELRC Working Paper 2003*. Geneva: International Environmental Law Research Centre.

Edquist, C. 1997, Introduction', in: C. Edquist (ed.) *Systems of Innovation: Technologies, Institutions and Organisations*. London: Pinter.

Fagerberg, J. *et al.*, 2005, *The Oxford Handbook of Innovation.* Oxford: Oxford University Press.

Freeman, C. 1987, *Technology Policy and Economic Performance: Lessons from Japan.* London: Pinter.

GoI, 2016. Intellectual Property Rights. Ministry of Commeres and Industry.

Kaufmann, A. and Todtling, F. 2001, 'Science-Industry Interaction in the Process of Innovation: The Importance of Boundary-Crossing Between Systems. *Research Policy*, 30, 791–804.

Kochhar, S. 2008. Institution and capacity building for the evolution of IPR regime in India: Protection of Plant Varieties and Farmers Rights. *Journal of Intellectual Property Rights*.Vol. 13, pp.51-56

Kumar, V. and Sinha, K. 2015. Status and Challenges of Intellectual Property Rights in Agriculture Innovation in India. *Journal of Intellectual Property Rights,* Vol 20, Issue 5, pp 288-296

Lundvall, B.-A. 1992, *National Innovation Systems: Towards a Theory of Innovation and Interactive Learning*. London: Pinter.

NAAS, "Intellectual Property Rights in Agriculture", *NAAS Policy Paper* No, 19, 2003, 1-10. National Academy of Agricultural Sciences, New Delhi.

Nelson, R. 1993, *National Innovation Systems: A Comparative Analysis. Oxford:* Oxford University Press.

Padolina, W.G. 2000. 'Plant Variety Protection for Rice in Developing Countries: Impacts on Research and Development'. *Limited Proceedings of the Workshop on the Impact on Research and Development of* Sui Generis *Approaches to Plant Variety Protection of Rice in Developing Countries.* 16–18 February 2000. IRRI, Los Banos, Laguna, Philippines.

Reilly, J. M., and Fuglie, K.O. 1998. Future Yield Growth in Field Crops: What Evidence Exists. *Soil and Tillage Research* 47: 275–90.

RIS. 2003. Cancun and Beyond. *World Trade and Development Report.* New Delhi: Research and Information System for Developing Countries.

Ruttan, W. Vernon. 1999. Biotechnology and Agriculture: A Skeptical Perspective. *AgBioForum* 2 (1): 54–60.

Singh, A. and Pal, S. 2015. Emerging Trends in the Public and Private Investment in Agricultural Research in India", *Agricultural Research,* Vol.4, No.2, pp.121-131.

WTO, 2016. Overview: the TRIPS Agreement. At: https://www.wto.org/english/tratop_e/trips_e/intel2_e.htm [Accessed on June 15,2016]

Chapter 19

Enhancement of Global Climate hange with Special Reference to Kyoto Protocol Backdrop

Rajendra Parikh[1] and Ketan Desai[2]

[1]*Faculty of Law, The Maharaja Sayajirao University of Baroda, Vadodara, Gujarat*
[2]*Faculty of Commerce, The Maharaja Sayajirao University of Baroda, Vadodara, Gujarat*
e-mail: [1]rajendraiparikh@gmail.com, [2]krshiv2006desai@gmail.com

ABSTRACT

'Climate change' refers to a change of climate which is attributed directly or indirectly to human economic activity that alters the composition of the global atmosphere. It is in addition to natural climate variability observed over a comparable time periods. Climate change has been described as defining issue for the twenty-first century. It is one of the most important challenges facing the international community today. An overwhelming amount of scientific evidences has attributed cause of the problem of climate change to the human activities and predicated that climate change has far reaching implications for ecosystems, including human beings. The scientific understanding of the issue of climate change, establishing the cause-effect relationship between increase in the earth's surface temperature and the human economic activities emitting greenhouse gases (GHG) through the physical process of enhanced greenhouse effect, necessitates the urgent need to control and limit anthropogenic GHG emissions. In fact, the increase in anthropogenic GHG emissions leads to increase in GHG concentration in the atmosphere which results in enhanced greenhouse effect. This enhanced greenhouse effect causes the increase in the surface temperature of the earth, thereby results in climate change. In this regard, the theory of greenhouse effect is a well established scientific theory. The IPCC reports have attributed the cause of the climate change to human activities. IPCC has played significant role in formulating evidence-based climate policy by providing an assessment of the existing scientific knowledge of the climate change. The IPCC also prepares Special Reports and Technical Papers on topics for which independent scientific information and advice is deemed necessary, and it supports the United Nations Framework Convention on Climate Change (UNFCCC) through its work on methodologies for National Greenhouse Gas Inventories. The Kyoto Protocol to the convention was negotiated under the Berlin Mandate and subsequently adopted in 1997.

This chapter focuses on the mitigation of global climate change in the framework of UNFCCC and the Kyoto Protocol. The mitigation of climate change has significant impact on socio-economic policies including equity, development and sustainability. However, differences in the distribution of technological and financial resources within developed and developing countries, as well as differences in mitigation costs are some of the key factors in the legal analysis of climate change mitigation.

In this respect, coordinated actions among countries are likely to facilitate reduction in cost of mitigation. The chapter focuses of the following questions. Firstly, what is the international legal response to the issue of global climate change? Secondly, after adapting Kyoto protocol framework what were the legal issues in governmental process? Thirdly, regarding legal issues raised by the developing countries contribution in the climate change regime?

Keywords: *Kyoto protocol, Climate Change, Greenhouse effect, Greenhouse Gas, Carbon dioxide.*

Introduction

Climate change has been represented as process issue for the 21st century. It's one among the foremost necessary challenges facing the international community nowadays. An awesome quantity of scientific evidences has attributed reason behind the matter of global climate change to the human activities and predicated that climate change has comprehensive implications for ecosystems, as well as human beings.

It generates very complex and multidimensional global issues in the context of its implications for the global environment and human beings. Many pollution problems give rise to impact on different social systems-social groups, countries, or regions-and on different natural ecosystems. What distinguishes climate change is the nature and potential seriousness of its human impacts, which transform the issue from a purely environmental problem into an environment and development-related one.

The scientific understanding of the difficulty of global climate change, establishing the cause-effect relationship between increase within the layer temperature and also the human economic activities emitting greenhouse gases (GHG) through the physical process of increased impact (atmospheric phenomenon), necessitates the pressing got to management and limit anthropogenic GHG emissions. Infact, the rise in phylogeny GHG emissions leads to increase in GHG concentration within the atmosphere which ends in increased greenhouse effect. This increased atmospheric phenomenon causes the rise within the surface temperature of the world, thereby ends up in global climate change. So this regards to, the idea of greenhouse effect could be a well established theory. The IPCC reports have attributed the reason for the global climate change to human activities.

Attribution of climate change to the human activities in turn transforms the issue of climate change from a scientific inquiry into a problem to be addressed at the political level by the international community of States. This is because both cause and effect of climate change are anthropocentric. Further, controlling and limiting anthropogenic GHG including carbon dioxide emissions resulting from human activities imply need to regulate the human activities related to GHG emissions within a legal framework. In fact, the international community has responded to the threat of climate change by adopting a legal regime through negotiation process. The present climate change regime is embodied in the UNFCCC and the Kyoto Protocol.

In 1988, shortly before the Toronto Conference, international community took the first step to address the climate change issue by requesting the WMO and the UNEP to establish the Intergovernmental Panel on Climate Change (IPCC).[1] Accordingly, IPCC was established by the WMO and the UNEP in 1988. It has been the assigned role of assessing the scientific, technical and socioeconomic information relevant for understanding the risk of human induced climate change.

IPCC has played significant role in formulating evidence-based climate policy by providing an assessment of the existing scientific knowledge of the climate change. A main activity of the IPCC is to provide on a regular basis an assessment of the state of knowledge on climate change. The IPCC also prepares Special Reports and Technical Papers on topics for which independent scientific information and advice is deemed necessary, and it supports the United Nations Framework Convention on Climate Change (UNFCCC) through its work on methodologies for National Greenhouse Gas Inventories.

The Kyoto Protocol to the convention was negotiated under the Berlin Mandate and subsequently adopted in 1997. Under the Kyoto Protocol, annex I developed countries have legally binding commitments to reduce greenhouse gas emissions, as inscribed in its annex B, with a view to reducing their overall emissions of such gases by at least 5 per cent below 1990 levels in the commitment period 2008-212.[2] Non-annex I developing countries are exempted from binding commitments. For providing flexibility to annex I developed countries in meeting their legally binding targets, the Kyoto Protocol provides three innovative market-based mechanisms - joint implementation; Clean Development mechanism (CDM); and carbon emission trading. These flexibility mechanisms are collectively known as the Kyoto Protocol Mechanisms.

Lawful Structure for Global Climate Change

Climate change is perceived as an enormous environmental concern and a potentially dangerous phenomenon which by its very nature is global in its scope. It involves a complex interplay of natural, ecological, physical, human, and climate systems transcending national boundaries. Therefore, both its causes and effects are stretched all over the world. According to the IPCC report, the world is already experiencing the effects of rising temperatures and extreme weather. [3]This necessitates that it should be addressed with all seriousness in a global framework.

---

1 See WMO, Report of the Thirty-Ninth Session of the Executive Council, *WMO Doc. 682,* 1987; UNEP, Report of the Governing Council, *UN Doc. A/42/25,* 1987

2 See, the Kyoto Protocol, art.3(1).

3 IPCC, *Climate Change 2001: Impacts, Adaptation and Vulnerability- Contribution of Working Group II to the Third Assessment Report* (Cambridge: Cambridge University Press, 2001).

Thus, the legal basis for international action to address the climate change problem is embedded in the United Nations Framework Convention on Climate Change (UNFCCC) and it's implementing Kyoto Protocol.[4] The Kyoto Protocol provides legally binding quantified emission limitation and reduction (QELAR) targets, enshrined in its annex B, for annex I developed countries to reduce their GHG emissions cumulatively by 5.2 per cent of the 1990 emission levels. [5] This legal framework also provides three Kyoto mechanisms under the Kyoto Protocol in order to facilitate annex I developed countries complying with their mandatory QELAR targets (inscribed in Annex B).

Salient Features of the United Nations Framework Convention On Climate Change (UNFCCC)

Framework Convention-Protocol Approach

The framework-protocol approach is one of the methods of international environmental law-making. [6] It is an important legal tool that the States may find helpful in building consensus over time on the appropriate means of addressing an environmental problem.[7] The law-making process, under the framework-protocol approach, comprises an initial agreement, a so-called 'Framework Convention' which lays down the general objective, goals and principles of cooperation, to be followed up with specific agreement called protocols in which details and specific issues are sought to be addressed. In fact, negotiations for a protocol take place within the framework of the legal and institutional arrangements established under the 'framework convention' In case of climate change, the design of international regime for addressing the climate change followed framework convention-protocol approach. Accordingly, under the review provision of Article 4(2) (d), the first Conference of the Parties (COP-1) initiated intergovernmental negotiations for adoption of a protocol to strengthen the mitigation commitments of Annex I developed countries within the framework of the 'Berlin Mandate'[8] subsequently, the Kyoto Protocol was adopted by the third Conference ofthe Parties (COP-3) in 1997.

Multilateral Framework/or Climate Change

The need to regulate and limit the anthropogenic greenhouse gas emissions is sought to be addressed in a legal framework that is sufficiently comprehensive

---

4 For a detailed analysis of the UNFCCC, see Daniel Bodansky, "The Framework Convention on Climate Change: A Commentary", *Yale Journal of International Law,* Vol.I8, 1993, p. 451-558.

5 This is calculated on the basis of the first communication report submitted by the Annex I parties in accordance with Article of the UNFCCC.

6 For details, see Bharat H. Desai, *Institutionalizing International Environmental Law* (New York: Transnational Publishers, 2004); Allyn Taylor and Daniel Bodansky, *The Development of the WHO Framework Convention on Tobacco Control: Legal and Policy Considerations,* WHO Background Paper, November, 1998

7 See, *ibid.*

8 See UNFCCC, "The Berlin Mandate: Review of the Adequacy of Article 4(2) (A) And (B) of the Convention, Including Proposals Related to a Protocol and Decisions on Follow-Up", *Decision I ICP. I, FCCC/CP/199517/Add.I,* 1995, p.4.

enough to incorporate a magnitude of relevant aspects, concerns and issues to deal with complexity of the climate change issue. The UNFCCC reflects the consensus to address climate change within its legal framework. In this regard, the UNFCCC sets an overall legal framework for international efforts to grapple with the challenge of climate change. The UNFCCC has got near universal membership.[9]

Accordingly, the developed countries are required to bear a greater burden of mitigation costs than the developing countries. The UNFCCC requires all countries parties to develop inventories of anthropogenic emissions and measures to mitigate climate change and send report on emissions in their national communication to the secretariat of the UNFCCC. However, actions of all the country parties for mitigating GHG emissions are voluntary.

Right to Sustainable Development

The Rio Earth Summit was a significant milestone in the further development of the principle of sustainable development in the field of international environmental law. The Rio Declaration emphasized that that the protection of the environment and social and economic development are fundamental to sustainable development. Further, the Rio Summit adopted a work programme for action entitled Agenda 21 to achieve sustainable development objective.

The Kyoto Protocol

The 1992 UN Framework Convention on Climate Change FCCC is generally considered to an important starting point to address the climate change. However, it seemed to be inadequate to achieve the ultimate objective of stabilizing greenhouse concentration in the atmosphere. Thus, it can be considered as a modest achievement in terms of addressing the climate change issue.[10] This was because of its failure to set clear GHG emission reductions targets

It is pertinent to point out here that all countries' commitments and actions to reduce greenhouse gas emissions were general and voluntary under the UNFCCC. In furtherance of the objective of the UNFCCC, the Kyoto Protocol became the first legal instrument to provide quantified emissions limitation and reduction (QELAR) targets. It laid down specific and legally binding QELAR targets for annex I developed countries for reductions in greenhouse gas concentrations in the global atmosphere. [11]

An interesting feature of the Kyoto Protocol is that annex I developed countries can meet their obligations both "individually" as well as "jointly."[12] In other words,

---

9 As of 15 July, 2007, 192 countries have ratified it.

10 See, Daniel Bodansky, "The Framework Convention on Climate Change: A Commentary",. *Yale Journal of International Law,* Vol. IS, 1993, pp. 451-558, at p. 554.

11 On the negotiations leading to the adoption of commitments under annex B, see Joanna Depledge, "Tracing the Origins of the Kyoto Protocol: An Article-by-Article Textual History," *UN Doc. FCCC/TP/2000/2,* 25 November 2000, paras. 295-306.

12 See, the Kyoto Protocol, art. 3(1).

Annex I developing countries can, in addition to making domestic efforts to reduce their emission levels, also meet part of their obligations by taking mitigation action together with other countries. This concept of joint implementation recognizes that climate change is a global problem. Thus, as a corollary to this concept, it could be argued that it is immaterial where emissions reductions are achieved. The Protocol supports the application of this concept by providing for three Kyoto mechanisms.[13] The main objective of the Kyoto mechanisms is to assists annex I developed countries in complying with their legally binding QELAR targets in a cost-effective manner. The regulatory framework of the Kyoto mechanisms also allows private legal entities to participate in the implementation of Kyoto Protocol under these mechanisms with the approval of the country parties concerned.[14] However, the Kyoto Protocol only makes provision for the first commitment period, *i.e.* 2008-2012. 149 Thus, the first commitment period will expire at the end of the year 2012. In this connection, the negotiations for the post-Kyoto framework are going on at present under the Bali Roadmap.

Salient Features

Cost-Effectiveness

The Kyoto mechanisms address the issue of cost-effectiveness in climate mitigation efforts. The use of these mechanisms is intended to reduce operational cost of mitigation of the carbon emissions from the various sources, which are based on the use of carbonintensive fossil fuels. These mechanisms have the potential to reduce the cost of meeting the Kyoto targets. In effect, they could enable annex I developed countries (with their respective targets in Annex B) to meet their emissions limits in a cost effective manner. These Mechanisms enables cost-effectiveness in fulfilling mandatory emission reduction target by an annex I developed country through the market mechanism by allowing trade in emissions reductions or sink enhancements[15] with other countries parties including non-annex- I developing countries at the market determined price

Flexibility in Mitigation Efforts

The Kyoto Protocol sets greenhouse gas (GHG) emissions limits for the annex I developed countries as their commitments are listed in its Annex B.[16] The Protocol provides different GHG emission targets for each annex I developed country under Annex B, taking into account scope and differences in the cost of achieving those reductions. The limits cover emissions of six greenhouse gases by all anthropogenic sources during the period 2008-2012. Under the Protocol, each annex I party must

---

13 See, the Kyoto Protocol, arts. 6, 12, 17.

14 See, Kyoto Protocol, Articles 6(3), 12(9); see also, in the Marrakesh Accords, Decision 16/CP.7, Annex, para.29; Decision 17/CP.7, Annex, para. 33; and Decision 18/CP.7, Annex, para. 5.

15 Sink enhancements are human activities, such as planting trees that absorb greenhouse gases.

16 See, the Kyoto Protocol, art. 3(1).

not exceed its total assigned amount of GHG emissions over the first five-year commitment period.[17]

Supplementarity

The Kyoto Protocol also deal with the issue of supplementarity by clearly providing the requirement that Annex I developed countries may use the Kyoto mechanisms to comply with only part of their commitments enshrined in annex B. The supplementarity requirement puts a cap on the use of the Kyoto mechanisms.

Additionality

It is pertinent to note that all types of emissions mitigations project activities are not considered as generating the emission reduction to be used by the annex I developed countries to comply with their binding commitments under the Kyoto Protocol. In fact,qonly the projects which satisfy the additionality requirement are useful for the purpose ofq, complying with the commitments under the Kyoto Protocol.

Article 12(5) of the Kyoto Protocol provides that only emissions reductions "additional" to those that would anyway have occurred can be certified emissions reductions under Clean Development Mechanism projects by the operational entity.[18] Similarly, emission reduction units can only be generated under the joint implementation (JI) if such emission reduction is in additional to those that would have occurred without JI project.[19]

Legal Framework of the Sustainable Development

The Brundtland Report

Since the end of the 1980s the term 'sustainable development' has dominated international activities in the field of environmental protection. The concept of sustainable development has its roots in the idea of a sustainable society[20] and in the management of renewable and non-renewable resources. The concept was introduced in the world conservation strategy by the International Union for the Conservation of Nature (IUCN).[21] The World Commission on Environment and Development (WCED) adopted the concept and put the idea of sustainable development on the international political agenda with their report *Our Common Future*.[22]

---

17 See, *ibid.*

18 See, *ibid.*, article 12(5).

19 See, *ibid.*, article 6(I)(b).

20 See, L. Brown, *Building a Sustainable Society* (Washington, D.C., Worldwatch Institute, 1981).

21 See, IUCN, *World Conservation Strategy: Living Resources Conservation for Sustainable Development* (Gland: IUCN, 1980).

The Rio Earth Summit

The 1992 UN Conference on Environment and Development (UNCED), also Known as Rio Earth Summit, played an important role in the evolution of the legal framework of sustainable development. It was held in the context of the UN General Assembly resolution to tackle the effects of environmental degradation by taking national and international action to promote sustainable and environmentally sound development in all countries.[23]

Post-Rio Developments

Since the Rio Earth Summit, there is general consensus that sustainable development requires the adoption of a comprehensive and integrated approach to economic, social and environmental processes.[24] Thus, the principles of sustainable development have progressively been internalized in various national and international legal instruments.[25] Growing numbers of international treaties, particularly in the fields of international environmental law including the UNFCCC, address sustainable developmental goals and instruments.[26] These treaties generally refer to sustainable development as a fundamental principle by which they must be interpreted. But they generally do not provide specific contents of sustainable development. The UN Framework Convention on Climate Change, for example, includes in its principles the right to promote sustainable development, but does not elaborate modalities for doing so.[27]

Legal Status

Although, the principle of 'sustainable development' has been recognized in international environmental law, still legal scholars continue to debate its legal and normative status.[28] Judge Weeramantry in his separate opinion in *Gabeikovo-*

---

22 See, The World Commission on Environment and Development, *Our Common Future* (Oxford: Oxford University Press, 1987) [hereinafter the "Brundtland Report"].

23 UNGA Res./44/228, 1989, para. 3, availableat <http://www.environment.fe:ov.be/Root/tasks/atmosphere/klim/pub/int/unga/44-228 en.htm>.

24 M. Munasinghe, *Environmental Economics and Sustainable Development* (Washington D.C.: The World Bank 1992).

25 see, A. Boyle and D. Freestone, *International law and sustainable development: past achievements and jitture challenges* (Oxford:University Press, 1999)

26 See P. Sands, *Principles of International Environmental Law,* 2"d Edition, (New York: Cambridge University Press, 2003), p. 252.

27 See, the UNFCCC, article 3(4).

28 See V. Lowe, "Sustainable Development and Unsustainable Arguments", in: Alan Boyle and David Freestone (eds.): *International Law and Sustainable Development: Past Achievements and Future Challenges* (Oxford: Oxford University Press, 1999), p. 23. See, A.B.M. Marong, "From Rio to Johannesburg: Reflections on the Role of International Legal Norms in Sustainable Development", *The Georgetown International Environmental Law Review,* Vol. 21, 2003, pp. 57. See also P. Sands, Principles of International Environmental Law, 2"d Edition, (New York: Cambridge University Press, 2003), p. 255. P. Birnie and A. Boyle, *International Law and the Environment* (Oxford: Oxford University Press, 2002), p. 122. See Case Concerning the Gabeikovo-Nagymaros Project (Hungary/Slovakia), *ICJ Rep.* 7, 1997, para. 140.

Nagymaros Project case considers the concept of sustainable development as having customary law status. Thus, there is a need to analyze the status and meaning of sustainable development in the on text of international law. In fact, the Rio Declaration and Agenda 21 provide the essential basis for identifying and assessing principles of international law for sustainable development. Further, the concept of sustainable development is considered as an appropriate framework for environment and development decision-making.

Developing Countres' Participation in the Climate Change Regime

Implications of Climate Change for Developing Countries

Developing Countries and Climate Change

Global problems require global solutions. The challenges presented by climate change provide the ultimate demonstration of global interdependence.[29] It is pertinent to note that though all countries are going to be affected by the physical phenomenon of climate change, but the developing countries are particularly vulnerable to the impacts of climate change.[30] Among the developing countries, the least developed countries (LDCs) and small island developing states (SIDS) are considered as being the most vulnerable countries to the adverse impacts of climate change. [31] This is a result of a number of factors, including their relative exposure to the adverse physical impacts of climatic changes such as sea level rise and increased temperatures; as well as their relatively high dependence on economic sectors that are climate sensitive.

Thus, the setting of legally binding target has become the bone of contention between the rich developed countries and the developing countries. It seems that this issue can not be quickly resolved as it goes beyond the climate diplomacy and gets involved with the issues the related to the traditional conflict of political and economic interests among the developed and developing countries of the world.

Developing Countries' Perspective

In the light of stark differences between the developed and developing countries, there is also a sharp divide in terms of their standpoint regarding international environmental policy. [32] In the case of climate change, countries have

---

29 See Peter Slinn, "Development Issues: The International Law of Development and Global Climate Change," In: Robin Churchill and David Freestone, *International Law and Global Climate Change* (London: Graham and Trotman, 1991), Chapter 5, p. 76.

30 Vulnerability in this context is defined as, "the degree to which a system is susceptible to, or unable to cope with, the adverse effects of climate change, including climate variability and extremes" See, IPCC, Climate Change 2001: Impacts, Adaptation and Vulnerability (Cambridge: Cambridge University Press, 2001).

31 See, the UNFCCC, Articles 4(8) and 4(9).

32 See, O. P. Dwivedi and Dhirendra K. Vajpeyi, eds., *Environmental Policies in the Third World: A Comparative Analysis* (Westport: Greenwood Publishing, I995), p.5.

different perspectives which are rooted in their economic development, energy structure, industrial structure and the anticipated impacts of climate change.[33] In fact, during initial climate change negotiations, the developing countries made clear that North-South issues would play a prominent role in the negotiation. In this regard, the Noordwijk Declaration recognizes the North-South dimension of the climate change issue and included a number of provisions sought by developing countries.

An important dimension of the climate change challenge is its global scale. It follows that no one country can solve the problem of climate change acting alone. Thus, it seems collective action is not an option but an imperative. In this context, it is pertinent to note that participation of the developing countries is critical for tackling the challenge of climate change, which is possible only when concerns and interests with regard to climate change are adequately addressed. The present trend of increasing GHG emissions in the developing country is driven by development imperatives - in particular, the need for economic development and eradication of poverty. In the context of the current debate about climate change, the developing countries are taking considerable domestic measures in terms of policies and programmes. Further, technology transfer can speed up this process and additional funds can accelerate these initiatives in energy conservation to tackle climate change.

Conclusion

Climate change' refers to a change of climate which is attributed directly or indirectly to human economic activity that alters the composition of the global atmosphere. It is in addition to natural climate variability observed over a comparable time periods. The state of the climate has been identified by scientists in terms of changes in the mean value of climate parameters like GHG concentration in the atmosphere, surface temperature and their variability. Climate change is due to internal atmospheric processes which are a result of highly complex interplay of natural, physical, ecosystems, human and atmospheric system. The scientific basis of this complex phenomenon of climate change has been explained through the theory of natural greenhouse gases effect.

Thus, there is a human dimension to the climate change. It is not natural, but anthropogenic. The root causes of the problem are the human economic activities including industrial production, change in land use and the like. Current concentrations of greenhouse gases in the atmosphere are primarily the result of economic activities in the developed countries since the industrial revolution. Therefore, in order to solve the problem of climate change, there is a need to change the human behavior and attitude towards adopting the less carbon intensive economic activities. The essence of this aspect then is the concern of legal, institutional, economic and social aspects of the issue of climate change. Thus, there is need to employ the insights and tools of social science to deal with the issue of anthropogenic climate change.

---

33 Qin Tianbao, "China's Peaceful Development and Global Climate Change: A Legal Perspective", *Law, Environment and Development Journal*, Vol.3, No. I, 2007, pp.54-69.

In this regard various studies have been undertaken in the field of social science, especially international law, economics, international relations, sociology, geography to develop a broad understanding of the issues arising out the problem and to make suggestions for human response to the problem through climate change policies. On this basis, the issue of climate change has been liked to sustainable development, trade, eradication of poverty, transfer of technology, financial assistance, equity, principle of international environmental law including the common but differentiated responsibility.

Viewing climate change in the context of sustainable development has a number of implications. Such an approach means that poverty eradication and socio-economic development are necessary for combating climate change. The critical effort of developing and diffusing clean energy technologies needs to be stepped up. At the same time, enhanced access for the poor to modern services also needs to be vigorously pursued. Incorporating climate change response measures into development planning, including national sustainable development strategies, could contribute to achieving the objectives of both the Climate Change Convention and the sustainable development goals. For instance, integrating adaptation measures into development planning could contribute to poverty eradication, while at the same time reducing the vulnerability of the poorest communities to climate variability and climate change.

The UNFCCC and its Kyoto Protocol provide the legal framework which is basis of collective action undertaken by the international community of sovereign States to tackle the challenge of climate change at the international level. This international legal regime of climate change have also established an institutional framework including the COP/MOP to facilitate the cooperation and participations through negotiations process on the issues related to implementation of the regime in order to achieve the ultimate objective of the UNFCCC. The UNFCCC and Kyoto Protocol have already created a strong system for estimating and reviewing emissions according to standard guidelines.

Chapter 20

Impacts of Climate-Smart Agricultural System on Food Security: A Case Study of Institutional Policy Recommendations and Challenges in Nigeria

EZEKIEL, Ayinde Alani

Department of Agricultural Economics, Ladoke Akintola University of Technology, P.M.B. 4000, Ogbomoso, Oyo State, Nigeria.
e-mail: aaezekiel@lautech.edu.ng

ABSTRACT

Climate simply refers to the average weather conditions in a certain place over many years. In recent times, a major concern to the scientists is the rapidly increasing average temperature of the earth, amongst other weather elements. Such increment is alarming and requiring urgent attention, so as to alleviate the undesirable effects on agricultural production and human welfare. However, climate change is a significant and lasting change in the statistical distribution of weather patterns spanning decades. It may be a change in average weather conditions, or in the distribution of weather around the average conditions. The causes of climate change involve biotic processes as well as variations in solar radiation received by the earth, plate tectonics and volcanic eruptions. Climate-Smart Agriculture is a welcome development in Agriculture which reasonably improves agricultural production practices, particularly integrated crop management, conservation agriculture, intercropping, improved seeds and fertilizer management, improved livestock management, improved grazing land management, agroforestry, as well as supporting increased investment in farming systems. Climate-Smart Agriculture (CSA) contributes to increase in sustainable productivity, incomes, strengthen farmers' resilience, reduce agriculture greenhouse gas emissions and increase carbon sequestration. It strengthens food security and delivers environmental benefits. It is broader than adaptation, and calls for more innovation and pro-activeness in changing the way farming is done in order to adapt and mitigate climate change while sustainably increasing productivity. Climate-Smart Agriculture practices propose the transformation of agricultural policies and agricultural systems to increase food productivity and enhances food and nutrition security while preserving the environment and ensuring resilience to a changing climate. CSA practices and technologies in Nigeria Climate-Smart Agriculture practices and technologies that are being promoted, adopted and implemented in Nigeria include conservation agriculture, use of crop residues for manure, green manure crops, agroforestry and planting of drought tolerant varieties. This study was used to develop a methodology for obtaining different types of data to build an evidence base on CSA practices, including incentives/barriers to adoption, mitigation-adaptation-food security synergies and trade-offs of different practice options (based on identification of food security and adaptation benefits, climate change indicators, mitigation potential and least-cost-investment options). In Nigeria, this combined data has shown that some farmers face difficulties in adopting conservation agriculture (CSA) practices, which potentially have productivity, adaptation and mitigation benefits. In some holdings, crop residues are needed for animal feed instead of soil cover and some households are too poor to wait several seasons for the benefits to materialize. However, CSA appears to be used as an adaptation response in areas of pronounced climate variability. The findings also indicate entry points for agricultural policies to increase food security under climate change and for extension services. The mapping of agricultural and climate change policy instruments, stakeholders/institutions and policy formulation and implementation processes is also being carried out with a view to enable greater policy alignment and more coordinated institutional arrangements.

Keywords: *Climate-smart, Agriculture, Institution, Policy recommendation.*

Introduction

The concept of Climate-Smart Agriculture

Climate-Smart Agriculture (CSA) aim at increase agricultural productivity, profits, improves farmers' resilience, reduce farm produce waste, minimize agriculture greenhouse gas emissions and soar carbon sequestration. It fortifies food security and utter environmental benefits. Climate-Smart Agriculture advocate agricultural best practices, it restore crop management, conservation agriculture, intercropping, improved seeds and fertilizer management, improved livestock management, improved grazing land management, agroforestry, as well as supporting grow investment in agricultural research. It is broader than adaptation, its calls for innovation and in changing the way farming is done in order to adapt and mitigate climate change to sustainably increase productivity. Climate-Smart Agriculture practices propose the transformation of agricultural policies and systems to increase food productivity and augment food and nutrition security while preserving the environment and ensuring resilience to a changing climate.

Climate-smart agriculture (CSA) gives opportunity of tackling threats of climate change on global food security; it's the origin of greenhouse gases. With the help to understand the conditions for agricultural innovation and adoption, the CGIAR Research Program on Climate Change, Agriculture and Food Security (CCAFS) describes the concept of climate-smart agriculture (CSA) in 2012 with a global research program to characterize and scale climate-smart agriculture practices. Different methods for scaling CSA practices are now beginning to develop based on practiced research and innovation. Currently, arable crops such as rice, maize and cassava, system of Rice Intensification and Alternate Wetting and Drying, with triple benefits of adaptation, mitigation, and increased productivity, have seen rapid large-scale uptake. In contrast, smallholders with more diverse land uses require more interventions in the sense of biophysical suitability and market opportunities. There was an argument that the slow uptake depends on CSA being perceived as too technology and knowledge intensive. The stress on CSA has being subject of discussion that looks contradict the notion of CSA as a scalable practice. One specific CSA-practice that frequently meets such criticism is agroforestry. Despite complex livelihood, adaptation and mitigation benefits, low autonomous adoption of agroforestry was describes by farmers who prioritised food security that perceived the period for return-on-investment being too long, markets uncertainty and short-term loans offering by the banks.

Research Questions

Therefore, the following questions are fundamental to this study:

1. What are the impacts of climate-smart agriculture system on food security?
2. What are the suggesting actions that can be taken to increase agricultural productivity?
3. What are the building resilience, and reduce GHG emissions through enhancing CSA, both in policies and practices?

General Objective of the Study

This study examined the impacts of Climate-Smart Agricultural System on Food Security.

Objectives of the study are to

1. Examine the impacts of climate-smart agriculture system on agriculture, food production and security,
2. Suggest actions that can be taken to increase agriculture productivity.
3. Build resilience, and reduce GHG emissions through enhancing CSA, both in policies and practices.

Justification of the Study

This study discovered that many are ready to practice climate-smart agricultural system; if there will be proper training from the extension officers. Climate-Smart Agriculture practices and technologies that are being promoted in Nigeria are conservation agriculture, use of crops residual manure, agroforestry, planting of drought tolerant varieties and the new practice of planting crops residue into the soil to yield soil fertility with the aim to also reduce soil acidity.

Literature Review

Theoretical and Conceptual Framework

Simelton, Dam (2015) opined a gradual transition towards promoting integrated systems in order to avoid lost through application of modern technology, he gave advice on adoption of change crops *or* the management rather than changing both at the same time. He identified problems and made difference between 'generic' and CSA complex interventions, that is, agroforestry, He divided practices into *technologies* - how things are grown, and *components* – he then asked a question on what is grown? Whereby the former can be applied broadly and the latter is context-specific. Furthermore, agroforestry/contour planting can be practiced anywhere, trees and crops in that system would depend on soil fertility. At this level there is needed to consider the framework that focused on participatory solutions at the field to landscape scale. Simlton didn't consider factors that enable or limit scalability at district or region, such as policy support and market potential or risk for market saturation. Though he taught on innovation in CSA, that farmer might have been practicing much climate-smart system and the innovative aspect may simply be making stakeholders to have knowledge on how farming practices can be improved to embraced climate or economic changes, and how to assess the progress towards such climate-smart objective. In 2014, four climate-smart agriculture systems were selected in Ogbomoso and its environment: home garden, livestock, agriculture intensification, and forestry. Hence, this study categorised common practices and purposive steps towards 'climate-smart Agriculture interventions, and to identify opportunities for scaling-out climate-smart agriculture practices in Northern and South-Western Nigeria. The ambition was to apply a pragmatic participatory methodology which farmers on minor budgets might be able to use, and with a considered scaling out potential beyond the scoping area itself. Agriculture has been recognized as one of the biggest drivers of environmental change (Smith *et al.*, 2007). Agricultural lands occupy about 50 to 60 per cent of the land surface (Smith *et al.*, 2007). It is estimated that agriculture is responsible for about three-quarters of tropical deforestation. (Wollenberg *et al.*, 2012) accounts for about 10 to 12 per cent of the total global anthropogenic emissions of greenhouse gases (GHGs). (Smith *et al.*, 2007) said that the world needs more food than ever before to sustain the people living in extreme poverty, especially in Africa where about 70 per cent of the people are engaged in some sort of agricultural activity (AMAF: ASEAN, 2015).

Lessons learnt will aid the future adoption of climate-smart agriculture in the study areas and serve as practical guidance for the implementation of agricultural emissions reduction initiatives, based on the knowledge and best practices. The ultimate purpose is to accelerate efforts towards mitigating agriculture-based climate change while at the same time enhancing livelihoods and food security (Adam *et al.*, 1997)

Benefits of Using Animal Manure

About 75 per cent of farmers in Nigeria are using animal manure (Crops Residue Manure) for crop and vegetable fertility. While 25 per cent use a combination of animal manure and inorganic fertiliser. There are about 300,000,000 cattle in Nigeria with a human population of about one sixty million (160,000,000) a ratio of about 3:1. Other farmers applied goat manure on high value crops such as vegetables. The advantages of using organic manure include addition of natural nutrients to the soil, in order to improve soil fertility and pH, and the sequestration of carbon dioxide thus reducing its adverse effects on global warming. Large quantities of crops residual manure are needed in the soil in order to yield fertility of the soil, the level of poverty of farmer has not allow them to have enough animals that can supply quantity number of manure needed to yield soil fertility, also lack of transport of manure to fields not close to homesteads is another factor (Below *et al.*, 2010)

Agroforestry

Conservation agriculture, such as agroforestry is an old land-use method practised by the farmers to yield soil fertility by relying of standing vegetation, use of trees by slash-and-burn shifting cultivation method in Nigeria. The common planted fruit trees are avocadoes, peaches, and mangoes to name a few. They also planted arable fields adjacent to homesteads where they can be monitor and protected from unauthorised harvesting. According to (Doan *et al.*, 2015) the most common fruit trees that grown and ploughed into lands to serve as manure are: malura (*Slerocarya birrea*), water berries (*Syzigium cordatum*), figs (*Ficus* spp) and Velvet-Wild-medlar (*Vangueria infausta*)

Institutional Setup for Addressing CSA Issues

The Ministry of Agriculture perform the responsibility of ensuring food security in the Nigeria. they developing and promoting appropriate technologies such as CSA. The departments and sections within the ministry that are relevant to climate smart agriculture are the Agricultural Research and Specialists Services, the Department of Veterinary and Livestock Production Services, and Agricultural and Extension Services. The Department of Agricultural Research and Specialists Services is responsible for identification of adaptable crop varieties that can be grown in the different parts of the country, as well as developing appropriate water management practices. The department of Veterinary and Livestock Production Services plays a major role in improving livestock and grazing land management. The Agriculture and Extension Services is responsible for promoting crop production and providing agricultural extension services in farming systems and technologies that will assure increased and resilient food production.

The four organization that were created by the MOA to complement it in fulfilling its mandate are National Agricultural Marketing Boards (NAM Board), National Maize Corporation (NMC), Nigeria Water and Agricultural Development Enterprise (NWADE) and Nigeria Dairy Board (NDB). Non-Government Organizations also provide extension services to complement the government extension service. They include WVI, IRD, ACAT and Caritas.

Climate Data

Report of daily rainfall, minimum and maximum temperatures of meteorological department (FCT, Abuja) for the period 1980-2016 were tested for conventional trend and variability analysis using Stata 11. To indicate future rainfall and temperature trends and assess the potential risk to cropping system in five local government of Ogbomoso, South-Western Nigeria We applied the analysed climate change scenario RCP8.5 for Northern Region for 2003-2020. The meteorological department is located in the state secretariat of each study area. The climate change scenarios were updated. While some specific details were updated for temperature (increase

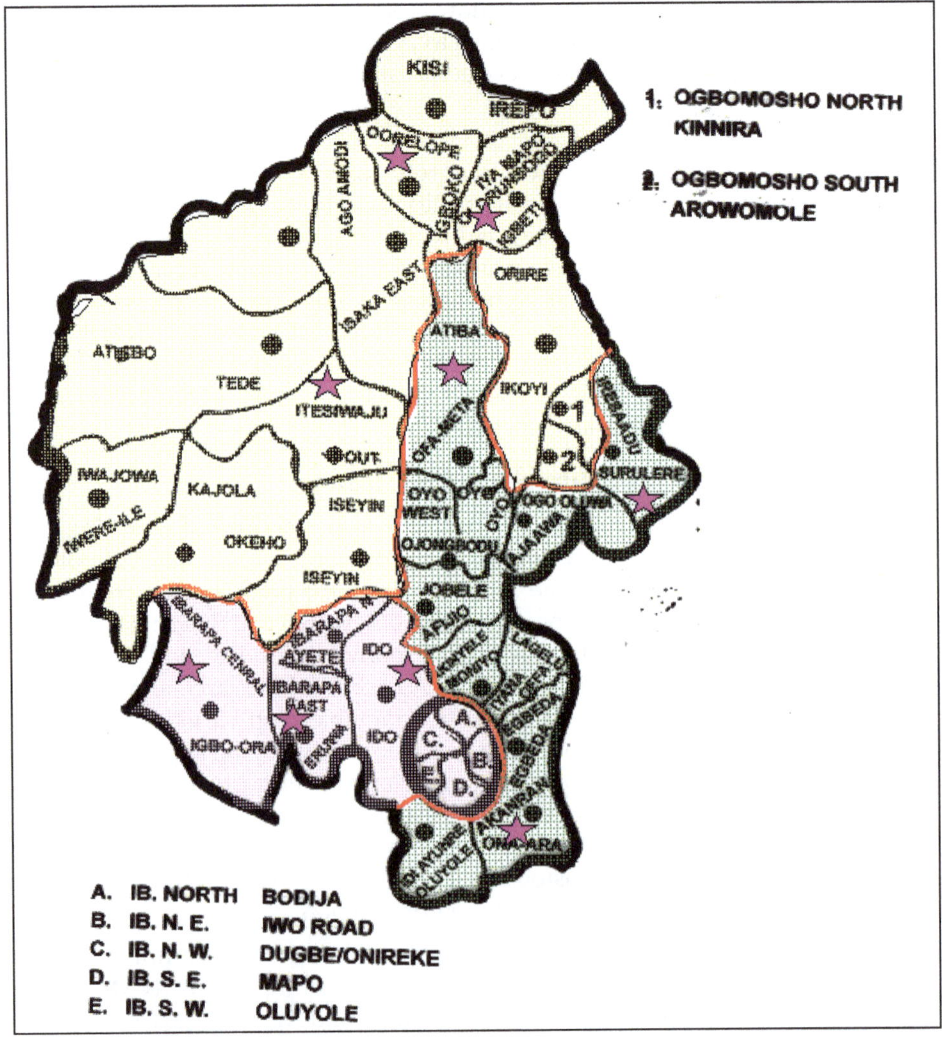

Figure 20.1: Map of Nigeria Showing Ogbomoso where Parts of the Study were Located.

projection) and rainfall (higher variability), the crude qualitative scenarios used in this study indicate little difference up to the 2020s.

Research Methodology

Study Area

The study was carried out in Oyo State and Katsina State of Nigeria. These two states are an inland state in both Northern Region and South-Western Nigeria with its capital at Katsina and Ibadan respectively. Oyo state is bounded in the North by Kwara state, in the East by Osun State, in the South by Ogun state and in the West partly by the Republic of Benin. It was formed in 1976 from the former Western

State, and originally included Osun State, which was split off in 1991. Oyo state is homogenous, mainly inhabited by the Yoruba ethnic (Wikipedia, 2007).

The indigenes mainly comprise the Oyo State, the Ibadan and Ibarapa, all belonging to Yoruba family and speaking the same Yoruba language. The state consists of thirty three (33) Local Governments Areas with a total population of 6,617,720 inhabitants (Census, 2006). The capital, Ibadan is reported to be the largest city in Africa, South of Sahara other notable cities and towns in Oyo State include Oyo, Ogbomoso, Iseyin, Kisi, Okeho, Saki, Eruwa, Lanlate, Awe and Igbo Ora. The climate in the state favours the cultivation of crops like maize, yam, cassava, millet, rice, plantain, cocoa tree, palm tree and cashew. Oyo State is located within longitude 8° and latitude 3° 28E with annual rainfall of 1247mm (Wikipedia, 2007).

The study area lies in the rainforest zone of Nigeria and this has made about 80 per cent of the inhabitants to engage in agriculture. There are two distinct seasons, rainy and dry season. The rainy season starts in Oyo State during the first week of March and lasts till the Month of October, while the dry season lasts November – March, all things being equal. The low rainfall is marked by the period of August break in August. Mean temperature varies from daily minimum of 25^{oC} to a daily maximum of 35°C. Humidity is quite high in Oyo State. Relative humidity in the State is around 70 per cent with a minimum of about 60 per cent in the evening and a maximum of around 80 per cent in the morning, (Wikipedia, 2007).

It was estimated that 75 per cent of the landed property in Nigeria belongs to the Northern region of the country (Fanen *et al.*, 2004). This region lies between latitudes 06° 27I N to 14° 00I N and between longitudes 02° 44I E and 14° 42I E, mostly occupied by farmers, engaged in arable crops farming and cattle rearing. This served as means of livelihood for the majority of the people. The people of this region are generally regarded to be poor, financially and educational terms, compared with other parts of the country (Omonona, 2009). The three climatic in northern Nigeria are: Guinea Savannah, Sudan Savannah and Sahel Savannah. Rainfall and temperatures varies across January to December (Akor, 2012). According to the Nigerian Meteorology Agency (NIMET)(2009), the northern region was experiencing lower rainfall but progressively became wetter than normal in the year 2011. The annual rainfall in the region ranges from 400 to 1000 mm. Further evidence suggested that climate change is more complex in this area. A comparison of average temperatures of previous years from 1941 to 2002 was investigated and showed the evidence of long-term temperature increased across the country, especially in the North Nigerian Meteorology Agency (NIMET, 2009). The most significant increase recorded was in the North with average temperature rising by 1.4 to 1.9°C. Comparison of rainfall from 1972 to 2001, by taken the record of combination of the late onset and early experience of rainfall shows that the length of the rainfall is shortened in most parts of the country (Building Nigeria's Response to Climate Change (BNRCC), 2012). This study discovered that between 1942 and 2001, the annual rainfall in most parts of Nigeria was decreased by 3 to 9 mm. The dry season, almost lasts for ten months, while rainfall only occurred seasonally but is often intensive, making it necessary for farmers to practiced soil moisture conservation methods. Dutsin-Ma Local Government Area (LGA) in

Katsina State, Northern Nigeria was considered in the Northern Region for this study. The majority of the inhabitants there are poor, living below the 500 Naira per person per day threshold. The Local Government Area has a population of 169,829 in about 18,800 households with ecological zones. Generally speaking, the mean monthly maximum temperature varies between 28 and 40°C. In the semi-arid zones comprising the Sudan and Sahel, the maximum temperatures could be as high as 40°C between March and May while at the lower end the maximum temperatures of 28°C are experienced between December and January.

Agriculture Census Data

Land use and agriculture production estimates for 2016 were taken from the annual social-economic report, including soil type, cropland area, yield, pest, cultivation techniques. For scaling potential, we consulted the provincial Master plan and land use plans for 2016-2020

Qualitative Data

Participatory focus group activities in each village of the local government areas resulted in detailed information: (i) Timeline of major development trends and extreme weather events in the village; (ii) Annual calendar of farming systems and natural hazards; (iii) Village sketch maps of actual land use, soil, and natural hazards to complement the low resolution (topography, soil, land use) maps and agriculture census data. Villages in Vietnam rarely have defined borders, however if such can be established the village maps can be transferred a commune map; (iv) Transect walks with key informants were used to assess current farming systems and start discussing potential interventions in the field. Three half-day focus group discussions were conducted in each village. The fieldwork was conducted between May 2015 and July 2016, the effective time estimated for the fieldwork was three weeks. Some information has been re-confirmed in 2017.

Climate Smart Agriculture Indicators

Drawing on the information generated in steps i-iii above, the participatory CSA prioritisation can be summarised in the following steps: (1) Description of the farming system(s), what crops are grown, and how they are managed (Baseline characterization); (2) Decide what problems to solve (Problem identification and target indicators from the CSA long list); (3) Design a farming system that aims to be climate-smart within 5-10 years, (Plan and design the system). Step (4) includes implementation, testing and adjustment, though it is not included in the scope of this study. In consultation with key informants, the following shortlist of CSA indicators was selected:

Food Security and Livelihoods

Crop yields (ton ha^{-1} $year^{-1}$), income from agriculture products sold (million VND ha^{-1} $year^{-1}$) and costs for labour and agriculture inputs, such as seed, fertiliser and herbicide (million VND ha^{-1} $year^{-1}$). Profit (million VND ha^{-1} $year^{-1}$) is calculated as costs subtracted from revenue.

Adaptation

The risk of crop failure was assessed through participatory ranking and mapping exercises, where farmers were asked to evaluate potential extreme weather event(s) and prioritise appropriate interventions, as to avoid overestimating the ability of any single practice to mitigate all risks. Yield stability and the added risks when accounting for the climate change scenarios were not rated but based on local perceptions and discussed in qualitative terms.

Mitigation Potential and Ecosystem Services

Farmers generally have a clearer understanding of environmental functions than greenhouse gas emissions. Here, a combined assessment of an intervention's contributions to environmental services as temporal duration (months year^{-1}), canopy strata (number of vertical layers), and vegetation cover (per cent canopy cover per unit area annually). Longer planting periods and higher vegetation cover are assumed to reduce negative environmental effects, although this is debated in the case of clear-felling. Soil nutrient status is viewed as ability to reduce soil degradation (erosion and/or nutrient depletion). Due to the apparent misuse of inorganic pesticides and herbicides which had resulted in reduced soil organic matter and hardpans, local authorities requested the research team to also recommend feasible alternatives.

Scaling Potential of the Practice

The household's preference for a farming system was based on farmers' qualitative assessment of its compatibility with their needs, capacity and desire to expand the practice. Desire is influenced by farmers' (realistic and unrealistic) perceptions of market opportunities. The market and spatial scaling potential at the commune or district levels were based on land use plans, supporting policies and consultations with expert representatives from Farmer's Union, Department of Agriculture and Rural Development (DARD), agriculture university and research institutes (representing an agronomist, forester, mitigation expert, and ecosystem assessment model).

Results and Discussion

Assessment of Climate-Smart Agriculture Sustainability (ACSAS)

Descriptive statistics such as frequency and percentage distribution mean and standard deviation was used to assess the level of sustainability of CSA in Nigeria. The assessment of modern Technologies gave better understanding of CSA framework, It was judged from the literature review, personal knowledge and observations from the field. Though it was not tested practically to ascertain information presented in the available sources systematically, we strictly obtained good results were based on data presented in different sources.

Securing Mankind's Existence

Five major steps were followed in order to achieve sustainability under securing mankind's existence, they are: (1) human health protection (2) satisfaction of human basic needs (3) encouraging self-support (4) sharing of opportunities for using natural resources (5) and appreciation differences in income and wealth. CSA gives knowledge of risk management; it ensures maximum protection against dangers and unbearable risks for human health due to polluted environmental factors. This steps needs to be emphasis so as to underscore its importance. Presently, ecosystem health case was emphasized and concluded that it could be diminished if there is proper monitoring. This step is important in Nigeria because of the increasing concern for heavy metal generating acidity content of agricultural lands under long-term application of both inorganic fertilizers and organic wastes, which also has dangerous effects on human health (Agbenin, 2002). Achieving these steps will surely help to reduce risks and deaths from agricultural land contaminations. The second goal is about the contribution of CSA to secure the basic human needs. CSA is meant for the provision of food and other basic needs, for example shelter and clothing. It is true that 'food is not only a basic need', but the fact is that no agriculture, no food, no life. It is important to maintain livelihood. In Africa, people believe that the inner peace will be disturbed when the external appearance is weak. In addition, adequate clothing and shelter will help men to protect themselves against health challenges, for example farmers contacting water-borne diseases because they lack shoes and being denied of access to source of good water. Achieving self-support autonomy is the third rule. CSA educate farmers to be aware of their environment by sending their children to school. It is important to emphasise preparation for ageing populations, in order to gain the conscience of the young one to participate in farming, so that they can support elderly farmers in their old age. The need to ensure a just distribution of opportunities for using natural resources is another rule for sustainability. CSA raises the need to ensure the fair and equitable sharing of benefits arising from the use of genetic resources. What has been left out is emphasis on the need of initiative to ensure that people's access to the necessary resources is assured. Currently, this step is often being satisfied through the traditional ownership structure. When this, however, is unsure by the formal state institutions, farmers can be denied access to their farm lands under the Land Use Act of 1978, which nationalised all land and vested its management to the state. The law said that occupancy can be revoked if the land is required for other activities. This is often done without compensation of the owners. The last step, linked to the previous to ensure appreciate the extreme differences in income and wealth. This is to guarantee that farmers who experience loss of profits are not left out, but are compensated to reduce disparity among them. There is little or no mention of this step in CSA; however, the methods emphasized payments for environmental services (PES), as a means for compensating farmers for maintaining ecosystem services.

Table 20.1: Sustainability Assessment in Northern and South-Western Nigeria

Aims	*Steps*	*Standardized as a Sustainable Strategy*	*Comments*	*Predicates in the African context*
	Health protection	xxx	Raised alongside ecosystem health	It can help reduce risk from misapplication of fertilisers
	Securing the satisfaction of basic needs	xx	Emphasis on food with little mention of shelter and clothing	Ensures food security and reduces risk of sickness from inadequate clothing and shelter
Securing mankind's existence	Autonomous self-support	x	Little emphasis on preparation for old age in the face of rapid flow of youths in urban areas	Prepares support for farmers in their old age
	Just distribution of opportunities for using natural resources	xx	Raised on benefit and cost sharing, but less on access to resources	There are changes needed to formal laws in order to reduce usurpation of farmlands for other uses
	Appreciation of extreme differences in income and wealth	x	Emphasis on payment for ecosystem services and little or no mention of compensation for income differentials	Decrease exploitation among farmers
	Sustainable use of renewable resources	xxx	Emphasises efficiency of available energy, as well as increasing the proportion of renewable energy	Can help create a good balance between increasing emphasis on fertilisers and organic manure through mixed farming
	Sustainable use of non-renewable resources	xx	Advocates reducing reliance on non-renewable external inputs	Attempts to stem the tide of possible move from renewable to non-renewable resources
Upholding society's productive potential	Sustainable use of the environment as a sink	xxx	Emphasises role of aquatic ecosystem, forests and tree planting as environmental sinks	Can aid conservation of wetlands, which are often cleared in many African societies. Also serves as a good platform to encourage tree planting
	Avoidance of unacceptable technical risks	xx	Emphasis centres on concerns with long-term potential impacts of biotechnology	With the rapid uptake of biotechnology, directs emphasis to negative impacts

Aims	*Steps*	*Standardized as a Sustainable Strategy*	*Comments*	*Predicates in the African context*
	Sustainable development of real, human and knowledge capital	xxx	Integrate systems that incorporate scientific and local knowledge sources	Promote indigenous knowledge
	Equal access to education, information and occupation	xxx	Emphasises social protection including access to social services for education, health, nutrition	Helps enhance societal organisation through reduction in disparity between rich and poor in society
Keeping options for development and action open	Participation in societal decision-making processes	xxx	Emphasises the need to broaden stakeholder participation with due consideration to cross-sectorial negotiations and planning processes	Ensures local people have a say in their development
	Conservation of nature's cultural functions	x	Less emphasis placed on cultural factors	May lead to a situation where culture is seen as entirely 'good' or completely 'bad'
	Conservation of 'social resources	x	Emphasises the interactions between sectors.	Need to encourage inter-personal interactions especially among farmers.

Agricultural Practice and Environmental Change in Northern and South-Western Nigeria

The commonly practiced agricultural system in Northern and South-Western Nigeria has been traditional farming system, such as, crop rotation, farm rotation, bush fallowing and crop residual cultivation (Adams and Mortimore, 1997), the practice involve farmer cultivates land, usually for one (1) to three (3) years, abandons it for period of years to fallow the plot fertility. Increase in population growth has result in land shortage, which has drastically reduced the amount of arable land available to farmers and reducing fallow periods. Farmers engaged in cutting down the vegetation on plots and setting fire on the remaining foliage, with the act of using the ashes to provide nutrients to the soil for planting food crops. This system of agriculture is deforestation that causes draught, desertification and climate change Nigeria. This led to overgrazing of lands by nomadic Fulani moving to South-Western Nigeria from the North the Sahara Desert. The rate of desert encroachment in the region is put at 0.7 km per annum while the rate of deforestation is about 400,000 ha p/a (Federal Ministry of Environment (FME), 2000). The fact is that, the agriculture practiced in the region contributes to climatic change (Oladipupo, 1993).

Nigerian governments have tried to mitigate the effects of climate change and desertification in the region by creating and implementing policies. Recent policies include: National Erosion and Flood Control Policy; National Environmental Sanitation Policy; National Forestry Policy; National Drought and Desertification Policy and the National Policy on E-Waste Control and Management (Oladipupo, 1993). These policies, have failed to yield results. The following reasons were alleged to explain the failure of the past policies. Firstly, the policies only focused on mitigating the immediate effects of desertification without addressing it source, not thinking of the causes of desertification, which include over-exploitation of natural resources, *i.e.*, natural vegetation and water sources for domestic and commercial purposes (Lasco *et al.*, 2015), and unsustainable agricultural practices which result in decreased crop productivity and emission of greenhouse gases (Luedeling *et al.*, 2012). Secondly, the issue of lack of provision for long-term measures and opportunities for the people and in particular the most vulnerable groups, such as women and children, in the region to cope with the effects of climate change and desertification (Simelton *et al.*, 2017). Lastly, there was an inadequate of incorporation of indigenous livelihood practices and initiatives in agricultural policies, for example, those aimed at struggling with climate change and desertification phenomena in the region (Von *et al.*, 1999). Therefore, any agricultural development policy to address the problem of desertification with climate change in Nigeria will require a broad approach that incorporates the abilities to increase agricultural productivity and incomes sustainability in Nigeria; remodel and construct resilience to climate change and reduces or removes greenhouse gases emissions using local knowledge and initiatives.

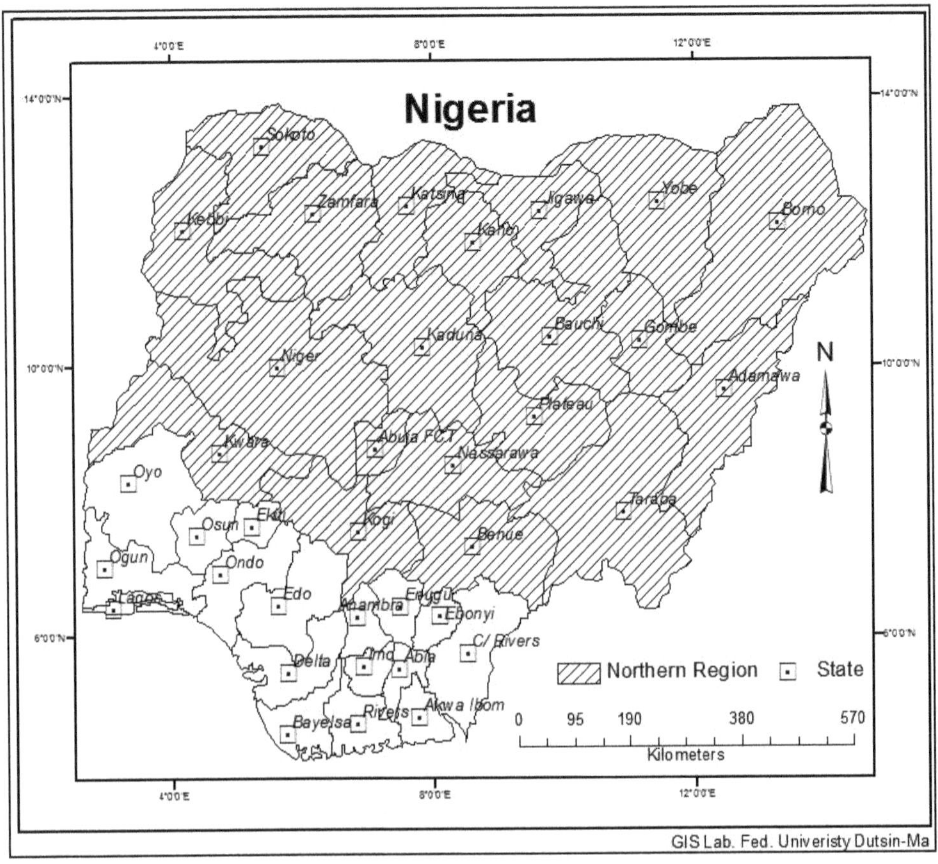

Figure 20.1: Map of Nigeria that Shows Northern Region of the Country.

How to Achieve Food Security with Climate-Smart Agricultural System

The global warming rate is progressing, aggravate by humans' past and present unsustainable practices which result in human and environmental-induced effects and risks. Any attempt toward sustainable development models will involve significant paradigm shifts, for example, the current economic models, presumed that a society can only develop by effectively expanding its use of resources and increasing per capita consumption patterns, despite the related long term negative effects. In this context, and since climate change is generating risks and opportunities for agriculture, which is the main part of development strategies in many Southern countries, climate-smart agriculture (CSA) has recently emerged as an important option in multilateral climate change debate. This option is believed to produce enormous benefits both in terms of adaptation, mitigation, and food security enhancement, improving preparedness of stakeholders to engage in well-informed actions. This first decade of the third millennium has gained rapid international recognition, leading to global consensus that the global warming rate is accelerating, exacerbated by humans' past and present unsustainable practices. These practices, including those responsible for large volumes of greenhouse gas (GHG) emissions, deforestation, excess consumption of finite resources, reducing global biodiversity and contamination of water supplies, result in human-induced effects and risks that negatively impact on our quality of life. Politically, most countries agree that the debate about global warming is over, that climate change is a key symptom of how humans have impacted on planetary systems and that it is time for serious collaboration to help transform our institutional and individual practices, if next generations are to inherit a sustainable future. This concern and call for concerted action to tackle impacts of climate change, duly recognizing the environmental and related social problems, are reflected in the rising numbers of academic papers and popular literature articles since the 1960s. In general terms, transformation of global societies from mainly unsustainable practices to a more sustainable way of living will involve significant paradigm shifts, particularly from the current economic paradigm, in which it is presumed that a society can only develop by expanding its massive use of resources and increasing per capita consumption patterns, despite the long term negative effects of this behavior (Daly 1996).

In this context, many researchers, decision-makers, land use planners and civil society actors increasingly believe that the interaction between climate change and food security will be one of the biggest challenges for the coming decades. By the year 2025, 83 per cent of the expected global population of 8.5 billion will be living in developing countries, where most of the poor are living, and the resources are vulnerable to climate change. Yet the capacity of available resources and technologies to meet the demands of growing population remains uncertain. Presently, close to one billion people are already suffering from hunger worldwide and the future is daunting too: food needs are projected to increase by 70 per cent by 2050 when the global population reaches nine billion, while climate change is projected to reduce global average yields, among other severe consequences. Within this perspective, many believe that agriculture must become central to future climate-change and food security governance. This is on account of at least three important interrelated aspects: Firstly, agriculture is the sector most vulnerable to climate change and many threats, including the reduction of agricultural productivity, production stability and incomes in many areas of the world already characterized by high levels of 28 M. (Smith *et al.*, 2008) food insecurity and limited means of coping with adverse climate impacts. Moreover, climate change will affect agriculture through higher temperatures, greater crop water demand, more variable rainfall and extreme climate events such as heat waves, floods and droughts. Many impact studies point to severe crop yield reductions in the next decades without strong adaptation measures, especially in areas where rural households are highly dependent on agriculture and farming systems are highly sensitive to inclement climate; Secondly, agriculture contributes a "significant" proportion of global carbon dioxide and nitrous oxide emissions (about 14 per cent of emissions according to current estimations) (Wright 2010); and Thirdly, agriculture can be a major part of the solution: helping people to feed themselves and adapt to changing conditions while mitigating impacts of climate change (carbon sequestration). This mitigation potential can be largely achieved in developing countries. The need to tackle climate change while producing more food to feed the world's growing population means that "climate-smart agriculture" (CSA) is one of the advocated ways forward. This approach primarily defends agriculture that sustainably increases productivity, resilience (adaptation), reduces/removes GHGs (mitigation). This will simultaneously help meet the goals of food security and overall development. This also envisions transformation of agriculture to feed a growing population in the face of a changing climate without corroding the natural resource base significantly and mitigate the negative effects of climate change. However, more productive and resilient agriculture will need better management of natural resources, such as land, water, soil and genetic resources through practices such as conservation agriculture, integrated pest management, agroforestry and sustainable diets. This study aims examined the impact of climate agriculture, food production and securities, and what actions can be taken to increase agriculture productivity, build resilience to tackle the negative impacts of climate change, and reduce GHG emissions through enhancing CSA – both in policies and practices. Given the inter-linkages between climate change, food security and agriculture policies, a governance approach has been recommended in this chapter. Some of the most important guiding principles include equal emphasis on the management of natural resources, appropriate institutional and financial mechanisms and improving preparedness of stakeholders to engage in well-informed actions.

Agriculture at the Intersection of Climate Change, Food Security, and Poverty Alleviation, as mentioned above, climate change is one of the main challenges facing our globalized world today since the science clearly indicates that a global temperature rise of 2°C above pre-industrial levels may change the face of the world from Achieving Food Security in a Changing Climate: Furthermore, this challenge is increasingly considered as a 'threat multiplier' since it increases a range of livelihood threats and vulnerabilities, rather than being an isolated specific risk (UNCTAD, 2011). The poor population in developing countries will be particularly impacted by this delicate environmental problem, of which developed – and currently emergent – countries are the major drivers. In addition, food security, poverty and climate change are closely linked challenges and should not be considered separately. In countries where the economic and human development strategies are heavily based on agriculture, the development of agricultural sector, with a clear redistribution potential, remains an efficient poverty reduction policy. Yet agricultural expansion for food production and economic development which comes at the expense of soil, water, biodiversity or forests, environment, conflicts with other global and national goals, often compromises production and sound development in the longer term. It is true that over the past six decades world agriculture has become considerably more efficient, especially in the 1960s through green revolution. Improvements in production systems and crop and livestock breeding programs have resulted in a doubling of food production while increasing the amount of agricultural land by 10 per cent. However, projections based on population growth and food consumption indicate that agricultural production will need to increase substantially to meet future demands. Most estimates also indicate that climate change is likely to reduce agricultural productivity, production stability and incomes in some areas already suffering from food insecurity, high rates of poverty, and feeble adaptive capacities to cope with adverse climate impacts. Preliminary estimates for the period up to 2080 suggest a decline of some 15–30 per cent of agricultural productivity in the most climate change-exposed developing country regions – Africa and South Asia (UNCTAD 2011). Hence, climate change is expected to exacerbate and multiply the existing challenges faced by agriculture and human security. It is also true that human societies, over the centuries, have developed the capacity to adapt farming practices to environmental change and climate variability. These adaptations include, among others, practicing shifting cultivation, adopting high yielding, and new crop varieties tolerant to salts and drought and modifying grazing patterns. But today the speed and intensity of climate change are outpacing autonomous actions and threaten the ability of poor smallholders and rural societies to cope. For most of the one billion extremely poor and hungry people who live in the rural areas of major developing countries, agriculture remains the principal income source. These people are already vulnerable, and climate change will in most cases deepen their vulnerability. More specifically, and in countries most reliant on rainfed agriculture and natural resources, poor rural women, who are often the primary food producers, have fewer assets and less decision-making power, are even more exposed than men (UNCTAD, 2911). Therefore, ensuring food security under a changing climate should be considered as one of the major challenges of our era, especially that many countries' agriculture is highly vulnerable to negative impacts of climate change. Even using optimistic lower-end projections of temperature rise, climate change may reduce 30 M. Simelton *et al.* (2015) calculated crop yields to be between 10–20 per cent by the year 2050s, with more severe losses in some regions. (Smith *et al.*, 2008) opined that World food prices for some of the main grain crops are likely to rise sharply in the first half of the twenty-first century, unlike the price declines witnessed in the twentieth century. Projections of price rises range from about 30 per cent for rice to over 100 per cent for maize, with about half or more than half of this rise due to climate change. Under a pessimistic high-end projection of temperature rise, the impacts on productivity and prices are even greater. Moreover, increasing frequencies of heat stress, drought and flooding events, not factored into the projections mentioned above, will result in further deleterious effects on productivity. It is likely that price and yield volatility will continue to rise as extreme weather continues. Climate change will also impact agriculture through effects on pests and disease. These interactions are complex and the full implications in terms of productivity are still uncertain (BNRCC, 2011). While agriculture is the most vulnerable sector, it is also a major cause of climate change, directly accounting for about 14 per cent of GHG emissions, and indirectly much more as agriculture is an important driver of deforestation and land-use change responsible for another 18 per cent of global emissions (IPCC 2007). Even if emissions in all other sectors were eliminated by 2050, growth in agricultural emissions in a business-as-usual (BAU) scenario, world with a near doubling in food production would perpetuate climate change. Therefore, while trying to cope with the effects of a changing climate, agriculture is simultaneously facing two other challenges: increasing food production in developing countries to meet population increases and dietary changes whilst remaining central to mitigation efforts (IFAD 2010).

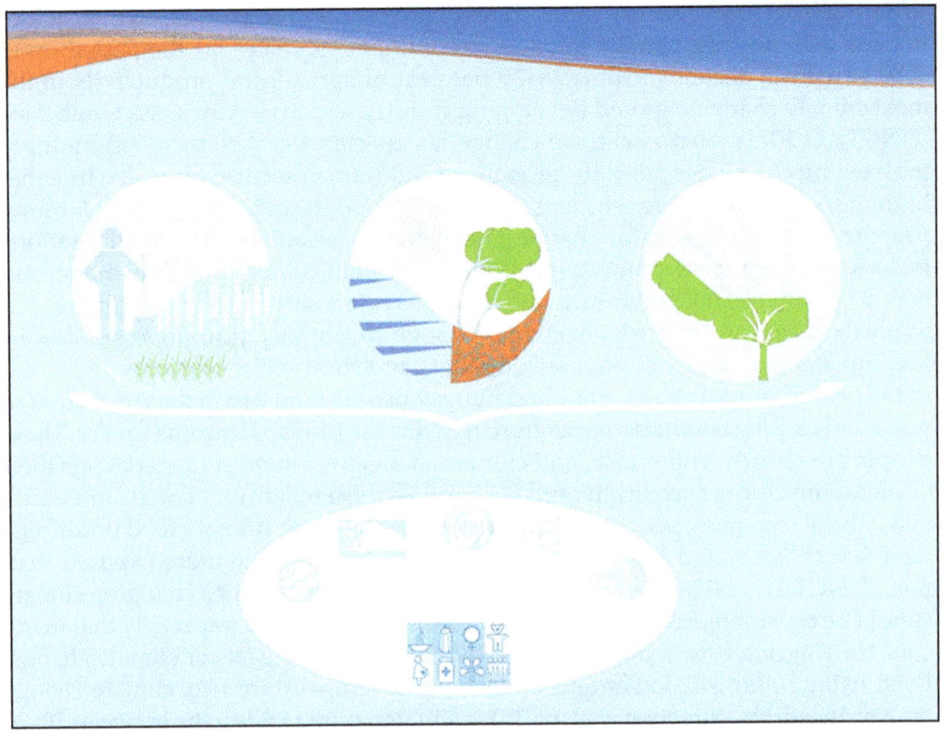

Figure 20.2: Potential of Climate-Smart Agriculture (CSA) (*Source*: FAO 2010).

Climate-Smart Agriculture: A 'Triple Win' Approach

A range of mitigation solutions is needed to tackle impacts and reduce the buildup of GHGs with implications on the 2° C limit. The need for "no regret measures", and more precisely a truly sustainable and climate-friendly agricultural development, is currently less controversial than before. A glance at global mitigation potential shows that changes in agriculture and land use, including deforestation in tropical areas, presently account for one-third of global GHG emissions. Increasingly, therefore, agriculture is being recognized as part of the problem in global climate governance. While developed countries' emissions result mostly from industry, energy consumption and transport, the Food and Agricultural Organization figures reveal that 74 per cent of all agricultural emissions originate in developing countries, and 70 per cent of the agricultural mitigation potential can be realized in these same countries. For example, about half of the 47 African countries that have recently submitted Nationally Appropriate Mitigation Action (NAMAs) have included agriculture-related actions (Fanen *et al.*, 2014). In general terms, agriculture has much to contribute to a low emissions development strategy. It can mostly contribute to mitigation (Smith *et al.*, 2008) in three ways: avoiding further deforestation and conversion of 2 Achieving Food Security in a Changing Climate: The Potential of Climate change have effects on grasslands and wetlands; increasing the carbon sequestration by vegetation and soil; and reducing current, and avoiding future, increases in emissions from nitrous oxide (from fertilizer use and soil organic matter breakdown) and from methane (from livestock production and rice cultivation) through appropriate cross-cutting and mutually enforcing policies, plans, programs and local initiatives. Could agriculture therefore be part of the solution, particularly in developing countries? Globally, three-quarters of all malnourished people depend on agriculture and would be directly affected by international mitigation agreements aimed at agriculture. Various "climate-friendly" agricultural solutions have already been proposed. They include CSA, which has been advocated during the last climate negotiations in Durban (2011) as instrumental in achieving many aims. CSA can be defined as an approach which seeks to increase productivity in an environmentally and socially sustainable way, strengthen farmers' resilience to climate change, and reduce agriculture's contribution to climate change by reducing GHG emissions and increasing carbon storage on farmland. Climate-smart agriculture includes proven practical techniques – such as mulching, intercropping, conservation agriculture, crop rotation, integrated crop-livestock management, agroforestry, improved grazing, and improved water management – but also innovative practices such as better weather forecasting, early warning systems and.

Reduces Agriculture's Contribution to Climate Change

Greenhouse gas emissions + carbon storage on farmlands is the Potential of climate-smart agriculture (CSA) M. Le *et al.* (2015). It is about getting existing technologies off the shelf and into the hands of farmers and developing new technologies such as drought or flood tolerant crops to meet the demands of the changing climate. It is also about creating and enabling policy environment for adaptation (Below *et al.*, 2010). The CSA approach neatly combines the twin goals of today's climate negotiators, helping to prevent climate change while at the same time adapting farms to inevitable change. It incorporates practices that increase productivity, efficiency, resilience, adaptive capacity, and mitigation potential of production systems (*i.e.* carbon sequestration). However, CSA requires more careful adjustment of agricultural practices to natural conditions, a knowledge-intensive approach, huge financial investment, and policy and institutional innovation.

Institutional and Policy Options

Ensuring food security and development under climate change will involve increasing yields, income and production, which can generally be expected to lead to increased aggregate emissions. While agricultural production systems will be expected first and foremost to increase productivity and resilience to support food security, there is also the potential for enhancing low emission development trajectories without compromising development and food security. To meet these multiple challenges, it has been suggested that a major transformation of the agriculture sector will be necessary and this will require institutional and policy support. Better aligned policy approaches across agricultural, environmental and financial boundaries and innovative institutional arrangements to promote their implementation will be needed. This section covers summarily the required critical adjustments to support the shift toward CSA: Enabling an Integrated Policy

Environment Key requirements for an enabling policy environment to promote climate-friendly agricultural transformations are greater coherence, coordination and integration between climate change, agricultural development and food security processes. Inter-sectorial approaches and consistent policies across these areas are necessary at all levels. Such policies have both impacts on smallholder production systems and on GHG emissions. Lack of coherence can prevent synergy capture and render the pursuit of the stated policy objectives ineffective and costly. At the national level, climate change policies are generally expressed through the National Action Plan for Adaptation (NAPAs) and the Nationally Appropriate Mitigation Actions (NAMAs) as well as through national and regional strategies. Agriculture and food security plans are generally expressed in national development and poverty reduction strategies. Better alignment of the technology approaches envisioned in these different policy frameworks, and in particular better integration of sustainable land and water management factors into mainstream agricultural development planning will facilitate a more holistic approach to considering agricultural development, adaptation and mitigation. In addition, better integration of food security nets and adaptation policies offers the potential to reap significant benefits. Better use of climate science information in assessing risks and vulnerability and then developing the safety nets and 2 Achieving Food Security in a Changing Climate: The Potential of Climate change is insurance products as an effective response is already being piloted in some areas with fairly positive results. Policies related to price stability are also key to both adaptation and food security. At the international level, better integration of food security, agricultural development and climate change policies and financing is also needed. Two parallel global dialogues on reducing food insecurity and responding to climate change have until now had little substantive integration of issues under consideration. Likewise, the agriculture community has only recently become active in the discussions and negotiations of international climate change policies that could have profound impacts on the sector. The creation of mechanisms that allow dialogues between food security, agricultural development and climate change policy-makers seems fundamental and imposing.

Conclusion

We have argued that introducing noble approaches as though giving orders to a subordinate is not what is needed for sustainable development in Africa. There is need to ensure that the approach is apt and has potential for success. In this line of thought we have argued for the sustainability of Climate-Smart Agriculture for adaptation in Northern Nigeria. Climate-Smart Agriculture has been proposed as an approach that can combat climate change and desertification comprehensively by emphasising adaptation to climate change. Having assessed the approach through the prism of the SAET framework, we found that broadly speaking it fits with what can be termed as a sustainable technology. Admittedly, there are many aspects, such as the emphasis on cultural functions that will need to be addressed. CSA in societies like Nigeria where the poor are often cheated out of programmes should integrate all the needs of the disadvantaged into the policy before its final adoption. Such a review has become necessary because the approach, as currently conceived, does not do enough justice to some of the critical issues in the agricultural sector in Nigeria. There is need for an all-inclusive approach that would not only enhance environmental protection for the country but also respect social values. The outcomes of some of the current practices adopted to manage adverse environmental impacts were found to provide coping strategies that fit with the concepts of CSA. These, however, are still not very widespread. Specifically, farm management and technology practices such as the use of cover crops, crop rotation and inter-cropping, the use of improved seed varieties, tillage systems, water harvesting and management systems, improved pasture management systems and agroforestry are recommended. It is expected that, if consciously adopted by farmers in the region, the adverse impact of climate change and desertification on the people shall be greatly mitigated. Secondly, CSA shall enable farmers in the region to adapt effectively to the adverse impacts of climate change and desertification and hence, improve the wellbeing of rural farm households (which constitute the majority population) and help Northern Nigeria attain food security and sustainable development.

REFERENCES

1. AMAF, *ASEAN Regional Guidelines for Promoting Climate Smart Agriculture (CSA) Practices* 2015, ASEAN Meeting on Agriculture and Forestry 7: Philippines.
2. Adams WM, Mortimore MJ (1997). Agricultural Intensification and Flexibility in the Nigerian Sahel. The Geogr. J. 163:150-160. Available online at: http://dx.doi.org/10.2307/3060178 http://dx.doi.org/10.2307/3060178.
3. Below T, Artner A, Siebert R, Sieber S (2010). Micro-level practices to adapt to climate change for African small-scale farmers: A review of selected literature. Environment and Production Technology Division.
4. Building Nigeria's Response to Climate Change [BNRCC] Project (2011). National Adaptation Strategy and Plan of Action on Climate Change for Nigeria (NASPA-CCN). Federal Ministry of Environment Special Climate Change Unit.
5. Doan, T.T.U., *et al., Case study: Huong Khe district, Ha Tinh province, Viet Nam. Characterising agro-ecological zones with local knowledge*, in *ICRAF Working Paper No 2012*015, World Agroforestry Centre: Bogor.
6. Fanen Terdoo and Olalekan Adekola (2014) Assessing the role of climate-smart agriculture in combating climate change, desertification and improving rural livelihood in Northern Nigeria African Journal of Agricultural Research.
7. Le, V.H., M.T. Duong, and E. Simelton, *Situation analysis and needs assessment report for My Loi village and Ha Tinh province - Viet Nam (VN02)*, in *CGIAR Research Program on Climate Change, Agriculture and Food Security (CCAFS)* 2015: Copenhagen, Denmark. p. 44.
8. Lasco, R.D., *et al., Climate risk adaptation by smallholder farmers: the roles of trees and agroforestry.*Current Opinion in Environmental Sustainability, 2014. 6: p. 83-88.
9. Luedeling E, Sileshi G, Beedy T, Dietz J (2012). Carbon Sequestration Potential of Agroforestry Systems in Africa. In: Kumar, B. M. and Ramachandran Nair, P.K. (eds). Carbon Sequestration Potential of Agroforestry Systems: opportunity

and challenges. Advances in Agroforestry 8:61-84. Available online at:http://dx.doi.org/10.1007/978-94-007-1630-8.

10. Omonona BT (2009). Quantitative Analysis of Rural Poverty in Nigeria. Nigeria Strategy Support Programme (NSSP) Background Paper 9, International Food Policy Research Institute, Washington D.C.
11. Oladipo E (1993). A Comprehensive Approach to Drought and Desertification in Northern Nigeria. Natural Hazards, 8:235-261. Available online at: http://dx.doi.org/10.1007/BF00690910. http://dx.doi.org/10.1007/BF00690910
12. Simelton, E., B.V. Dam, and D. Catacutan, *Trees and agroforestry for coping with extreme weather events - experiences from northern and central Viet Nam* Agroforestry Systems, 2015. 89(6): p. 1065-1082.
13. Simelton, E., *et al., Factors constraining and enabling agroforestry adoption in Viet Nam: a multi-level policy analysis.* Agroforestry Systems, 2017. 91(1): p. 51-67.
14. Smith P, Martino D, Cai Z, Gwary D, Janzen H, Kumar P, McCarl B, Ogle S, O'Mara F, Rice C, S choles B, Sirotenko O, Howden M, McAllister T, Pan G, Romanenkov V, Schneider U, towprayoon S, Wattenbach M, Smith J (2008) Greenhouse gas mitigation in agriculture Philos Trans R Soc B 363:789–813.
15. UNCTAD (2011) Assuring food security in developing countries under the challenges of climate change: Key trade and development issues of a fundamental transformation of agriculture http;//archive, unctad.org/templates/page.asp?intItemID=2101 and lang=I
16. Von Storch, H. and F. Zwiers, *Statistical Analysis in Climate Research*1999, Cambridge: Cambridge University Press.
17. Wollenberg E, Higman S, Seeberg-Elverfeldt, C, Neely C, Tapio-Biström ML, Neufeldt H (2012). Helping Smallholder Farmers Mitigate Climate Change. CCAFS Policy Brief 5: 1-6. CGIAR Research Program on Climate Change, Agriculture and Food Security (CCAFS). Copenhagen, Denmark. Available online at: ccafs.cgiar.org/resources/reports-and-policy-briefs.

www.ingramcontent.com/pod-product-compliance
Ingram Content Group UK Ltd.
Pitfield, Milton Keynes, MK11 3LW, UK
UKHW021010290726
14059UKWH00001BA/51

9 789388 173940